W9-ARG-923

Long-Term Effects of Stroke

NEUROLOGICAL DISEASE AND THERAPY

Advisory Board

Additional Volumes in Preparation

Long-Term Effects of Stroke

edited by

Julien Bogousslavsky

*University of Lausanne and
Centre Hospitalier Universitaire Vaudois
Lausanne, Switzerland*

MARCEL DEKKER, INC.   NEW YORK · BASEL

BS

ISBN: 0-8247-0624-2

This book is printed on acid-free paper.

Headquarters
Marcel Dekker, Inc.
270 Madison Avenue, New York, NY 10016
tel: 212-696-9000; fax: 212-685-4540

Eastern Hemisphere Distribution
Marcel Dekker AG
Hutgasse 4, Postfach 812, CH-4001 Basel, Switzerland
tel: 41-61-261-8482; fax: 41-61-261-8896

World Wide Web
http://www.dekker.com

The publisher offers discounts on this book when ordered in bulk quantities. For more information, write to Special Sales/Professional Marketing at the headquarters address above.

Current printing (last digit):
10 9 8 7 6 5 4 3 2 1

PRINTED IN THE UNITED STATES OF AMERICA

4/14/03

With compassionate dedication to all future stroke victims,
and in the memory of Aron Bogousslavsky and Jean Belime,
two grandfathers who had to cope with the consequences of a stroke.

Series Introduction

The past quarter century has seen a virtual revolution in the ability of physicians to learn more about their stroke patients. Modern brain imaging now has the ability to show quickly and safely whether strokes are hemorrhagic or ischemic, and to define the location and extent of the brain injury. Even more importantly, modern diagnostic technology can also define the underlying cardiac, hematological, and cervicocranial cerebrovascular lesions that cause the stroke and threaten to cause subsequent strokes and further brain injury.

This technological revolution has allowed physicians to define and quantitate neurological damage much better than in the past. Now they are able to add neuroimaging and cardiovascular imaging results to their customary detailed neurological examinations. Neurological scales that quantitate neurological signs and functional capabilities have also been introduced widely into stroke care. This quantification of clinical neurological abnormalities and brain and vascular findings allows doctors to render a more reliable prognosis than at any time in the past. Knowing what is wrong with the patient also allows much more logical selection of treatment than in the era before modern technology.

Patients and families as well as caring physicians want to know: What is wrong with the patient? What is the outlook? What can be done to help improve the natural course of the condition or illness? Central to these queries is information about the usual and natural course of a condition. Hippocrates, the Greek physician often lauded as the father of medicine, developed his reputation almost solely on the basis of his ability to describe diseases and to prognosticate. The rendering of an accurate prognosis is a very important core function for treating physicians and researchers alike. After all, the aim of treatment is to improve the natural course. Without knowing the natural course, how can the effect of treatment be analyzed?

Correlation of neurological abnormalities with the brain and vascular imaging data, and knowledge from follow-up care, have only recently taught physicians who care for stroke patients a great deal. Although the ability of stroke experts to prognosticate and treat has vastly improved, much of this knowledge is not currently available in the medical and neurological literature. Julien Bogousslavsky, a master clinician and skilled writer and editor, has compiled in this volume the work of impressive group of international chapter authors. The contributors are among the most experienced stroke doctors in the world. The chapters in this volume cover most of the essential bases concerning long-term effects of stroke and the prognoses of various neurological deficits and handicaps. This material is essential for physicians who care for patients after stroke. This information is also important if physicians are to understand rehabilitation, recovery, and treatment after stroke. The book should prove very useful for a wide array of health care providers who care for patients during and after stroke.

Louis R. Caplan, M.D.
Professor of Neurology
Harvard Medical School
Boston, Massachusetts

Preface

Stroke is the third most common cause of death and the first leading cause of acquired handicap in adults. Each stroke costs a mean of $80,000 in medical expenses. If one realizes that over 700,000 people in the United States and over 700,000 Europeans are the victims of a first stroke each year, it is easy to imagine that stroke not only is a major burden to patients and their families, but also represents a global health and social issue—the "burden" of stroke.

In the past decade, major advances were made in acute stroke management, including fibrinolysis, and in stroke prevention (treatment of risk factors, antiplatelet/antithrombotic agents, carotid surgery, etc.). However, despite these achievements, strokes continue—and will continue—to occur, with potentially devastating consequences that include impairment or loss of brain functions, inability to resume previous activities, social changes, decreased quality of life, depressed mood or loss of drive, various handicaps, and increased risk of death. A higher risk of developing a new stroke and other vascular events, including myocardial infraction, must also be emphasized.

In the first part of this book, definitions and assessment of outcome, handicap, disability, and quality of life after stroke are presented. Mortality and stroke recurrence are also addressed. The following chapters cover specific dysfunctions that are particularly common and disabling after stroke, including motor impairment, neurobehavioral changes, cognitive loss, emotional disorders, and dementia. Finally, emerging issues are presented, including the complex problem of cost vs. benefit of poststroke management. Since a discussion of rehabilitation issues and programs could fill an entire book in itself, we have decided not to cover this field, in which several controversies remain. Instead, we have focused the book on the best possible update of what is known about prognosis after stroke.

In order to provide the reader with representative worldwide opinions, we have attempted to put together a truly international panel of experts covering views from America, Europe, and Australia. Indeed, many aspects of rehabilitation after stroke are still flavored with local traditions, which should be clearly recognized as such. While national or regional secularities should be taken into account, it is important to differentiate them from scientific data, especially when poststroke management programs are initiated at individual centers.

With the general aging of the Western population, the aftermath of stroke is likely to be one of the major health care issues of the 21st century. This book attempts to summarize what we currently know on the evolution and prognosis of patients who have suffered a stroke.

Julien Bogousslavsky

Contents

Contributors

A. T. Al-Khodairy, M.D. Department of Neurological Rehabilitation, Clinique Romande de Réadaptation, Sion, Switzerland

Kjell Asplund, M.D. Departments of Medicine, University Hospital, Umeå, Sweden

Monica Åström, M.D. Departments of Psychiatry, University Hospital, Umeå, Sweden

Ferdinand Binkofski, M.D. Department of Neurology, University Hospital Lübeck, Lübeck, Germany

Julien Bogousslavsky, M.D. Department of Neurology, University of Lausanne and Centre Hospitalier Universitaire Vaudois, Lausanne, Switzerland

Antonio Carota, M.D. Department of Neurology, University of Lausanne and Centre Hospitalier Universitaire Vaudois, Lausanne, Switzerland

K. Diserens, M.D. Department of Neurology, University of Lausanne and Centre Hospitalier Universitaire Vaudois, Lausanne, Switzerland

José M. Ferro, M.D., Ph.D.   Department of Neurology, Hospital Santa Maria, Lisbon, Portugal

Seth P. Finkelstein, M.D.   Department of Neurology, Massachusetts General Hospital and Harvard Medical School, and ViaCell Neuroscience, Boston, Massachusetts

Hans-Joachim Freund, M.D., F.R.C.P.   Department of Neurology, University Hospital Düsseldorf, Düsseldorf, Germany

J. Ghika, M.D.   Department of Neurology, University of Lausanne and Centre Hospitalier Universitaire Vaudois, Lausanne, Switzerland

Graeme J. Hankey, M.B.B.S., M.D., F.R.C.P., F.R.C.P. (EDIN), F.R.A.C.P. Stroke Unit, Department of Neurology, Royal Perth Hospital and University of Western Australia, Perth, Western Australia, Australia

Sofia Madureira, PsyD.   Department of Neurology, Hospital Santa Maria, Lisbon, Portugal

Jorge Moncayo-Gaete, M.D.   Service de Neurologie, Eugenio Espejo Hospital, Quito, Ecuador

Rüdiger J. Seitz, M.D.   Department of Neurology, University Hospital Düsseldorf, Düsseldorf, Germany

P. Vuadens, M.D.   Department of Neurological Rehabilitation, Clinique Romande de Réadaptation, Sion, Switzerland

Philip A. Wolf, M.D.   Department of Neurology, Boston University School of Medicine, Boston, Massachusetts

Dileep R. Yavagal, M.D.   Department of Neurology, Massachusetts General Hospital and Harvard Medical School, Boston, Massachusetts

Long-Term Effects of Stroke

1

Definition and Measurement of Outcome

P. Vuadens
Clinique Romande de Réadaptation, Sion, Switzerland

I. INTRODUCTION

Stroke is considered the most prevalent disabling disorder requiring neurorehabilitation. The cost of care is directly dependent on the ability of patients to return home. It is estimated that approximately 60% of stroke survivors are expected to recover independence, and 75% to walk independently (1). Whether or not neurorehabilitation is efficacious is still controversial because of different variables that contribute to stroke outcomes: severity of neurological deficit, comorbidity, and psychosocial factors (2–4). However, outcome measures are becoming more and more important, especially to assess the efficacy of pharmacological interventions and quality of care provided for stroke patients. To meet these needs a growing number of outcome measures are available. To use them to their best effect, it is important to know their strengths and weaknesses.

In neurorehabilitation the correct measurement of outcomes is not based on a single factor and the use of less than optimal scales for measuring outcome may cause problems. Conflicting results can be observed when the outcome measures vary. In fact, in terms of neurorehabilitation, different outcomes such as returning home or working can be evaluated. Usually, people dealing with stroke rehabilitation are more concerned with adaptation to disability and ability to perform activities of daily living (ADL), because the major goal of stroke rehabilitation is to return to independence in ADL. This goal needs specific scales for assessing effectiveness of therapeutic or institutional programs (5). Other outcome measurements include measure of ambulation, motor abilities, and overall quality of life (6). So applications of outcome measurements can focus on the

1

patient needs or on larger applications such as health care needs, efficacy of treatment or therapy, and quality of life.

To measure the outcomes of neurorehabilitation programs entails evaluating the impact of disability across different functions, especially concerning the person and societal level (7). Therefore, it seems necessary to work within a framework to determine or classify what might be analyzed. In this way, under the leadership of Nagi and Wood, a framework for rehabilitation concepts has been described and developed over many years (8–10). Finally, based on the concepts of impairment, disability, and handicap, the World Health Organization (WHO) published an international classification of the consequences of any diseases (ICIDH) in 1980 (11). Later, Granger proposed to organize these concepts across three levels: organ, person, and society (12). Each one can result in either impairment, disability, or handicap. All organic dysfunctions determine impairment, while performance defects or difficulty in coping with daily tasks within the physical and social environment correspond to disability. Handicaps are represented by all social limitations or disadvantages, especially influenced by social rules and policy. In reality, each impairment can create limitations in function, such as using skills, performing activities, or fulfilling social roles. Contextual factors are also determinants.

Therefore, to provide health outcomes in terms proposed by Granger, the WHO revised its system and proposed a revised version of the International Classification of Impairments, Disabilities, and Handicaps (ICIDH-2) in 1999 (13). The terminology had to be changed and the terms "disability" and "handicap" were replaced by "limitations in activities" and "restriction in participation." This new version also includes contextual factors (personal experiences, physical environment, and social environment).

Outcomes measures can have different goals and according to the WHO classification, they may be measured at different levels. The first goal is to provide the results that measure not only therapeutic or technical success of rehabilitation but the patient's satisfaction, as well as the patient's ability to function physically, emotionally, and socially. Outcome measures can be a study of cohorts of stroke patients in order to understand the clinical evolution of patients treated by specific drugs or techniques. Administrative data can also be useful for clinical research on effectiveness or efficacy. Finally, outcome measures can help to diffuse information and develop guidelines for clinical practice.

So in selecting an outcome measure, it is necessary to define clearly the functional attribute of interest: a global outcome measure or an assessment of partial function. Jette suggested that functioning can be divided into physical, mental, emotional, and social performance (14). Usually patients are more concerned with activity. In addition, the items in any outcome measure ought to relate to only one single level within the ICIDH because of the difficulty in analyzing results from a measure that reflects more than one level (15).

II. OUTCOME MEASURES SELECTION

There is no single correct measurement of outcome for stroke patients. The choice of a particular scale depends on the type of underlying condition and the specific motive for obtaining the measure. Moreover, an outcome measure can be appropriate for a patient or group of patients at one stage of the evolution but not at another stage. In fact, given the natural history of stroke, change may continue over months and the proportion of change may vary between the different levels of the ICIDH (16). Usually outcome scales are based on the classification of the WHO and attempt to assess impairment, disability, handicap, or quality of life. However, the choice of a scale requires scales that can provide standardization among different examiners and institutions. Two elements are important for selecting an outcome scale. First, the criteria in the scale must correspond with the user's purpose (17,18). The wrong choice can lead to erroneous results or information. Second, the scale must be reliable, valid, and appropriately responsive (17,19–21).

Consequently, outcome measure must consider the timing of any assessment, and the factors that can impact on the chosen outcomes. The method of statistical analysis must also suit the chosen outcome.

III. RELIABILITY

Reliability corresponds with the property of reproducibility, in other words if the variance in scoring is minimal on an unchanged population. A scale is reliable when any differences over time reflect true change and not random fluctuation (18). Reliability can be assessed in different ways. Test-retest reliability (intrarater reliability) is evaluated by repeated measures under the same conditions at different stages in time. An interval of 2–14 days is usually recommended (22). Enough time allows one to minimize the effects of memory, but too much time may change the phenomenon under study significantly. Therefore, only experience may sometimes determine whether the reliability of a scale is adequate or not. In addition, the reliability of scale scores tends to be higher than that of individual items.

Interrater reliability represents the level of agreement between different examiners who evaluate the same patient or group of patients at the same stage in time (23–25). Good interrater reliability is an essential quality in selecting a scale.

Reliability of a scale is evaluated with k-statistics and with weighted k for ordinal scales. A k-value of 0 signifies a chance agreement. Almost perfect reliability is accepted for k-values of 0.81–1.00 and substantial reliability for k-values of 0.61–0.80 (24–26).

Internal consistency is an estimate of the homogeneity of the items and the mean correlations between them (23). It measures the strength of the relationships between the items of the scale. In other words, internal consistency allows one to judge whether the items of a scale being grouped together measure a unified domain. It is estimated by Cronbach's alpha coefficient and item-total correlations, e.g., Kuder-Richardson 20 (23,27). To consider good internal consistency, it is necessary that Cronbach's alpha coefficient should be higher than 0.7 and that item-total correlations should exceed 0.2 (22,28).

IV. VALIDITY

Validity means that a scale must indeed evaluate and measure what it proposes to do (17,21). It is different from reliability but it cannot be obtained without reliability.

Validity can be estimated when a "gold standard" exists with which to compare a mean measure. In fact, such estimation is difficult when validity is applied to variables such as behavior. There are three main types of validity: content, construct, and discriminant.

A. Content Validity

This relates to a scale that includes all the relevant, appropriate, and representative aspects of what is being evaluated (23). It supposes that all relevant concepts are present in the scale. Unfortunately, there is no statistical test to quantify content validity. Usually, it is based on systematic use of expert opinion (21,29).

B. Criterion Validity

By comparing the relationship between the scale and other tests or scales, construct validity is accepted if expected patterns of relationships are observed. If the examined scale measures the same construct, convergent validity is admitted. On the other hand, discriminant validity maps the correlations between measures of different constructs (29,30).

V. RESPONSIVENESS OR SENSITIVITY

To establish comparisons between patients, doctors, or institutions, discriminative scales are required (31). In fact, the term "sensitivity" describes good discriminatory power of a scale that allows detection of clinical differences between individuals or groups at a given point in time. On the other hand, responsiveness is the property of being able to detect clinical change over time. It is the power of a test to detect the smallest difference for evaluative indices. This aspect is difficult to establish, and approaches to measuring responsiveness are still uncertain (32). So in selecting a scale, it is important to choose one that has been designed to detect meaningful change. Moreover, many scales are responsive to change only in the midportion of the scale. Therefore, they must not be applied to patients who are at one extreme of the scale (33).

A scale can be unresponsive to change for different reasons. First, the selected instrument may not contain the specific items for a particular group of patients. Second, the presence of static items reduces responsiveness, as well as the inclusion of single global questions, or the use of only broad response categories. Third, ceiling and floor effects can also alter responsiveness. Ceiling effect means that improvement or modifications cannot be detected in patients included with a maximal pretreatment score. Floor effect means the contrary: a deterioration in patient conditions cannot be noticed in patients with minimal pretreatment scores.

VI. STATISTICAL CONSIDERATIONS

A stroke scale is composed of several items with scores that highlight different degrees of dysfunction and the results correspond to the order of the qualitative responses. There are four main types of scales.

A nominal scale classifies the construct according to different possibilities: presence/absence, yes/no, or different types of stroke for example. Ordinal scales establish a hierarchy, e.g., maximal to minimal dependency. In interval scales, the difference between adjacent levels of an ordinal scale is constant, while a ratio scale is an interval scale with an absolute zero point (time required to complete a task for example).

Ordinal and nominal scales cannot be subjected to parametric statistics. In fact, the difference between two scores on an ordinal scale is not necessarily more than the difference between two other scores. So the data are not true values but categories in a ranked grading system. Usually, the Mann-Whitney U-test is the most frequently used nonparametric test.

The range of values on a scale is also important to reflect relevant differences. Limited levels would probably be insufficiently discriminative, while numerous levels would be more sensitive but the differences between levels would become much less clear.

REFERENCES

1. Gresham GE, Phillips TF, Wolf PA et al. Epidemiologic profile of long-term stroke disability: the Framingham study. Arch Phys Med Rehabil 1979; 60:487–491.

2. Reding MJ, Potes E. Rehabilitation outcome following initial unilateral hemispheric stroke: life table analysis approach. Stroke 1988; 19:1354–1358.

3. Kotila M, Waltimo O, Niemi M, Laaksonen R, Lempinen M. The profile of recovery from stroke and factors influencing outcome. Stroke 1984; 15:1039–1044.

4. Lincoln NB, Blackburn M, Ellis S, Jackson J, Edmans JA, Nouri FM, Walrer MF, Haworth H. An investigation of factors affecting progress of patients on a stroke unit. J Neurol Neurosurg Psychiatry 1989; 52:493–496.

5. Good DC. Outcome assessment in chronic neurological disease. In: Good DC, Couch JR, eds. Handbook of Neurorehabilitation. New York: Marcel Dekker, 1994, pp 107–128.

6. Bergner M, Bobbitt RA, Carter WB, Gilson BS. The Sickness Impact Profile: development and final revision of a health status measure. Med Care 1981; 19:787–805.

7. Jette AM. How measurement techniques influence estimates of disability in older populations. Soc Sci Med 1994; 38:937–942.

8. Nagi SZ. Disability and Rehabilitation. Columbus: Ohio State University Press, 1969.

9. Nagi SZ. Some conceptual issues in disability and rehabilitation. In: Sussmann MB, ed. Sociology and Rehabilitation. Columbus: Ohio University Press, 1965.

10. Wood PHN. Classification of Impairment and Handicap. Document WHO/ICDP/REV-CONF/75.15. Geneva: World Health Organization, 1975.

11. World Health Organization. The International Classification of Impairments, Disabilities, and Handicaps. Geneva: World Health Organisation, 1980.

12. Granger CV. A conceptual model for functional assessment. In: Granger CV, Gresham GE, eds. Functional Assessment in Rehabilitation Medicine. Baltimore: Williams & Wilkins, 1984.

13. World Health Organization. ICIDH-2: International Classification of Functioning and Disability, Beta-2 Draft, Short Version. Geneva: World Health Organization, 1999.

14. Jette AM. Concepts of health and methodological issues in functional assessment. In: Granger CV, Gresham GE, eds. Functional Assessment in Rehabilitation Medicine. Baltimore: Williams & Wilkins, 1984.

15. Orgogozo JM. The concepts of impairment, disability, and handicap. Cerebrovasc Dis 1994; 4(suppl 2):2–6.

16. Jorgensen HS, Nakayama H, Pedersen PM, Kammersgaard L, Raaschou HO, Olsen TS. Outcome and time course of recovery in stroke. II. Time course of recovery: the Copenhagen Stroke Study. Arch Phys Med Rehabil 1995; 76:406–412.

17. Turner RR. Quality of Life Assessment in Clinical Trials. Spilker B ed. New York: Raven Press, 1990, pp 247–267.

18. Johnston MV, Keith RA, Hinderer SR. Measurement standards for interdisciplinary medical rehabilitation. Arch Phys Med Rehabil 1992; 73 (suppl):S3–S23.

19. Wade DT. Measurement in Neurological Rehabilitation. Oxford: Oxford University Press, 1992.

20. Applegate WB, Blass JP, Williams JF. Instruments for the functional assessment of older patients. N Engl J Med 1990; 322:1207–1214.

21. Lyden PD, Lau GT. A critical appraisal of stroke evaluation and rating scales. Stroke 1991; 22:1345–1352.

22. Streiner DL, Norman GR. Health Measurement Scales: A Practical Guide to Their Development and Use. Oxford: Oxford Medical Publications, 1989.
23. Nunnally JC. Psychometric Theory, 2d ed. New York: McGraw-Hill, 1978.
24. Feinstein AR. Clinimetrics. New Haven, CT: Yale University Press, 1987.
25. Kaplan RM. Basic Statistics for the Behavioural Sciences. Boston: Allyn & Bacon, 1987.
26. Landis RJ, Koch GG. The measurement of observer agreement for categorical data. Biometrics 1977; 33:159–174.
27. Cronbach LJ. Coefficient alpha and the internal structure of tests. Psychometrika 1951; 16:297–334.
28. Kline P. A Handbook of Test Construction. London: Methuen, 1986.
29. Cote R, Battista RN, Wolfson C, Boucher J, Adam J, Hachinski V. The Canadian Neurological Scale: validation and reliability assessment. Neurology 1989; 39:638–643.
30. Hanston L, De Keyser J. Neurological scales in the assessment of cerebral infarction. Cerebrovasc Dis 1994; 4(suppl 2):7–14.
31. Guyatt GH, Feeny DH, Patrick DL. Measuring health-related quality of life. Ann Intern Med 1993; 118:622–629.
32. Guyatt GH, Walters S, Norman G. Measuring change over time: assessing the usefulness of evaluative instruments. J Chronic Dis 1987; 40:171–178.
33. MacKenzie CR, Charlson ME. Standards for the use of ordinal scales in clinical trials. Br Med J 1986; 292:40–43.

2

Assessment of Disability After Stroke

P. Vuadens
Clinique Romande de Réadaptation, Sion, Switzerland

I. INTRODUCTION

According to the World Health Organization International Classification of Impairment, Disability, and Handicap, disability is "any restriction or lack (resulting from an impairment) of ability to perform an activity within the range considered normal for a human being." It concerns the consequence of the impairment at the personal level and it is the reflection of performances in activities of daily living (ADL) (1,2). The basic ADLs include all the self-care skills necessary for personal independence: feeding, dressing, bathing, grooming, toileting, continence, transfers, and mobility. So the different scales that attempt to evaluate these functional abilities must be able to assess patient progress with good reliability and validity. Since the late 1980s, many scales or indexes have been developed and used for outcome evaluation of stroke patients. They may assist not only clinical management but also research or medical audit. These scales are also useful for assessing outcome in many different conditions, especially the ability to live independently (3–5). Moreover, most of these scales measure independence in ADL in a similar manner (6,7). In this chapter we will describe the best-known and most extensively studied scales.

II. MEASURES OF GLOBAL DISABILITY

A. The Barthel Scale (Table 1)

Published by Mahoney and Barthel in 1965, the Barthel scale, or Barthel's Index, is a worldwide ADL scale used in stroke trial (8). In 1979 the number of items

Table 1   The Barthel Index

Bowels
   0 = Incontinent
   5 = Occasional accident (1 ×/week), or needs help with enema or suppository
   10 = Continent, able to use enema or suppository if needed
Bladder
   0 = Incontinent, or catheterized and unable to manage
   5 = Occasional accident (maximum 1 ×/24 hr)
   10 = Continent (>7 days), or able to manage collecting device if used
Grooming
   0 = Needs help with personal care
   5 = Washes face, combs hair, brushes teeth
Toilet use
   0 = Dependent
   5 = Needs help, but can do something alone
   10 = Independent (on and off, wiping, dressing)
Feeding
   0 = Unable
   5 = Needs help cutting, spreading butter, etc.
   10 = Independent if food provided
Chair/bed transfer
   0 = Completely bedridden, use of chair not possible
   5 = Able to sit, but needs major help (1–2 people) to transfer
   10 = Minor help (verbal or physical) to transfer
   15 = Independent, including locking wheelchair and lifting footrests
Mobility
   0 = Sits on wheelchair, but cannot propel it
   5 = Independent in wheelchair, including corners, etc., for 50 yd
   10 = Walks with help of one person (verbal or physical) for 50 yd
   15 = Independent, but may use any aid
Dressing
   0 = Dependent
   5 = Needs help, but can do about half unaided
   10 = Independent, including buttons, zippers, and laces
Stairs
   0 = Unable
   5 = Needs help (verbal or physical)
   10 = Independent up and down, but may use any aid
Bathing
   0 = Needs help
   5 = Independent (or in shower)

and the rating categories were increased and in 1988 Collin et al. simplified the scoring system of the original version (9–11). This index of ADL was initially developed to measure progress in self-care and mobility of patients in rehabilitation. Designed for use with patients with neuromuscular or musculoskeletal disorders, it has been rapidly applied to monitor stroke patients and it is an excellent scale to measure the outcome of stroke patients for long-term follow-up (12). It is recommended as the best measure available (13–15). In a critical review of over 20 ADL scales, Law and Letts analyzed the most appropriate function for each index and they recommended the Barthel Index over all others (16).

This scale consists of 10 items referring to incontinence for bowel and bladder, grooming, toilet use, feeding, transfer, mobility, dressing, stairs, and bathing. Patient performances are rated in three response categories: "dependent," "needs help," and "independent." The items are scored in five-point increments, based upon the amount of help needed and time taken in providing help. So the item scores may range from 0 (totally dependent) to 100 the maximal score indicating normal function. The modified version uses a range of 0–20. A score of 60 or more marks relative functional independence and with 75 points or more, patients can be considered considerably independent (9,17). A score over 60 is the cutoff point at which a stroke patient can live at home with the assistance of a spouse or caregiver (18,19). In acute stroke trials, there is often a difference in the definition of favorable outcome. According to Sulter et al., poor outcome can be defined if the end points are: death, institutionalization, Barthel's Index < 60 or modified Rankin scale >3 (20). A score of 100 points means that the patient is independent in daily activities but it does not necessarily mean that the patient can live alone. He may not be able to cook or keep house for example, but he is able to get along without attendant care.

As the scale evaluates the ability to perform ADL, guidelines are available that focus on actual, not potential, functioning (10). Moreover, this index is very useful for moderately to severely disabled patients. A ceiling effect can arise if patients are relatively independent and this may lead to underestimation of patients' and carers' needs in up to a third of patients (21).

Administration of the Index is very short (a few minutes) and can even be done by telephone (22,23). It can be made by anyone who is familiar with the patient's ADL or by self-report. A recent study that compared the Barthel Index scores between relatives and occupational therapists showed that the difference in total score was two points or less in more than 80% of the patients. This means an acceptable agreement between the raters. A moderate agreement has been reported for the items "grooming" and "bladder" and the probability of disagreement between raters may increase with the patient's age (24). In fact, the scale has a high test-retest reliability and interrater reliability (9,10,17). This advantage is also valid with the modified version. Examining the relations between this scale and other tests, numerous studies have demonstrated construct validity, and high correlation with the Katz ADL scale has been confirmed. Criterion validity was also revealed and the scale relates to many variables: survival, length of hospital stay, stroke severity, age, and others (11,13,25–27).

The disadvantage of this scale is that it does not take cognitive aspects, social functioning, or household activities into account. To assess the entire range of ADL, the Barthel Index can be combined with the Frenchay Activities Index (28).

B. The Functional Independence Measure (FIM) (Table 2)

The Functional Independence Measure is the functional assessment scale of the Uniform Data System for Medical Rehabilitation (UDS), which allows measuring disability and outcome rehabilitation (29–32). Sponsored by the American Academy of Physical Medicine and Rehabilitation, the UDS has been progressively developed (32) and rapidly became more and more frequently used in rehabilitation facilities for different reasons. First, this scale has expanded the number of categories found in earlier ADL scales and has increased the number of scoring possibilities for each category. More importantly, this scale has considerably improved the sensitivity of the measurement to small changes in function. It is used to assist and evaluate rehabilitation programs, to select patients for intensive rehabilitation, to assess outcomes of rehabilitation, and even to calculate the reimbursement for rehabilitation services based upon improvement in functions (33–37).

The FIM measures selected daily activities, incorporating additional items of cognitive and communication skills and social integration. In fact, 18 items explore motor activities (13 items) and mental functions and social interactions (five items). In addition, six general fields are explored: grooming, continence, mobility, transfer, communication, and social behavior. Each item is scored according to a scale from 1 to 7 points corresponding to complete dependence to total independence. Total score varies from 16 to 126 points. The score allows appreciating not only the improvement of patients but also the efficacy of rehabilitation (38). However, the same total score can describe two different patients. In fact, the global score does not determine the specific functions of ADL that have been improved. Subscores for motor or cognitive functions can be used (39).

Validity, reliability, and sensitivity have largely been evaluated (40–42). Validity is excellent. The FIM is more appropriate than the Barthel Index to explore the functions of grooming, transfer, locomotion, and the cognitive aspects (42). Construct validity is globally high for each item, except for locomotion (walk and stairs), which is more a handicap than a disability (43). Certain functions, such as feeding or grooming, are easier to be executed by patients than transfer or locomotion. Moreover, the score between 1 and 7 is not strictly linear for each item. Nevertheless, using Rasch analysis, it is possible to give the same

Table 2 The Functional Independence Measure (FIM)

Self-care	Follow up	
A. Eating	☐	
B. Grooming	☐	
C. Bathing	☐	
D. Dressing—upper body	☐	
E. Dressing—lower body	☐	
F. Toileting	☐	
Sphincter control		
G. Bladder management	☐	
H. Bowel management	☐	
Mobility		
Transfer:		
I. Bed, chair, wheelchair	☐	
J. Toilet	☐	
K. Tub, shower	☐	
Locomotion		
L. Walk/wheelChair	☐ W	☐ C
M. Stairs	☐	
Communication		
N. Comprehension (auditory, visual)	☐ A	☐ V
O. Expression (vocal, nonvocal)	☐ V	☐ N
Social cognition		
P. Social interaction	☐	
Q. Problem solving	☐	
R. Mcmory	☐	
Total FIM (maximum 126)	☐	

No help	7 Complete independence 6 Modified dependence (device)	L
With help	*Modified dependence* 5 Supervision 4 Minimal assistance (subject ≥ 75%) 3 Moderate assistance (subject ≥ 50%) *Complete dependence* 2 Maximal assistance (subject ≥ 25%) 1 Total assistance	E V E L S

importance to each item and then the interval between each notation becomes similar. So the FIM scale is actually one of the most reliable scales (44–46). Reliability is good with test/retest coefficient between 0.86 and 0.96: total score = 0.96, cognitive score = 0.91, and motor score = 0.96 (47,48). Median and mean reliability coefficients for FIM motor items are higher than for cognitive or communication items. In a meta-analysis of 11 published studies, the majority of the reliability values (81%) are from interrater reliability studies (48).

The sensitivity of the FIM scale has been compared with that of the Barthel Index and the FIM was considered to be more valid than the Barthel Index. In a cohort of 25 patients, 14% significantly improved on the FIM scale without any modification on the Barthel Index (42).

The difference of scores between admission and discharge of patients is indicative of improvement, prognosis of stroke patients, and efficacy of rehabilitation (49–51). The score at admission is also useful for predicting discharge destination of stroke patients (52,53). However, familial and environmental factors interfere with the chances of home discharge when the FIM score is between 50 and 80. According to Galin et al., a score < 50 at admission predicts a 25–30% chance to be discharged home, while 40–80% of patients will return home when the score is between 50 and 80, and 80–90% of patients if the FIM score is greater than 100 (54).

The FIM score at discharge is less predictive of the destination of patients. Nevertheless, if the score is less than 50, patients will be discharged to a nursing home. On the other hand, discharge home can be planned when the score is greater than 100 (55,56).

Thus the FIM scale fits well for stroke patients. It allows prediction of the prognosis of patients, the length of hospital stay, and evaluation of the care needs before discharge.

C. The Katz Index of ADL

Used in orthopaedic and elderly patients by Katz et al. in 1963, this index measures independence in ADL (57). It is one of the earliest and most widely used scales of functional independence and it has been used in a variety of settings and populations (58–62). It is not copyrighted and is available in many languages.

This evaluation assumes that the abilities recover in a predictable order, and with hierarchical scoring it evaluates six basic functions (bathing, dressing, toileting, transfer, continence, and feeding) on a three-point scale. It omits mobility, wheelchair skills, grooming, and the use of stairs. The ratings of each function are dichotomized to "independence" and "dependence" and converted into a graded index from A to G. A is the most independent grade and G the most dependent grade.

Patient performance rather than ability is measured. For example, a patient who refuses to perform a function is considered as not performing the function, even though he is deemed able to do so.

In the original article, agreement between raters occurred in 19 of 20 cases, but test-retest reliability has not been reported yet. However, reproducibility of the index is admitted (63,64). It has a construct validity to predict outcomes, such as mortality and discharge status (58,59,63). There is a high degree of agreement between the scores on the Barthel Index and on the Katz Index of ADL (Kappa Coefficient of Agreement, K = 0.77) and internal consistency is excellent (11,65).

D. PULSES Profile

This acronym means: P = physical condition, U = upper-limb functions, L = lower-limb functions, S = sensory components (speech, vision, hearing), E = excretory functions, S = mental and emotional status.

First introduced by Moskowitz and McCann in 1957 to evaluate fitness for military duty, this index was modified in 1975 by Granger et al. (66,67). Each section is graded from 1 (normal) to 4 (severe abnormalities, complete dependence), with scores ranging from 0 to 24. It is a scale designed to evaluate the consequences of disease and usually used by a community rehabilitation network (68).

E. The Frenchay Activities Index

Developed in 1983 for use with stroke patients by Holbrook and Skilbeck, this index aims to provide detail on the premorbid lifestyle of patients and to measure modifications in daily activities following a stroke (69). A revised coding and a simplification of the scoring system were presented in 1985 (70). This version, easy to understand, offers an extensive list of instructions, which are not copyrighted. It takes 5 min to score and can be completed by interview or be used as a mail questionnaire. Fifteen items referring to activities both within and outside the home are rated on a four-point scale. The activities were chosen to reflect lifestyle, e.g., hobbies, shopping, social activities, and they are scored according to the frequency with which they are performed. A total score of 0 corresponds to an inactive patient and the maximal score of 45 to a highly active patient. Bond et al. demonstrated a test-retest coefficient of 0.83 between two assessments with an interval of 9 months (71). Good interrater reliability and internal consistency were confirmed by others studies (70,72). Concerning the construct validity of this index, convergent and discriminant validity was confirmed with comparison with the Barthel Index and selected items form the Sickness Impact Profile (72,73). However, the responsiveness has yet to be established.

F. Nottingham Extended ADL Scale

This scale, developed by Nouri and Lincoln in 1987, is divided into four sections: mobility, kitchen, domestic, and leisure (74). It can be used as a mailed measure of instrumental ADL ability of stroke patients. In fact, this scale is appropriate for studies evaluating rehabilitation outcome and it is suitable for mail surveys. Its validity was examined in 303 stroke patients (75). It was confirmed that each section (mobility, kitchen, domestic, leisure) forms a unidimensional hierarchical scale and that the scores from the sections can be added to provide a global score (76). Usually it is used for following functional ability of stroke patients after discharge from hospital or rehabilitation center (77).

G. The Rivermead ADL Scale

Developed for evaluation of stroke patients in a rehabilitation center in 1980, this scale was revised 10 years later (78,79). The new version is valid for elderly stroke patients (aged > 64 years) and has improved reliability by using each item without an intermediate grade. The scoring ranges from 1 (dependent) to 3 (independent with/without aid). The scale assesses two main aspects of daily activities: self-care and household. Its major fault is not to evaluate continence.

III. GLOBAL OUTCOME SCALES

A. The Rankin Scale

The Rankin Scale was one of the earliest to be developed to evaluate the outcome of stroke patients. It has been found useful for evaluating outcome in many large clinical trials (80–84) (Table 3). The initial scale has five grades (1–5): 1 = no significant disability but symptoms only and 5 = severe disability: bedridden, incontinent, and requiring constant care with all activities. For trial purpose, an additional class (0) for no symptoms at all was used (85,86). More recently, a class for death has been included (87). Its good inter- and intrarater reliability has been confirmed by two studies (85,88). Moreover, even though the Rankin Scale mixes impairments and disabilities, it is not a measure of handicap.

B. The Glasgow Outcome Scale

The Glasgow Outcome Scale is used to evaluate the outcome after coma (89). It has five grades: 1 = death; 2 = persistent vegetative state; 3 = severe disability

Table 3 Rankin Scale

Grade	Description
0	No symptoms at all
1	No significant disability, despite symptoms; able to carry out all duties and activities
2	Slight disability; unable to carry out all previous activities but able to look after own affairs without assistance
3	Moderate disability; requiring some help, but able to walk without assistance
4	Moderately severe disability; unable to walk without assistance and unable to attend to own bodily needs without assistance
5	Severe disability; bedridden, incontinent, and requiring constant nursing care and attention

(conscious but dependent); 4 = moderate disability (independent, but disabled); 5 = good recovery. It is reliable and as sensitive as other stroke impairment scales to detect differences between treatment groups (90,91).

IV. MEASURES OF FOCAL DISABILITY

The evaluation of disability in one specific function or body part can also be important to plan treatment or care needs. So a number of scales have been designed to assess mobility, hand dexterity for example.

The Rivermead Mobility Index (RMI) has been developed to assess mobility specifically and was validated in the stroke population (92). Fifteen questions allow evaluation of such tasks as managing stairs, standing without aid, running, or turning in bed. The RMI is simple to use in hospital or at home and is reliable (93,94).

Time walking can quantify the patient's functional walking abilities in testing either speed or endurance with good reliability (95). However, endurance is more sensitive to change than speed in stroke patients (96). In a short period, the distance covered, velocity, or heart rate before and after the walk can be easily measured (97,98). Patients are asked to walk at a self-selected speed for a period of 2, 3, 6, or 12 min (95,97). Because a 12-min walk can be fatiguing to the patient and time-consuming, a study has confirmed that the 12-min test has good test-retest reliability; the 2-min test is equally reliable (95). To examine the patient's ability to adapt gait to changing locomotor demands the Duke Mobility Skills Profile is appropriate, according to Shummway-Cook and Woollacott (99).

Upper-extremity disability can be tested with simple scales. For example, the Purdue Pegboard Test is a time-based test of finger manipulation and dexterity

(100). It requires the placement of pins into holes, or the assembly of a group of pins, washers, and collars. In the same way, the Nine-Hole Peg Test measures the time necessary to place nine wooden dowels into holes drilled into a wooden base (101). These two tests are valid and reliable but they are insensitive to proximal arm dysfunction and not useful when impairment is severe (102,103).

The Jebsen Hand Function Test is a standardized test to assess especially hand functions: writing, picking up small items, card turning, simulated feeding, etc. (104,105). It is quick to administer (10–15 min) and has excellent test-retest reliability, except for writing and feeding subtests (106,107). In the same way, the Action Research Arm Test (ARAT) is a quantitative test for upper-extremity functions, divided into four subtests: grasp, grip, pinch, and gross movement. The original version (1965) was simplified by Lyle in 1981 (108,109). For each subtest, the items are hierarchically ordered so that if the first item, the most difficult of the subtest, is achieved, it is not necessary to pass the other items, which are easier. The ARAT takes only 10–15 min to be completed but it requires some equipment. It has excellent validity and reliability. The Frenchay Arm Test was a 25-item test that was also shortened to seven and then five items. It is simple, quicker than the ARAT, but focuses on proximal function (110,111). Its validity and reliability have been demonstrated (112).

REFERENCES

1. WHO MONICA Project Principal Investigators. The World Health Organization MONICA project: a major international collaboration. J Clin Epidemiol 1988; 41: 105–114.
2. International Classification of Impairments, Disabilities and Handicaps. Geneva: World Health Organization, 1980.
3. Reding MJ, Potes E. Rehabilitation outcome following initial unilateral hemispheric stroke. Life table analysis approach. Stroke 1988; 19:1354–1358.
4. Viitanen M, Fugl-Meyer KS, Bernsprang B, Fugl-Meyer AR. Life satisfaction in long-term survivors after stroke. Scand J Rehabil Med 1988; 20:17–24.
5. Granger CV, Hamilton BB, Gresham GE. The Stroke rehabilitation outcome study. Part I. General description. Arch Phys Med Rehabil 1988; 69:506–509.
6. Feinstein AR, Josephy BR, Wells CK. Scientific and clinical problems in indexes of functional disability. Ann Intern Med 1986; 105:413–420.
7. Gresham GE, Phillips TF, Labi MLC. ADL status in stroke: relative merits of three standard indexes. Arch Phys Med Rehabil 1980; 61:355–358.
8. Mahoney Fl, Barthel DW. Functional evaluation. The Barthel Index. MD State Med J 1965; 14:61–65.
9. Granger CV, Albrecht GL, Hamilton BB. Outcome of comprehensive medical rehabilitation: measurement by PULSES profile and Barthel Index. Arch Phys Med Rehabil 1979; 60:145–153.

10. Collin C, Wade DT, Davis S, Horne V. The Barthel ADL Index: a reliability study. Int Disabil Stud 1988; 10:61–63.

11. Wade D, Langton Hewer R. Functional abilities after stroke: measurement, natural history and prognosis. J Neurol Neurosurg Psychiatry 1987; 50:177–182.

12. Wilkinson PR, Wolfe CD, Warburton FG, Rudd AG, Howard RS, Ross-Russell RW, Beech R. Longer term quality of life and outcome in stroke patients: is the Barthel Index alone an adequate measure of outcome. Qual Health Care 1997; 6:125–130.

13. Gresham G, Phillips T, Labi M. Relative merits of three standard indexes. Arch Phys Med Rehabil 1980; 61:355–358.

14. Wade DT, Collin C. The Barthel ADL Index: a standard measure of physical disability? Int Disabil Stud 1988; 10:64–6722.

15. Wade DT. Measurement in neurological Rehabilitation. Wade DT, ed. New York: Oxford University Press, 1992, pp 70–82.

16. Law M, Letts L. A critical review of scales of activities of daily living. Am J Occup Ther 1989; 43:522–528.

17. de Haan R, Limburg M, Schuling J, Broeshart J, Jonkers L, van Zuylen P. Clinimetric evaluation of the Barthel Index: a measure of disability in the activities of daily living. Ned Tijdschr Geneeskd 1993; 137:917–921.

18. Granger CV, Hamilton BB, Gresham GE. The stroke rehabilitation study: general description. Part 1. Arch Phys Med Rehabil 1988; 69:506–509.

19. Granger CV, Dewis LS, Peters NC, et al. Stroke rehabilitation: analysis of repeated Barthel Index measures. Arch Phys Med Rehabil 1979; 60:14–17.

20. Sulter G, Steen C, De Keyser J. Use of the Barthel Index and modified Rankin Scale in acute stroke trials. Stroke 1999; 30: 1538–1541.

21. Wellwood I, Dennis MS, Warlow CP. A comparison of the Barthel Index and the OPCS disability instrument used to measure outcome after acute stroke. Age Ageing 1995; 24:54–57.

22. Shinar D, Gross C, Bronstein K, et al. Reliability of the Activities of Daily Living Scale and its use in the telephone interview. Arch Phys Med Rehabil 1987; 68: 723–728.

23. Korner-Bitensky N, Wood-Dauphinee S. Barthel Index information elicited over the telephone. Is it reliable? Am J Phys Med Rehabil 1995; 74:9–18.

24. Wyller TB, Sveen U, Bautz-Holter E. The Barthel ADL Index one year after stroke: comparison between relatives' and occupational therapist's scores. Age Ageing 1995; 24:398–401.

25. Granger C, Hamilton B, Gresham G, Kramer A. The Stroke Rehabilitation Outcome Study. Part II. Relative merits of the total Barthel Index score and four-item subscore in predicting patient outcomes. Arch Phys Med Rehabil 1989; 70:100–103.

26. Granger C, Dewis L, Peters N, Sherwood C, Barrett J. Stroke rehabilitation: analysis of repeated Barthel Index measures. Arch Phys Med Rehabil 1979; 60:14–17.

27. Brown EB, Tietjen GE, Deveshwar RK, Ramadam NM, Levine SR, Dietrich Kl, Nazareno F, Welch KMA. Clinical stroke scales: an intra- and interscale evaluation. Neurology 1990; 40(suppl 1):352.

28. Hsieh CL, Hsueh IP. A cross-validation of the comprehensive assessment of activities of daily living after stroke. Scand J Rehabil Med 1999; 31:83–88.

29. Jette AM. Physical disablement concepts for physical therapy research. Phys Ther 1994; 74:380–386.
30. State University of New York. Guide to the Use of the Uniform Data Set for Medical Rehabilitation Including the Functional Independence Measure. Version 3.1 Buffalo, NY: SUNY, 1990.
31. State University of New York. Guide to the Use of the Uniform Data Set for Medical Rehabilitation Including the Functional Independence Measure. Version 4.0. Buffalo, NY: SUNY, 1994.
32. Granger CV, Hamilton BB, Keith RA, Zielezny M, Sherwin FS. Advances in functional assessment for medical rehabilitation. Topics Ger Rehabil 1986; 3:59–74.
33. Merbitz C, Morris J, Grip JC. Ordinal scale and foundations of misinference. Arch Phys Med Rehabil 1989; 70:308–312.
34. Applegate WB, Blass JP, Williams TF. Instruments for the functional assessment of older patients. N Engl J Med 1990; 322:1207–1214.
35. Carey RG, Posavac EJ. Program evaluation of physical medicine and rehabilitation unit: a new approach. Arch Phys Med Rehabil 1978; 59:330–337.
36. Johnston MV, Keith RA, Hinderer SR. Measurement standard for interdisciplinary medical rehabilitation. Arch Phys Med Rehabil 1992; 73(suppl):S3–S23.
37. Wilkerson DL, Batavia AI, DeJong G. Use of functional status measures for payment of medical rehabilitation services. Arch Phys Med Rehabil 1992; 73:111–120.
38. Minaire F. La MIF: historique, présentation, perspectives. J Réadapt Méd 1991; 3:168–174.
39. Linacre JM, Heinemann AW, Wright BD, Hamilton BB, Granger CV. The structure and stability of the FIM. Arch Phys Med Rehabil 1994; 75:127–132.
40. Brosseau L, Philippe P, Dutil E, Boulanger Y. Mesure d'indépendance fonctionnelle: recension des écrits. J Réadapt Méd 1996; 1:9–21.
41. Fourn L, Brosseau L, Dassac C, Dutil E. Validation factorielle de la MIF auprès des personnes atteintes de scléroses en plaques. J Réadapt Méd 1994; 1:7–16.
42. Kidd D, Stewart G, Baldry J, Johnson J, Rossiter D, Petruckevitch A, Thompson AJ. The Functional Independence Measure: a comparative validity and reliability study. Disabil Rehabil 1995; 17:10–14.
43. Dodds TA, Martin DP, Stolov WC, Peyo RA. A validation of the FIM and its performance among rehabilitation inpatients. Arch Phys Med Rehabil 1993; 73:531–536.
44. Granger CV, Cotter AC, Hamilton BB, Fiedler RC. Functional assessment scales: a study of persons after stroke. Arch Phys Med Rehabil 1993; 74:133–138.
45. Heinemann AW, Linacre JM, Wright BD, Hamilton BB, Granger CV. Relationship between impairment and physical disability as measured by the FIM. Arch Phys Med Rehabil 1993; 74:566–573.
46. Stineman MG, Shea JA, Jette A, Tassoni CJ, Ottenbacher KJ, Fiedler R, Granger CV. The functional independence measure: tests of scaling assumptions, structure, and reliability across 20 diverse impairment categories. Arch Phys Med Rehabil 1996; 77:1101–1108.
47. Hamilton BB, Laughlin JA, Fiedler RC, Granger CV. Inter-rater reliability of the seven levels of the FIM. Scand J Rehabil Med 1994; 26:115–119.

48. Ottenbacher KJ, Hsu Y, Granger CV, Fiedler. The reliability of the functional independence measure: a quantitative review. Arch Phys Med Rehabil 1996; 77:1226–1232.

49. Gresham GE, Granger CV, Linn RT, Kulas MA. Status of functional outcomes for stroke survivors. Phys Med Rehabil Clin North Am 1999; 10:957–966.

50. Giaquinto S, Buzzelli S, Di Francesco L, Lottarini A, Montenero P, Tonin P, Nolfe G. On the prognosis of outcome after stroke. Acta Neurol Scand 1999; 100:202–208.

51. Werner RA, Kessler S. Effectiveness of an intensive outpatient rehabilitation program for postacute stroke patients. Am J Phys Med Rehabil 1996; 75:114–120.

52. Mauthe RW, Haaf DC, Hayn P, Krall JM. Predicting discharge destination of stroke patients using mathematical model based on six items from the Functional Independence Measure. Arch Phys Med Rehabil 1996; 77:10–13.

53. Oczkowsky WJ, Barecca S. The Functional Independence Measure: its use to identify rehabilitation needs in stroke survivors. Arch Phys Med Rehabil 1993; 74:1291–1294.

54. Galin LC, Rode G, Soler-Michel P, Eysette M, Boisson D. Intére//t de l'étude de la MIF dans l'évaluation de la rééducation des sujets hémiplégiques âgés de plus de 60 ans. Ann Réadapt Méd Phys 1994; 37:281–290.

55. Granger CV, Byron B, Hamilton BB, Fiedler RC. Discharge outcome after stroke rehabilitation. Stroke 1992; 23:978–982.

56. Barrois B, Ribinik P, Aranda B. Analyse comparative de l'indice de Barthel et de la MIF à l'entrée et à la sortie d'un service de réadaptation. Application sur l'avenir des patients. In: Actualités en rééducation fonctionnelle 18 ème série. Paris: Masson, 1993, pp 55–57.

57. Katz S, Ford AB, Moskowitz RW, et al. Studies of illness in the aged. The Index of ADL: a standardized measure of biological and psychosocial function. JAMA 1963; 185:914–919.

58. Katz S, Downs TD, Cash HR, et al. Progress in the development of the Index of ADL. Gerontologist 1970; 10:20–30.

59. Katz S, Apkom CA. A measure of primary sociobiological functions. Int J Health Serv 1976; 6:493–507.

60. Sauvel C, Barberger-Gateau P, Dequae L, et al. Facteurs associés à l'évolution à un an de l'autonomie fonctionnelle des personnes a//gées vivant à leur domicile. Rev Epidémiol Santé Publique 1994; 42:13–23.

61. Winblad I. Comparison of the prevalence of disability in two birth cohorts at the age of 75 years and over. J Clin Epidemiol 1993; 46:303–308.

62. Schütte T, Summa JD, Platt D. Zur rehabilitativen Behandlung von zerebralen apoplektischen Insulten in höhere Lebensalter und ihrer Effizienbeurteilung-Ergebnisse eines Modelprojekts. Z Gerontol 1984; 17:214–222.

63. Brorsson B, Asberg KH. Katz index of independence in ADL: reliability and validity in short-term care. Scand J Rehabil Med 1984; 16:125–132.

64. Spector WD, Katz S, Murphy JB, et al. The hierarchical relationship between activities of daily living and instrumental activities of daily living. J Chronic Dis 1987; 40:481–489.

65. Lindmark B. Evaluation of functional capacity after stroke with special emphasis on motor function and ADL. Scand J Rehabil Med 1988; 21S:1–40.
66. Moskowitz E, McCann CB. Classification of disability in the chronically ill and aging. J Chronic Dis 1957; 5:342–346.
67. Granger CV, Greer DS, Liset E, et al. Measurement of outcomes of care for stroke patients. Stroke 1975; 6:34–41.
68. Caroll RA, Borstein SS, Hoffman SG. Rehabilitation networking: a solution for the future. In: Granger CV, Gresham GE, eds. Functional Assessment in Rehabilitation Medicine. Baltimore: Williams & Wilkins, 1984, pp 364–377.
69. Holbrook M, Skilbeck CE. An activities index for use with stroke patients. Age Ageing 1983; 12:166–170.
70. Wade DT, Legh-Smith J, Langton Hewer R. Social activities after stroke: measurement and natural history using the Frenchay Activities Index. Int Rehabil Med 1985; 7:176–181.
71. Bond MJ, Harris RD, Smith DS, et al. An examination of the factor structure of the Frenchay Activities Index. Disabil Rehabil 1992; 14:27–29.
72. Schuling J, de Haan R, Limburg M, et al. The Frenchay Activities Index: assessment of functional status in stroke patients. Stroke 1993; 24:1173–1177.
73. Cockburn J, Smith PT, Wade DT. Influence of cognitive function on social, domestic, and leisure activities of community-dwelling older people. Int J Disabil Stud 1990; 12:169–172.
74. Nouri FM, Lincoln NB. An extended activities of daily living scale for stroke patients. Clin Rehabil 1987; 1:301–305.
75. Gladman JR, Lincoln NB, Adams SA. Use of the extended ADL scale with stroke patients. Age Ageing 1993; 22:419–424.
76. Lincoln NB, Gladman JR. The Extended Activities of Daily Living scale: a further validation. Disabil Rehabil 1992; 14:41–43.
77. Gladman JR, Lincoln NB, Barer DH. A randomised controlled trial of domiciliary and hospital-based rehabilitation for stroke patients after discharge from hospital. J Neurol Neurosurg Psychiatry 1993; 56:960–966.
78. Whiting S, Lincoln N. An ADL assessment for stroke patients. Br J Occup Ther 1980; 43:44–46.
79. Lincoln NB, Edmans JA. A re-validation of the Rivermead ADL scale for elderly patients with stroke. Age Ageing 1990; 19:19–24.
80. Rankin J. Cerebral vascular accidents in patients over the age of 60. Part 2. Prognosis. Scott Med J 1957; 2:200–215.
81. Candelise L for the Italian Acute Stroke Group. Haemodilution in acute stroke: results of the Italian Haemodilution Trial. Lancet 1988; 1:318–321.
82. Goslinga H, Eijjzenbach V, Heuvelmans JA, van de Lann de Vries E, Melis VMJ, Schmid-Schönbein H, Bezemer PD. Custom-tailored haemodilution with albumin and crystalloids in acute ischemic stroke. Stroke 1992; 23:181–188.
83. Limburg M, Hijdra A. Flunarizine in acute ischemic stroke: a pilot study. Eur Neurol 1990; 30:121–122.
84. Kaste M, Fogelholm R, Erilä T, Palomäki H, Murros K, Rissanen A; Sarna S. A randomized, double-blind, placebo-controlled trial of nimodipine in acute ischemic hemispheric stroke. Stroke 1994; 25:1348–1353.

85. van Swieten JC, Visser MC, Schouten HJA, van Gijn J. Interobserver agreement for the assessment of handicap in stroke patients. Stroke 1988; 19:604–607.
86. UK-TIA Study Group. The UK-TIA aspirin trial: Interim results. Br Med J 1988; 296:316–320.
87. Hacke W, Kaste M, Fieschi C, Toni D, Lesaffre E, von Kummer R, Boysen G, Bluhmki E, Höxter G, Mahagne M-H, Hennerici M for the ECASS Study Group. Intravenous thrombolysis with recombinant tissue plasminogen activator for acute hemispheric stroke. The European Cooperative Acute Stroke Study (ECASS). JAMA 1995; 274:1017–1025.
88. Wade DT, Langton Hewer R, Skilbeck CE, et al. A critical approach to diagnosis. Treatment and management. In: Wade DT LHR, Skilbeck CE, et al, eds. A Critical Approach to Diagnosis, Treatment and Management. London: Chapman & Hall, 1985, pp 139–140, 153–156.
89. Jennett B, Bond M. Assessment of outcome after severe brain damage. Lancet 1975; 1:480–484.
90. Mass A, Braakman R, Schouten H, Minderhoud J, van Zomeren A. Agreement between physicians on assessment of outcome following severe head injury. J Neurosurg 1983; 58:321–325.
91. Wahlgren NG, Romi F, Wahlberg J. Glasgow Outcome Scale and Global Improvement Scale were at least as sensitive as the Orgogozo, Mathew and Barthel scales in the Intravenous Nimodipine West European Stroke Trial (INWEST). Cerebrovasc Dis 1995; 5:235.
92. Collen FM, Wade DT, Bradshaw CM. Mobility after stroke: reliability of measures of impairment and disability. Int Disabil Stud 1990; 12:6–9.
93. Collen FM, Wade DT, Robb GF, Bradshaw CM. The Rivermead Mobility Index: a further development of the Rivermead Motor Assessment. Int Disabil Stud 1991; 13:50–54.
94. Forlander DA, Bohannon RW. Rivermead Mobility Index: a brief review of research to date. Clin Rehabil 1999; 13:97–100.
95. Butland RJA, Pang J, Gross ER, Woodcock AA, Geddes DM. Two, six, and twelve minute walking test in respiratory disease. Br Med J 1982; 284:1604–1608.
96. Satta NJ, Benson SM, Reding MJ, Sagullo C. Walking endurance is better than speed or functional independence measure walking subscore for documenting ambulation recovery following stroke. Stroke 1995; 26:157.
97. McGavin CR, Gupta SP, McHardy GJR. Twelve minute walking test for assessing disability in chromic bronchitis. Br Med J 1976; 1:822–823.
98. Brandstater M, de Bruin H, Gowland C, Clark B. Hemiplegic gait: analysis of temporal variable: Arch Phys Med Rehabil 1983; 65:583–587.
99. Shumumway-Cook A, Woollacott M. Motor Control. Theory and Practical Applications. Baltimore: Williams & Wilkins, 1995, pp 319–322.
100. Tiffin J. Purdue Pegboard Examine Manual. Chicago: Science Research Associates, 1968.
101. Mathiowetz V, Weber K, Kashman N, Volland G. Adult norms for the nine-hole peg test of finger dexterity. Occup Ther J Res 1985; 5:24–37.
102. Desrosiers J, Hebert R, Bravo G, Dutil E. The Purdue Pegboard Test: normative data for people aged 60 and over. Disabil Rehabil 1995; 17:217–224.

103. Reddon JR, Gill DM, Gauk SE, Maerz MD. Purdue Pegboard: test-retest estimates. Percept Mot Skills 1988; 66:503–506.
104. Jebsen RH, Taylor N, Trieschmann RB, Trotter MJ, Howard L. An objective and standard test of hand function. Arch Phys Med 1969; 50:311–319.
105. Agnew PJ, Maas P. Hand function related to age and sex. Arch Phys Med Rehabil 1982; 63:269–271.
106. Stern EB. Stability of the Jebsen-Taylor hand function tests across three test sessions. Am J Occup Ther 1992; 7:647–649.
107. Linch KB, Bridle MJ. Validity of the Jebsen-Taylor hand function test in predicting activities of daily living. Occup Ther J Res 1989; 5:316–318.
108. Carroll D. A quantitative test of upper extremity function. J Chronic Dis 1965; 18: 479–491.
109. Lyle RC. A performance test for assessment of upper limb function in physical rehabilitation treatment and research. Int J Rehabil Res 1981; 4:483–492.
110. De Souza LH, Langtom-Hewer R, Miller S. Assessment of recovery of arm control in hemiplegic stroke patients. Arm function test. Int Rehabil Med 1980; 2:3–9.
111. Wade DT, Langton-Hewer R, Wood VA, Skilbeck CE, Ismail IM. The hemiplegic arm after stroke: measurement and recovery. J Neurol Neurosurg Psychiatry 1983; 46:521–524.
112. Berglund K, Fugl-Meyer AR. Upper extremity function in hemiplegia: a cross-validation study of two assessment methods. Scand J Rehabil Med 1986; 18:155–157.

3

Handicap and Quality of Life After Stroke

Monica Åström and Kjell Asplund
University Hospital, Umeå, Sweden

I. HANDICAP—DEFINITION AND ASSESSMENT

In the World Health Organization's (WHO) model, any illness can be considered at four levels: pathology, impairment, disability, and handicap (1). Handicap is defined as "the social disadvantage for a given individual, resulting from an impairment or a disability, that limits or prevents the fulfillment of a role that is normal (depending on age, sex, social, and cultural factors) for that individual" (1).

Handicap relates to social roles that the individual no longer can fulfill, such as parenthood, being the breadwinner of the family, ability to run the home, etc. It refers to the social disadvantage that may arise from disability. A minor injury can handicap a violinist but may not restrict, or even be recognized by, someone else. The environment has a major impact upon handicap. The International Classification of Impairments, Disabilities, and Handicaps (ICIDH) suggests six areas of handicap, called "survival roles":

orientation
physical independence
mobility
occupation of time
social integration
economic self-sufficiency

A nine-point scale of severity and a description of the grading are presented in the ICIDH but reliability and validity have not been studied. Impairment and disability are more distinctly conceptualized than handicap that contains many disability-related elements (e.g., mobility, physical independence) rather than the level of social disadvantage conferred by the disability.

There are a few other handicap measures (2–4) and among them the Rankin Scale is the most well known in stroke outcome research. The original scale has been modified and the word "disability" was replaced by "handicap" and the word "lifestyle" was included in the descriptions of scoring categories (5). de Haan et al. (6) have investigated the clinical meaning of the Rankin Scale, and conclude that it should not be used as a handicap measure but rather as a global functional health index with a strong emphasis on physical disability. As such, it is useful in large multicenter studies because it is simple, reliable, and well tested.

As handicap arises from an interaction between the disability and the patient's external environment, environmental factors should also be assessed. These include physical, social, cultural, and economic conditions affecting the patient's life, e.g., appropriateness of housing, accessibility of a wheelchair in public buildings, financial allowances, availability of meals-on-wheels, etc. Clinically, a simple checklist can identify problem areas where changes can reduce handicap. Because assessment of handicap is so complex, several authorities have suggested that when medical treatments for stroke patients are evaluated, focus should not be on handicap as a primary outcome but rather on more tangible manifestations of disease such as disability (7,8).

However, the extent to which a disabled stroke patient can fulfill expected social roles and relate adequately with his social environment is of major importance for his overall quality of life. The concept of "quality of life" (QL) does not feature within the ICIDH model. In this context, Wade (8) proposes that handicap could be seen as probably synonymous with QL.

In 1997, WHO made a revision of the ICIDH model called the ICIDH-2 (9). The terms "disability" and "handicap" are replaced by the more positive terms "activity" and "participation" (e.g., in society). According to this classification, impairments, activity limitations, and participation restriction are the negative poles of these dimensions and describe the disablement of a person. The contextual factors consist of external environmental and internal personal factors that interact to form the level of disablement. The ICIDH-2 is aimed at field trials and is yet not implemented in clinical practice and research.

Clearly, more patient-centered outcomes are needed. In a 1998 meta-analysis based on the Cochrane Stroke Group's database, handicap or QL was assessed as clinical outcome in only 2% of acute stroke trials (use of the Rankin Scale excluded) (10). Most measures were inadequate in terms of their content, reliability, validity, and statistical analysis, and were of insufficient relevance to patients. The authors state that phase III trials in acute stroke ought to concentrate on measurement of disability, handicap, or health-related QL. More than a decade earlier, Seale and Davies (11), after an examination of representative articles in stroke rehabilitation research, reached the same conclusion.

II. QL—METHODOLOGICAL CONSIDERATIONS

A. Theoretical Aspects

Fifty years ago, WHO defined health as not merely the absence of disease but also physical, mental, and social well-being (12). Since then, QL aspects have become steadily more important in health care and research, being used to sum up various health-related components centered around the patient's point of view. Health status, life satisfaction, and QL are concepts that have been used interchangeably.

Valued aspects of life exist, which are not considered as "health," but they are mostly used by social scientists in population studies. As we here focus on QL after stroke, we restrict the term to health-related quality of life (HQL). HQL is conceptualized as the physical, psychological, and social aspects of health, seen as distinct areas influenced by a person's experience, beliefs, expectations, and perceptions (13). These core aspects of life are thought of as affected by changes in health states filtered through the person's values, personality, coping strategies, etc. The importance of measuring outcome of stroke in this more holistic way has become increasingly recognized.

When the HQL concept is considered unidimensionally and globally (e.g., "How would you rate your quality of life?"), it becomes vague and ambiguously defined. Nevertheless, a global rating by the patient of his or her "overall" HQL is a valuable and recommended part of a more extensive HQL measurement (14).

Today, there is a broad consensus on the multidimensionality of the HQL concept. The number of domains and the extent to which they are covered vary between instruments (Table 1). Dimensions such as self-care, mobility, sexuality, activity level/work are often added. The physical dimension refers to disease- and treatment-related symptoms. Central components of the psychological life domain are emotional and cognitive status, general well-being, life satisfaction, or happiness. The social dimension includes social integration and contacts. Health profiles are descriptive and attempt to measure all important aspects of HQL. Thus, differential effects on specific dimensions of HQL are possible to detect. Well-known examples of this type of scales are shown in Table 1.

B. Generic and Disease-Specific Scales

HQL measures can be differentiated into:

> generic ("broad-spectrum") scales
> disease-specific scales
> scale batteries

The generic scales are applicable across different diseases, as they are not developed for a specific target population. Thus, they allow comparison of HQL results across patient populations or different diseases. Generic instruments include

Table 1 Generic HQL Instruments Used in Stroke Research: A Comparison

Instrument (ref. to early version)	Selected refs.	Studies in stroke (ref.)	Reliability	Validity	No. of items	No. of domains (incl global health)	Domain[a]							Comments
							Physical health	Functional health (incl. ADL activity, etc.)	Psychological/ emotional	Social	Pain	Sleep	Energy	
SIP (16)	(16, 29)	(7, 21, 29)	++	++	136	12	X	X	X	X		X	X	Also "change in health"
SF-36 (31)	(31, 32, 81)	(32–35)	++	++	36	8	X	X	X	X	X		X	
NHP (15)	(15)	(37)	+	+	45	6 (part 1)	X	(part 2)	X	X	X	X	X	Part 2 includes effects on 7 life areas
EuroQOL (38)	(38)	(39–40)	+	+	6	6	X	X	X	X	X			Also global health

SIP = Sickness Impact Profile (16)

SF-36 = Short Form-36 (31)

NHP = Nottingham Health Profile (15)

EuroQOL = EuroQOL Quality of Life Scale (38)

[a] As domains differ in content and labeling, this is a simplified comparison.

health profiles and utility measures of HQL. For example, the Nottingham Health Profile (15), as shown by its name, contains a profile consisting of 13 component dimensions (subscales). Some instruments, such as the Sickness Impact Profile (SIP) (16), report results either as a profile or as a single aggregated score, or both. Examples of other instruments often used in stroke research emerge from Table 1.

In utility measures of HQL, a single summary score is obtained. The single score is thought of as representing the net impact on quality and quantity of life. By comparing alternative treatments, HQL-based cost-utility analyses are an integral part of pharmacoeconomic evaluations and have been used as a basis for allocation of limited health care resources. There is an ongoing debate regarding standards and guidelines in this expanding field.

Generic scales are not always sufficiently focused on the specific problems of interest. The disease-specific scales assess HQL with questions and scales specific to a disease or condition. They often are more relevant to patients as the questions cover functions typically affected by that disease, e.g., stroke. These scales do not allow comparisons across diseases but are more sensitive to assess within-subject changes over time (e.g., in clinical trials) and can detect small changes in scores between experimental and control groups. Only a few disease-specific scales have been developed for stroke.

A battery of established scales can be selected for measuring the specific domains of interest, such as ADL, depression, cognitive and social functioning, etc. This approach gives good possibility to assess each relevant domain more in depth, and with high psychometric quality of data.

Each approach has its strengths and weaknesses and is suitable for different circumstances. A combination of generic and disease-specific measures may be used, especially in groups of patients in whom comorbidity is prevalent, such as among elderly stroke patients. However, substantial resources are needed for data collection, and a whole battery of tests can burden the patients too much.

C. Modes of Administration

Patients' self-reports are the basis for most of the available HQL instruments. Structured interviews or written questionnaires for self-administration are used for data collection. The former method requires considerable resources, but gives better compliance and decreases misunderstandings and missing items. The latter approach is less expensive, but has a lower response rate. Both methods have weaknesses in studies of stroke patients, who often cannot read or write, have aphasia, and have cognitive disorders. These patients have often been excluded from HQL assessments. As this is a highly relevant subgroup of patients, many results cannot be generalized to the total stroke population. One solution has been to ask physicians to rate their patients' HQL. Studies have shown low interrater reliability and disagreement between physician and patient ratings (17,18).

Significant others, such as partners or children, are an alternative source of information. In this so-called proxy rating, the respondent is asked to answer the questions as he or she thinks the patient would. Evidence regarding the quality of proxy ratings is mixed (19,20). Sneeuw et al. (21) assessed HQL after stroke by means of the Sickness Impact profile (SIP). The proxies systematically rated patients as having more functional impairments than the patients had rated themselves. This is in agreement with other findings (19). Nevertheless, the authors conclude that the benefits of using proxy ratings, for noncommunicative stroke patients, outweigh their limitations (the difference was small). This is confirmed in a study of stroke patients and their caregivers, using the Health Utilities Index (22). The correlation between patient and proxy ratings was acceptable, also regarding more subjective domains of HQL, such as pain and emotion. Further, Robinson (23) found that valid social functioning assessment can be made by another person who is well acquainted with the patient.

Another approach to include as many noncommunicative patients as possible is to use a visual analogue scale (VAS) (24,25). It typically consists of a 10-cm line, where patients are asked to make a mark to reflect their current state between the two defined extremes of the line. Ahlsiö et al. found that VAS was a useful tool in stroke patients (24), but Kwa et al. remark that the VAS did not fulfill their expectations regarding an increase of the number of testable patients (25). Price et al. (26) investigated how stroke-related impairments could alter the ability of subjects to answer accurately on VAS, and concluded that many patients after a stroke are unable to successfully complete self-report measurement scales, including VAS.

D.   HQL as a Measure in Clinical Practice

Routine assessment of HQL in clinical practice could serve many purposes, e.g., to really assess the needs and concerns of one specific individual, to describe his or her overall state also regarding subjective matters, setting treatment goals in which the patient actively participates, monitoring treatment response, etc. A crucial question is: Can a change in a measure that has been shown meaningful in group terms be expected to have the same relevance on an individual basis? To be used at the individual-patient level, scales should meet several measurement standards, e.g., regarding reliability, range, and depth of health states (ceiling and floor effects), responsiveness, and validity. McHorney and Tarlov (27) concluded, after an examination of HQL instruments proposed for individual-patient application, that the tools available today are far from perfect for individual-patient assessment, and particularly so for longitudinal individual monitoring.

In clinical practice, HQL measures can be used as the first part of a screening process. Although imprecise, they can act as "flags" for problems (e.g., emotional, social, functional, etc.) that otherwise could be unrecognized. An example of an HQL instrument intended for routine clinical use is the COOP Chart system (28). It comprises nine simple charts, where a drawing illustrates the domains, such as perceived health and physical, emotional, and social functioning, along a five-point ordinal scale. The drawings make the charts "user-friendly." Mostly, it has been used in primary care. Its usefulness and psychometric properties in stroke patients have not been reported.

E. HQ Measures in Stroke Studies

Stroke studies have not used HQL measures until quite recently. The *Sickness Impact Profile* (SIP) has been used in a long-term follow-up study of stroke patients (29). A major disadvantage of SIP is its length. A shorter version is developed for use in stroke outcome research, and is called SA-SIP 30 (30). The authors conclude that it is a feasible and clinimetrically sound measure. However, its responsiveness is not known, and there is uncertainty if its yes/no format makes it less sensitive to within-patient changes.

The *Short Form 36* (SF-36) is rapidly becoming the generic HQL measure of choice for use in many settings (31), and is increasingly being used in stroke studies (32–35). Anderson et al. (32) explored its validity in stroke patients and found it to be high as regards physical and mental health but less valid in social functioning. They used an interview setting, and found low rates of missing data. Administration of SF 36 (as well as other HQL scales) by mail is not appropriate in elderly stroke patients. A shorter form, called SF-12, reproduces SF-36 scores (physical and mental subscales) without substantial loss of information in stroke patients capable of self-report (36).

The *Nottingham Health Profile* (NHP) is commonly used in many countries (15). NHP emotion scores are convergent with well-known depression scales (37), and might be a valid screening of depressed mood. Thus, patients with high NHP emotion scores should be questioned more closely about depression.

The *EuroQOL Instrument* was developed by a multidisciplinary group of European researchers (38). An advantage over the SF-36 is its simplicity. In the International Stroke Trial, patients were randomized to either the SF-36 or the EuroQOL (39). More patients provided complete data on the EuroQOL. This research group also has validated the EuroQOL for proxy completion (40). There is a continuing research agenda from the EuroQOL collaboration group, indicating that progress will continue to be made.

Two new stroke-specific measures of HQL, called *SS-QOL* (34) and *Stroke Impact Scale Version 2.0* (41), seem promising regarding reliability, validity, and responsiveness in mild to moderate stroke. The development of these scales, as well as SA-SIP 30 (30), is based on stroke patients who had the communication skills and cognitive function to participate. Further studies are required in larger and more heterogeneous stroke populations, and the feasibility and validity of proxy responses for more severely impaired patients have to be evaluated.

F.   Assessing QL in the Family

Means of assessing the QL of the total family system around the stroke patient need to be developed. However, there are special scales to estimate the burden of caregiving. The *Sense of Competence Questionnaire* (SCQ) has been developed and used to measure the burden in caregivers of dementia patients. At least one study has shown that SCQ has good psychometric properties for use in assessing the burden of caregiving in partners of stroke patients (42). The instrument may help to identify caregivers at risk for high levels of burden. Furthermore, the SCQ is able to identify the characteristics of caregiving that especially burden caregivers of stroke patients and thus give guidelines for interventions to provide support.

The *Caregiver Strain Index* (23) has been used to identify the strain perceived by caregivers of stroke patients (43). It is a short summary measure. Its validity was well tested in the original paper; however, not in stroke carers.

The burden of caregiving often leads to physical as well as psychological health problems, emotional distress, depression, and social isolation (44,45). Thus, the HQL concept might be relevant, and the ''broad-spectrum'' instruments recently described could be used as a screening device also in the carers. For instance, in a study of HQL in partners to patients after subarachnoid hemorrhage (46), the SF-36, the SIP, and a visual analogue scale were used. However, the psychometric properties for this purpose have not been reported.

Today, the most valuable instrument for assessing burden of caregiving as experienced by partners of stroke patients seems to be the multidimensional and specific SCQ (42). It might be suitable for use in clinical trials as well as in everyday clinical practice. Further studies are needed to explore the influence of partner characteristics on perceived burden.

III.   IMPACT OF STROKE ON QL AND HANDICAP

A.   Patients' Preferences for Various Outcomes of Stroke

Time tradeoff or standard gamble methods have been used to assess how people value life after stroke. On a scale with 0 as worst possible life and 1 as perfect health, life after a minor stroke scores 0.88–0.91 on average, whereas a major stroke scores 0.51–0.61 (47). Interestingly, stroke survivors assign considerably higher QL utilities than healthy people. Psychological mechanisms like inhibition (patients) and stigmatization (healthy people) may explain the differences in how the consequences of a stroke are perceived.

A U.S. study included patients who had suffered a stroke or were at particular risk. As many as 45% considered major stroke to be a worse outcome than death (48). Subjects who considered major stroke to have the greatest impact on HQL were older and perceived themselves to be in poorer health. Again, patients who already had had a stroke assigned higher values to life after stroke than asymptomatic patients at risk (48). In a similar study on preferences for life-sustaining treatment performed in Canada, 29% of patients who had suffered a stroke thought that a severe stroke was worse than death. This proportion was considerably lower than among older people without stroke (49%) (49).

Common to all studies, and perhaps the most striking finding, is that there is a wide variation in how people perceive life after stroke (47,48,50). Nevertheless, the studies uniformly show that people who have experienced a stroke assign higher values to life after stroke than healthy individuals do.

B. Reduced QL as Predictor for Stroke

Psychosocial factors have been shown to predict various manifestations of cardiovascular disease, including stroke. In a study focusing on QL as predictor in a cohort of treated hypertensive men, patients with poor contentment and/or poor vitality at entry into the study had a significantly higher risk for stroke during more than 6 years of follow-up (51). The relationship persisted after adjustment for a large number of other possible determinants.

C. Quantification of QL Reduction After Stroke

Figure 1 shows the proportion of stroke patients who experience deterioration in QL at late follow-up (at least 1 year after stroke), in relation either to their prestroke situation or to nonstroke subjects of the same age. This proportion ranges from 44% to 60%. For five studies combined, the proportion with lowered QL or increased handicap is 54% (95% confidence interval 48–60%).

When quantified using various scales, usually the SIP or VAS, the mean or median reduction in QL is typically estimated at 20–35% (Table 2). When the extent of handicap is measured, a median reduction of approximately 60% has been reported (52).

D. QL Over Time After Stroke

Few studies have assessed how QL changes over time after stroke. Figure 2 shows the time profile in two such studies. In one of the studies, the patients were asked to relate their present QL to the situation before stroke. In the other study, the

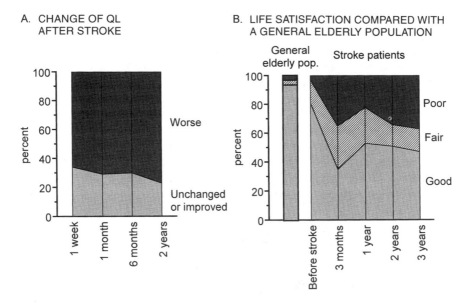

A. CHANGE OF QL
   AFTER STROKE

B. LIFE SATISFACTION COMPARED WITH
   A GENERAL ELDERLY POPULATION

Fig. 1 Longitudinal development of QL and life satisfaction. (Left) How patients rate their QL in relation to the situation before stroke. Data from Ahlsiö et al. (24). (Right) How stroke patients estimate their life satisfaction in comparison with a general elderly population. Adapted from Åström et al. (53).

Table 2 Quantitative Change as Measured by QL or Handicap Instruments (studies listed by number of patients)

First author, year (ref.)	Country	No. of patients	Time to follow-up	Percentage decline[a]
Hackett, 2000 (35)	New Zealand	639	6 years	−16%
de Haan, 1995 (57)	The Netherlands	441	6 mo	−24%
Sneew, 1997 (21)	The Netherlands	228	6 mo	−18%
Johansson, 1992 (60)	Sweden	224	6 mo	−22%
Ebrahim, 1986 (37)	UK	198	6 mo	−25%
Yoon, 1997 (61)	Korea	119	Not stated	−30%
Ahlsiö, 1984 (24)	Sweden	96	2 years	−24%
King, 1996 (55)	USA	86	1–3 years	−24%
Nydevik, 1991 (98)	Sweden	57	9 mo	−25%
Kim, 1999 (99)	Canada	50	1–3 years	−38%
Bethoux, 1999 (100)	France	45	6–26 mo	−44%
Jonkman, 1998 (101)	The Netherlands	35	1 year	−66%
Granger, 1993 (102)	USA	21	3–12 mo	−35%

[a] Calculated from various scoring systems with baseline = maximum points.

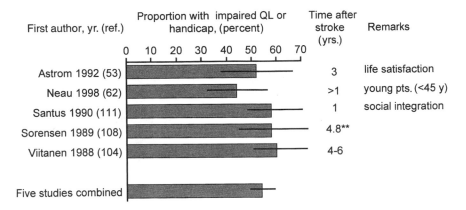

Fig. 2 Proportion of stroke patients with impaired QL, life satisfaction, or social integration (handicap) in five studies with follow-up performed at least 1 year after stroke (307 patients in total). The proportions relate either to the situation before stroke or to a reference population. Horizontal lines show 95% confidence intervals.

patients were asked if their QL was good, fair, or poor and the ratings were compared with a general elderly population. Both approaches show that there is little or no spontaneous improvement of QL late after the stroke event. The study by Åström et al. (53) also showed that life satisfaction was considerably lower in patients already before stroke compared to a general population of the same age (Fig. 2B).

E. Effects of Stroke on Dimensions of QL and Handicap

Several of the studies on QL after stroke have reported on the effects on various dimensions of QL and handicap. In general, physical, mental, as well as emotional dimensions and social functioning are profoundly affected (29,33,52,54–56). Stroke may also have severe impact on economic self-sufficiency (52,55). Figure 3 illustrates the profiles of deterioration in one large study on QL and one study on handicap after stroke.

F. Size, Localization, and Type of Brain Lesion

As shown in Table 3, large size of brain lesion, not unexpectedly, predicts poor QL at late follow-up. Patients with lacunar infarcts have better outcome in various dimensions of QL with the exception of emotional distress, which seems to be

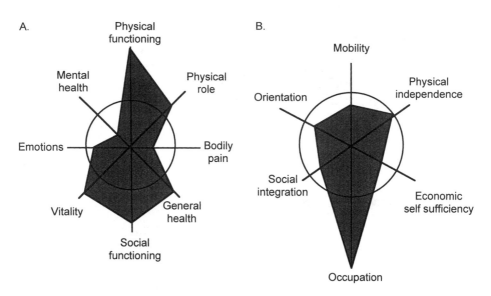

Fig. 3 Extent to which stroke affects various dimensions of QL and handicap. Circles denote a 10% reduction in a QL dimension (A) and a 25% increase in the degree of handicap (B). Based on data by Hackett et al. (35) (n = 639) and Harwood et al. (52) (n = 141).

as common as in patients with cortical or subcortical stroke (57). Left-sided and right-sided hemispheric lesions appear to have similar effects on the various QL dimensions at 6 months after stroke with one obvious exception: the dimension of communication is much more often impaired in patients with right-sided lesions (57).

Surviving patients with infarcts and cerebral hemorrhages seem to have similar QL outcome (Table 3). Survivors after a subarachnoid hemorrhage quite often experience substantial deterioration of QL (58), but direct comparisons suggest that they are better off than patients with ischemic stroke (54).

G. Other Determinants of QL

A large number of studies have attempted to identify determinants of handicap or poor QL after stroke (Table 4). Many of the studies included only a few patients and had low statistical power to detect possible determinants. A general picture emerges, with depression, stroke severity with impaired ADL functions, and poor social support as being very important determinants of poor QL. Depression is also closely related to loss of social activities (59), which may be seen

Table 3 Effect of Type, Size, and Localization of Brain Lesion on QL After Stroke (studies listed by number of patients)

First author, year (ref.)	Country	No. of patients	Time of follow-up	Type of stroke	Size of lesion	Localization
de Haan, 1995; Sneew, 1997 (21, 57)	The Netherlands	437–441	6 mo	Similar QL after infarcts and intracerebral hemorrhages	Relatively good QL after lacunar infarcts	Worse QL after supratentorial than after infratentorial infarcts
Kwa, 1996 (25)	The Netherlands	97	3 mc–4 years		QL worse after larger infarcts	No difference between right- vs. left-sided hemispheric or between supra- vs. infratentorial infarcts
Niemi, 1998 (54)	Finland	46	4 years	Worse QL after infarcts than after SAHs		Worse QL after hemispheric than after brainstem infarcts
Brilstra, 1997 (103)	The Netherlands	25	6 mo–6 years	No reduction in QL among survivors of perimesencephalic hemorrhage		

Table 4   Studies Aimed at Identifying Determinants of Poor QL or Handicap After Stroke (listed by number of patients studied)

Author, year (ref.)	Country	No. of patients	Time to follow-up	High age	Sex	Education, SES[a]	Social support, martial status	Motor dysfunction	ADL function	Depression	Cognitive impairment	Aphasia	Comorbidity
de Haan, 1995; Sneew, 1997 (21, 57)	The Netherlands	437–441	6 mo.	+								+	+
Duncan, 1997 (33)	USA	304	mean 535 days		−			+		+			
Harwood, 1994 (52)	UK	141	1 year						+	+		+	
Kwa, 1996 (25)	The Netherlands	129	3 mo.–4 years	−		−			+	+	+		−
Yoon, 1997 (61)	Korea	119	not stated				+	+					
Ahlsiö, 1984 (24)	Sweden	96	2 years	−	−	−			+	+			
Johansson, 1992 (60)	Sweden	90	1 year		−		+		+				
King, 1996 (55)	USA	86	1–3 years				+		+	+			
Åström, 1992 (64)	Sweden	80	3 mo.	−	−		−		+	+			
Viitanen, 1988 (104)	Sweden	62	4–6 years					+	+				
Wyller, 1997 (105)	Norway	60	1 year		−			+	−				
Nydevik, 1991 (98)	Sweden	57	9 mo.						+		−		
Åström, 1992 (53)	Sweden	50	3 years	+			+		+	+			
Kim, 1999 (99)	Canada	50	1–3 years				+		+	+			
Löfgren, 1999 (110)	Sweden	47	3 years							+			
Niemi, 1998 (54)	Finland	46	4 years	+	−			+	+	+			
Jonkman, 1998 (101)	The Netherlands	35	1 year								+		
Granger, 1993 (102)	USA	21	3–12 mo.						+	+	+		
Taylor-Sarno, 1992 (106)	USA	20	3 mo.							+		+	

[a] Socioeconomic status.

as a proxy for handicap. There is considerable, although somewhat weaker, support for high age, aphasia, and cognitive impairment as determinants of poor QL. Premorbid personality traits have occasionally been reported to influence QL after stroke (60,61). After adjustment for age, men and women seem to experience about the same deterioration in QL after stroke (Table 4).

H. Specific Aspects of QL and Handicap

1. Return to Work

The proportion of stroke patients who are able to return to their previous work obviously depends on age and type and severity of stroke. Most studies on work as an aspect of QL have reported that 54–73% of patients have been able to return to previous work, either full-time or part-time (Table 5). In a French study, patients who returned to full-time work did so at 4 months after stroke on average, whereas patients who could work only part-time or needed adjustments in their work returned at a mean of 18 months (62). In a multivariate analysis, stroke severity was the only independent determinant of return to work (62).

2. Leisure

Leisure is closely associated with life satisfaction (63). Even prior to stroke, the patients have reduced physical and social activities (64). They often fail to resume leisure activities that they had before stroke. The reduction in leisure pursuits caused by loss of physical ability is, even in young stroke patients, seldom replaced by new types of activities (65). Survivors of a subarachnoid hemorrhage often have a significant reduction in their leisure-time activities despite relatively few physical limitations (58,66).

Both the number of leisure activities and the frequency are reduced (65,67). Not only physical but also other activities like reading books diminish (64). The result is often a discontented and passive patient, with time spent alone or with the spouse (65). In fact, reduction in leisure activities contributes substantially to overall loss of QL after stroke (29). Improved leisure activity may be an important component of stroke rehabilitation but there are, as yet, no scientific studies to support the concept that this approach will improve overall life satisfaction among stroke patients (63). A small randomized trial failed to show any effects on QL of occupational therapy aimed at improving leisure-time activities (68).

3. Sexual Activity

Sexual activity is one component of QL that is seldom addressed in follow-up studies after stroke. It has, however, been shown that long-term survivors after stroke have a very marked decline in all sexual functions measured: libido, coital

Table 5 Return to Work Among Subjects Who Were Fully Employed Before Stroke (only studies on work as a component of QL, listed by number of included patients)

First author, year (ref.)	Country	No. of patients	Patient characteristics	Return to work, %		
				Full employment	Part-time or adjusted employment	No return to work
Lindberg, 1992 (66)	Sweden	296	Long-term survivors of SAH (2–13 years after the event)	60%		——40%——
Ogden, 1997 (107)	New Zealand	123	Survivors of SAH 4–7 years after the event	59%		——41%——
Soelberg-Sørensen, 1989 (108)	Denmark	102	Patients with ischemic events of < 72 hr duration		——62%——	38%
Neau, 1998 (62)	France	63	<45 years, brain infarct	54%	19%	27%
Niemi, 1998 (54)	Finland	39	<65 years, survivors at 4 years, all stroke subtypes		——54%——	46%

frequency, erectile and orgasmic ability, vaginal lubrication, and sexual satisfaction (69–71). Severe ADL dependency and impaired cutaneous sensibility has been identified as important determinants of loss of sexual activity (69). Fear that a new stroke may occur during intercourse may also contribute (70). Not only stroke patients but also their spouses report reduced libido, sexual activity, and satisfaction (71). Unsuccessful coping seems to be crucial for sexual dysfunction after stroke (69).

I. Impact of Stroke Interventions on QL

1. Organization of Stroke Services

The beneficial effects of dedicated stroke units on survival, disability, and need for long-term institutional care have been amply demonstrated (72). However, few of the 19 randomized trials included in the Stroke Unit Trialists' Collaboration studied QL as an end point. In a trial performed in Trondheim, Norway, improvement in several dimensions of QL (energy, physical mobility, emotions, social activities, and sleep) was observed as late as 10 years after stroke unit care (73). Another Norwegian trial, performed in Oslo, failed to confirm any effects of stroke unit management on HQL (74). A major difference between the Trondheim and the Oslo stroke units was that the former placed considerably more emphasis on early rehabilitation with longer hospital stay.

Not unexpectedly, a very modest intervention like distribution of an information pack to stroke patients at discharge from hospital had no measurable impact on any of the aspects of QL 6 months after stroke (75).

In randomized controlled trials of home rehabilitation versus conventional rehabilitation, QL has been measured as outcome in one trial (76) and handicap in one trial (77). Both studies failed to detect any significant differences in these outcomes. After having reviewed seven randomized trials on day-hospital rehabilitation, the evaluators concluded that, as of now, it has not been possible to prove beneficial effects of this form of rehabilitation (78).

2. Acute Stroke Treatment

In calculations of the cost-effectiveness of acute thrombolytic therapy in ischemic stroke, quality-adjusted life years (QALYs) gained have been calculated in the U.S. NINDS rt-PA trial. The estimated improvement in health outcome was approximately 0.5 QALYs saved per patient treated (79). It should be noted that these calculations are based on results from the single most successful trial of thrombolytic therapy, and that modeling, which included several imprecise assumptions, was used. The estimates of QALYs saved by thrombolytic therapy are therefore crude.

3. Antithrombotic Stroke Prevention

Time tradeoff and standard gamble methods have been applied to patients with atrial fibrillation to estimate the utilities of aspirin and warfarin in stroke prevention (80). Both antithrombotic strategies were found to have generally high utilities; i.e., the trouble of taking drugs and the risks involved by far outweigh the effects of a possible stroke as estimated by the patients. However, a small subgroup of patients with atrial fibrillation (16%) rated the utility of warfarin therapy so low that their quality-adjusted life expectancy would be greater with aspirin (80).

4. Surgery

In an uncontrolled study with methodological weaknesses, cerebral vascularization (extracranial-intracranial bypass) surgery in stroke patients was reported to improve QL and return to work (81). These beneficial results are yet to be confirmed in controlled trials. There seem to be no immediate adverse or beneficial effects by carotid endarterectomy on HQL (82). An exception may possibly be patients operated for carotid stenoses who have a contralateral carotid occlusion. In a small group of such patients, improvement in QL was reported at 3 months after the endarterectomy (82). Cognitive function has been reported to be close to normal 8–11 years after carotid endarterectomy, but nonoperated patients with carotid stenoses have the same good cognitive performance at late follow-up (83).

5. Acupuncture

Effects of acupuncture in the subacute phase of stroke on QL have been reported in four randomized control trials. Two early studies reported improved social situation and/or QL (84,112), whereas two subsequent trials failed to confirm any beneficial effects (85,86). Features of the two negative trials (as distinct from the positive ones) were that they included more patients and that subjects in the control group received the same attention and time as the intervention group.

6. Physiotherapy and Occupational Therapy

There is limited scientific information from controlled trials on the effects of physiotherapy, occupational therapy, and speech therapy on long-term QL and/or handicap. In a randomized trial of 101 severely disabled stroke patients, intensive training of leg or arm function was shown to give at least a temporary improvement in sickness impact (87). A program involving aerobic exercises and muscle strengthening has also been reported to improve quality of life, as measured by the Nottingham Health Profile (88).

In a British study randomizing stroke patients 1 month after the event, 5 months of occupational therapy at home was compared with no intervention. Occupational therapy significantly reduced handicap, measured by the London handicap scale, and also reduced cargivers' strain (89). In a similar randomized trial, a relatively brief (6 weeks) domiciliary occupational program improved overall patient satisfaction (but specific QL or handicap was not assessed) (90). An intense multifaceted rehabilitation program late (> 1 year) after stroke seemed to be beneficial after 3 months' intervention when compared with no treatment in a trial that was small and not strictly randomized (91). There is, as yet, no scientific support for an effect of specific speech therapy on QL or handicap (92).

Common to all rehabilitation programs that have reported beneficial effects on QL or handicap is that they have also had positive effects on determinants of QL such as physical performance, gait, or ADL proficiency.

J. QL of Caregivers

A meta-analysis published in 1999 identified 31 studies on QL of informal carers of stroke patients (93). Caregivers, most often the spouse, usually experience a considerable physical and emotional burden (22,94). This is so not only in carers of elderly stroke patients but also among partners of relatively young patients who have had a subarachnoid hemorrhage (46). The spouses rate their satisfaction with the marriage much lower after stroke compared with the situation before their partner was affected.

Coresident caregivers of stroke patients experience the same degree of burden and have the same high levels of psychological morbidity as the caregivers of demented patients (94). The patients' physical as well as mental impairments contribute to the burden placed on caregivers. Partners are especially burdened by the consequences of caregiving for their own personal life, e.g., the burden of continuously feeling heavily responsible and worried (42). Loss of the possibilities to travel seems to be particularly frustrating (95). Inappropriate expectations of what the stroke patient can do may lead to strained family relations (96). A substantial proportion of the carers who were working at the time the patient has his/her stroke give up there jobs during the subsequent year (97). Table 6 lists some of the determinants of poor well-being of carers of stroke patients.

Few interventions have been directed at improving carer outcomes and the studies have shown mixed results (93). Lack of information is only a weak predictor of poor QL in caregivers (42), and it is unlikely that better information alone will improve the well-being of caregivers. It has been suggested that use of positive coping strategies (93), sharing of responsibilities, and getting tempo-

Table 6 Determinants of Poor QL Among Caregivers of Stroke Patients

Patient characteristics	Caregiver characteristics
Extensive impairments (100,109) and severe handicap (42)	Degree of disability (109)
Poor QL (42,111)	Close relation to patient (111)
Impaired cognitive function (42)	Social isolation (109)
Degree of extraversion (111)	Emotional distress (109)
Behavior (e.g., demanding, irritable or depressed) (97)	Unrealistic expectations of what the patient can do (96)
	Unmet demands of psychosocial and physical support (109)

rary relief from caregiving (42) may be useful ways of supporting caregivers of stroke patients.

REFERENCES

1. WHO. Classifications of Impairments, Disabilities and Handicap. Geneva, Switzerland: World Health Organization 1980.
2. Holbrook M, Skilbeck C. An activities index for use with stroke patients. Age Ageing 1983; 12:166–170.
3. Harwood R, Roger A, Dickinson E, Ebrahim S. Measuring handicap: the London handicap scale, a new outcome measure for chronic disease. Qual Health Care 1994; 3:11–15.
4. Rankin J. Cerebral vascular accidents in patients over the age of 60. II: prognosis. Scott Med J 1957; 2:200–215.
5. Bamford J, Sandercock P, Warlow C, Slattery J. Interobserver agreement for the assessment of handicap in stroke (letter). Stroke 1989; 20:828.
6. de Haan R, Limburg M, Bossuyt P, van der Meulen J, Aaronson N. The clinical meaning of Rankin "handicap" grades after stroke. Stroke 1995; 26:2027–2030.
7. de Haan R, Aaronson N, Limburg M, Langton-Hewer R, Crevel H. Measuring quality of life in stroke. Stroke 1993; 24:320–327.
8. Wade DT. Measurement in Neurological Rehabilitation. New York: Oxford University Press, 1992.
9. WHO. International Classification of Impairments, Activities and Participation: A Manual of Dimensions of Disablements and Functioning. Beta-1 Draft for Field Trials. Geneva, Switzerland: World Health Organization, 1997.
10. Roberts L, Counsell C. Assessment of clinical outcomes in acute stroke trials. Stroke 1998; 29:986–991.

11. Seale C, Davies P. Outcome measurement in stroke rehabilitation research. Int Disabil Stud 1987; 9:155–160.
12. WHO. Constitution of the World Health Organization. Handbook of Basic Documents, 5th ed. Geneva, Switzerland: World Health Organization, 1952.
13. Testa MA, Simonson DC. Assessment of quality-of-life outcomes. N Engl J Med 1996; 334:835–840.
14. Gill TH, Feinstein AR. A critical appraisal of the quality of quality-of-life measurement. JAMA 1994; 272:619–626.
15. European Group for Quality of Life Assessment and Health Measurement. European Guide to the Nottingham Health Profile. Surrey: Brookwood Medical Publications, 1993.
16. Bergner M, Bobbitt RA, Carter WB, Gilson BS. The Sickness Impact Profile: development and final revision of a health status measure. Med Care 1981; 19:787–805.
17. Lomas J, Pickard L, Mohide A. Patient versus clinician item generation for quality-of-life measures. Med Care 1987; 25:764–769.
18. Hall JA, Epstein AM, McNeil BJ. Multidimensionality of health status on an elderly population: construct validity of a measurement battery. Med Care 1989; 27:S168–S177.
19. Sprangers MAG, Aaronson NK. The role of health care providers and significant others in evaluating the quality of life of patients with chronic disease. J Clin Epidemiol 1992; 45:743–760.
20. McCusker J, Stoddard AM. Use of a surrogate for the SIP. Med Care 1984; 22:789–795.
21. Sneeuw KCA, Aaronson NK, de Haan RJ, Limburg M. Assessing quality of life after stroke. Stroke 1997; 28:1541–1549.
22. Mathias SD, Bates MM, Pasta DJ, Cisternas MG, Feeny D, Patrick DL. Use of the Health Utilities Index with stroke patients and their caregivers. Stroke 1997; 28:1888–1894.
23. Robinson B. Validation of a caregiver strain index. J Gerontol 1983; 38:344–348.
24. Ahlsiö B, Britton M, Murray V, Theorell T. Disablement and quality of life after stroke. Stroke 1984; 15:886–890.
25. Kwa VIH, Limburg M, de Haan RJ. The role of cognitive impairment in the quality of life after ischaemic stroke. J Neurol 1996; 243:599–604.
26. Price CIM, Curless RH, Rodgers H. Can stroke patients use visual analogue scales? Stroke 1999; 30:1357–1361.
27. McHorney CA, Tarlov A. Individual-patient monitoring in clinical practice: are available health status surveys adequate? Qual Life Res 1995; 4:293–307.
28. Nelson E, Wasson J, Kirk J, Keller A, Clark D, Dietrich A, Stewart A, Zubkoff M. Assessment of function in routine clinical practice: description of the COOP Chart method and preliminary findings. J Chronic Dis 1987; 40(suppl 1):55S–63S.
29. Nydevik I, Hulter-Åsberg K. Sickness impact after stroke. A 3-year follow-up. Scand J Prim Health Care 1992; 10:284–289.
30. van Straten A, de Haan RJ, Limburg M, Schuling J, Bossuyt PM, van den Bos GAM. A stroke-adapted 30-item version of the Sickness Impact Profile to assess quality of life (SA-SIP 30). Stroke 1997; 28:2155–2161.

31. Ware JE, Sherbourne CD. The MOS 36-item short-form health survey (SF-36) I. Conceptual framework and item selection. Med Care 1992; 30:473–483.
32. Anderson C, Laubscher S, Burns R. Validation of the Short Form 36 (SF-36) Health Survey Questionnaire among stroke patients. Stroke 1996; 27:1812–1816.
33. Duncan PW, Samsa GP, Weinberger M, Goldstein LB, Bonito A, Witter DM, Enarson C, Matchar D. Health status of individuals with mild stroke. Stroke 1997; 28:740–745.
34. Williams L, Weinberger M, Harris LE, Clark DO, Biller J. Development of a stroke-specific quality of life scale. Stroke 1999; 30:1362–1369.
35. Hackett ML, Duncan JR, Anderson CS, Broad JB, Bonita R. Health-related quality of life among long-term survivors of stroke: results from the Auckland stroke study, 1991–1992. Stroke 2000; 31:440–447.
36. Pickard AS, Johnson JA, Penn A, Lau F, Noseworthy T. Replicability of SF-36 summary scores by the SF-12 in stroke patients. Stroke 1999; 30:1213–1217.
37. Ebrahim S, Barer D, Nouri F. Use the Nottingham Health Profile with patients after a stroke. J Epidemiol Commun Health 1986; 40:166–169.
38. EuroQOL Group. EuroQOL: A new facility for the measurement of health-related quality of life. Health Policy 1990; 16:199–208.
39. Dorman P, Slattery J, Farrell B, Dennis M, Sandercock P. Qualitative comparison of the reliability of health status assessments with the EuroQol and SF-36 questionnaires after stroke. United Kingdom Collaborators in the International Stroke Trial. Stroke 1998; 29:63–68.
40. Dorman PJ, Waddell F, Slattery J, Dennis M, Sandercock P. Are proxy assessments of health status after stroke with the EuroQol questionnaire feasible, accurate, and unbiased? Stroke 1997; 28:1883–1887.
41. Duncan PW, Wallace D, Lai SM, Johnson D, Emberton S, Laster LJ. The Stroke Impact Scale Version 2.0 Evaluation of reliability, validity, and sensitivity to change. Stroke 1999; 30:2131–140.
42. Scholte op Reimer WJM, de Haan RJ, Pijnenborg JMA, Limburg M, van den Bos GAM. Assessment of burden in partners of stroke patients with the Sense of Competence Questionnaire. Stroke 1998; 29:373–379.
43. Wilkinson PR, Wolfe CD, Warburton FG, Rudd AG, Howard RS, Ross-Russell RW, Beech RR. A long-term follow-up of stroke patients. Stroke 1997; 28:507–512.
44. Anderson CS, Linto J, Stewart-Wynne EG. A population-based assessment of the impact and burden of caregiving for long-term stroke survivors. Stroke 1995; 26:843–849.
45. Carnwath TCM, Johnson DAW. Psychiatric morbidity among spouses of patients with stroke. Br Med J 1987; 294:409–411.
46. Hop JW, Rinkel GJE, Algra A, van Gijn J. Quality of life in patients and partners after aneurysmal subarachnoid hemorrhage. Stroke 1998; 29:798–804.
47. Hallan S, Asberg A, Indredavik B, Wideroe TE. Quality of life after cerebrovascular stroke: a systematic study of patients' preferences for different functional outcomes. J Intern Med 1999; 246:309–316.
48. Samsa GP, Matchar DB, Goldstein L, Bonito A, Duncan PW, Lipscomb J, Enarson C, Witter D, Venus P, Paul JE, Weinberger M. Utilities for major stroke: results

from a survey of preferences among perons at increased risk for stroke. Am Heart J 1998; 136:703–713.

49. Patrick DL, Pearlman RA, Starks HE, Cain KC, Cole WG, Uhlmann RF. Validation of preferences for life-sustaining treatment: implications for advance care planning. Ann Intern Med 1997; 127:509–517.

50. Shin AY, Porter PJ, Wallace MC, Naglie G. Quality of life of stroke in younger individuals. Utility assessment in patients with arteriovenous malformations. Stroke 1997; 28:2395–2399.

51. Agewall S, Wikstrand J, Fagerberg B. Stroke was predicted by dimensions of quality of life in treated hypertensive men. Stroke 1998; 29:2329–2333.

52. Harwood RH, Gompertz P, Ebrahim S. Handicap one year after a stroke: validity of a new scale. J Neurol Neurosurg Psychiatry 1994; 57:825–829.

53. Åström M, Asplund K, Åström T. Psychosocial function and life satisfaction after stroke. Stroke 1992; 23:527–531.

54. Niemi ML, Laaksonen R, Kotila M, Waltimo O. Quality of life 4 years after stroke. Stroke 1998; 19:1101–1107.

55. King RB. Quality of life after stroke. Stroke 1996; 27:1467–1472.

56. Ljunggren B, Sonesson B, Saveland H, Brandt L. Cognitive impairment and adjustment in patients without neurological deficits after aneurysmal SAH and early operation. J Neurosurg 1985; 62:673–679.

57. de Haan RJ, Limburg M, van der Meulen JH, Jacobs HM, Aaronson NK. Quality of life after stroke. Impact of stroke type and lesion location. Stroke 1995; 26:402–408.

58. Hutter BO, Gilsbach JM, Kreitschmann I. Quality of life cognitive deficits after subarachnoid haemorrhage. Br J Neurosurg 1995; 9:465–475.

59. Feibel JH, Springer CJ. Depression and failure to resume social activities after stroke. Arch Phys Med Rehabil 1982; 63:276–278.

60. Johansson BB, Jadbäck G, Norrving B, Widner H. Evaluation of long-term functional status in first-ever stroke patients in a defined population. Scand J Rehabil Med 1992; 26(suppl):105–114.

61. Yoon II. Factors affecting quality of life of the Korean aged stroke patients. Int Aging Hum Dev 1997; 44:167–181.

62. Neau JP, Ingrand P, Mouille-Brachet C, Rosier MP, Couderq C, Alvarez A, Gil R. Functional recovery and social outcome after cerebral infarction in young adults. Cerebrovasc Dis 1998; 8:296–302.

63. Parker CJ, Gladman JRF, Drummond AER. The role of leisure in stroke rehabilitation. Disabil Rehabil 1997; 19:1–5.

64. Åström M, Adolfsson R, Asplund K, Åström T. Life before and after stroke. Cerebrovasc Dis 1992; 2:28–34.

65. Sjögren K. Leisure after stroke. Int Rehabil Med 1982; 4:80–87.

66. Lindberg M, Angquist KA, Fodstad H, Fugl-Meyer K, Fugl-Meyer AR. Self-reported prevalence of disability after subarachnoid haemorrhage, with special emphasis on return to leisure and work. Br J Neurosurg 1992; 6:297–304.

67. Drummond A. Leisure activity after stroke. Int Disabil Stud 1990; 12:157–160.

68. Jongbloed L, Morgan D. An investigation of involvement in leisure activities after a stroke. Am J Occup Ther 1991; 45:420–427.

69. Sjögren K, Fugl-Meyer AR. Adjutment to life after stroke with special reference to sexual intercourse and leisure. J Psychosom Res 1982; 26:409–417.

70. Monga TN, Lawson JS, Inglis J. Sexual dysfunction in stroke patients. Arch Phys Med Rehabil 1986; 67:19–22.

71. Korpelainen J, Kauhanen M, Kemola H, Malinen U, Myllyla V. Sexual dysfunction in stroke patients. Acta Neurol Scand 1998; 98:400–405.

72. Langhorne P, Dennis M, eds. Stroke Units: An Evidence-Based Approach. London: BMJ Books, 1998.

73. Indredavik B, Bakke, F, Slordahl, SA, Rokseth R, Haheim LL. Stroke unit treatment. 10-year follow-up. Stroke 1999; 30:1524–1527.

74. Ronning OM, Guldvog B. Stroke unit versus general medical wards. II. Neurological deficits and activities of daily living: a quasi-randomized controlled trial. Stroke 1998; 29:586–590.

75. Mant J, Carter J, Wade DT, Winner S. The impact of an information pack on patients with stroke and their carers: a randomized controlled trial. Clin Rehabil 1998; 12:465–476.

76. Widén Holmqvist L, von Koch L, Kostulas V, Holm M, Widsell G, Tegler H, Johansson K, Almazan J, de Pedro-Cuesta J. A randomized controlled trial of rehabilitation at home after stroke in southwest Stockholm. Stroke 1998; 29:591–597.

77. Rodgers H, Soutter J, Kaiser W, Pearson P, Dobson R, Skillbeck C, Bond J. Early supported hospital discharge following acute stroke: pilot study results. Clin Rehabil 1997; 11:280–287.

78. Dekker R, Drost EA, Groothoff JW, Arendzen JH, van Gijn JC, Eisma WH. Effects of day-hospital rehabilitation in stroke patients: a review of randomized clinical trials. Scand J Rehabil Med 1998; 30:87–94.

79. Fagan SC, Morgenstern LB, Petitta A, Ward RE, Tilley BC, Marler JR, Levine SR, Broderick JP, Kwiatkowski TG, Frankel M, Brott TG, Walker MD. Cost-effectiveness of tissue plasminogen activator for acute ischemic stroke. NINDS rt-PA Stroke Study Group. Neurology 1998; 50:883–890.

80. Gage BF, Cardinalli AB, Owens DK. The effect of stroke and stroke prophylaxis with aspirin or warfarin on quality of life. Arch Intern Med 1996; 156:1829–1836.

81. Stewart AL, Greenfield S, Hays RD, Wells K, Rogers WH, Berry SD, McGlynn AA, Ware JE. Functional status and well-bring of patients with chronic conditions: results from the Medical Outcomes Study. JAMA 1989; 262:907–913.

82. Vriens EM, Post MW, Jacobs HM, van Huffelen AC, Eikelboom BC. Changes in health-related quality of life after carotid endarterectomy. Eur J Vasc Endovasc Surg 1998; 16:395–400.

83. Sirkka A, Salenius JP, Portin R, Nummenmaa T. Quality of life and cognitive performance after carotid endarterectomy during long-term follow-up. Acta Neurol Scand 1992; 85:58–62.

84. Johansson K, Lindgren I, Widner H, Wiklund I, Johansson BB. Can sensory stimulation improve the functional outcome in stroke patients? Neurology 1993; 43:2189–2192.

85. Gosman-Hedström G, Claesson L, Klingenstierna U, Carlsson J, Olausson B, Frizell M, Fagerberg B, Blomstrand C. Effects of acupuncture treatment on daily

life activities and quality of life: a controlled, prospective, and randomized study of acute stroke patients. Stroke 1998; 29:2100–2108.

86. Johansson BB, Haker E, von Arbin M, Britton M, Långström G, Terent A, Ursing D, Asplund K. A randomized controlled trial of acupuncture after stroke. Stroke 2001; 32:707–713.

87. Kwakkel G, Wagenaar RC, Twisk JWR, Lankhorst GJ, Koetsier JC. Intensity of leg and arm training after primary middle-cerebral artery stroke: a randomised trial. Lancet 1999; 354:191–196.

88. Teixeira-Salmela LF, Olney SJ, Nadeau S, Brouwer B. Muscle strengthening and physical conditioning to reduce impairment and disability in chronic stroke survivors. Arch Phys Med Rehabil 1999; 80:1211–1218.

89. Walker MF, Gladman JR, Lincoln NB, Siemonsma P, Whyteley T. Occupational therapy for stroke patients not admitted to hospital: a randomised controlled trial. Lancet 1999; 354:278–280.

90. Gilbertson L, Langhorne P, Walker A, Allen A, Murray GD. Domiciliary occupational therapy for patients with stroke discharged from hospital: randomised controlled trial. Br Med J 2000; 230:603–606.

91. Werner RA, Kessler S. Effectiveness of an intensive outpatient rehabilitation program for postacute stroke patients. Am J Phys Med Rehabil 1996; 75:114–120.

92. Greener J, Enderby P, Whurr R, Grant A. Treatment of aphasia following stroke: evidence for effectiveness. Int J Lang Commun Disord 1998; 33(suppl 1):158–161.

93. Low JT, Payne S, Roderick P. The impact of stroke on informal carers: a literature review. Soc Sci Med 1999; 49:711–725.

94. Draper BM, Poulos CJ, Cole AM, Poulos RG, Ehrlich F. A comparison of caregivers for elderly stroke and dementia victims. J Am Geriatr Soc 1992; 40:896–901.

95. Mumma CM. Perceived losses following stroke. Rehabil Nurs 1986; 11:19–24.

96. Evans RL, Connis RT, Bishop DS, Hendricks RD, Haselkorn JK. Stroke: a family dilemma. Disabil Rehabil 1994; 16:110–118.

97. Brocklehurst JC, Morris P, Andrews K, Richards B, Laycock P. Social effects of stroke. Soc Sci Med 1981; 164:35–39.

98. Nydevik I, Hulter-Åsberg K. Subjective dysfunction after stroke. A study with Sickness Impact Profile. Scand J Prim Health Care 1991; 9:271–275.

99. Kim P, Warren S, Madill H, Hadley M. Quality of life of stroke survivors. Qual Life Res 1999; 8:293–301.

100. Bethoux F, Calmels P, Gautheron V. Changes in the quality of life of hemiplegic stroke patients with time. A preliminary report. Am J Phys Med Rehabil 1999; 78:19–23.

101. Jonkman EJ, de Weerd AW, Vrijens NLH. Quality of life after a first ischemic stroke: long term developments and correlations with changes in neurological deficit, mood and cognitive impairment. Acta Neurol Scand 1998; 98:169–175.

102. Granger CV, Cotter AC, Hamilton BB, Fiedler RC. Functional assessment scales: a study of persons after stroke. Arch Phys Med Rehabil 1993; 74:133–138.

103. Brilstra E, Hop J, Rinkel G. Quality of life after perimesencephalic haemorrhage. J Neurol Neurosurg Psychiatry 1997; 63:382–384.

104. Viitanen M, Fugl-Meyer K, Bernspång B, Fugl-Meyer A. Life satisfaction in long-term survivors after stroke. Scand J Rehabil Med 1988; 20:17–24.

105. Wyller T, Sveen U, Sodring K, Pettersen A, Bautz-Holter E. Subjective well-being one year after stroke. Clin Rehabil 1997; 11:139–145.

106. Taylor-Sarno M. Preliminary findings in a study of age, linguistic evolution and quality of life in recovery from aphasia. Scand J Rehabil Med 1992; 26(suppl):43–59.

107. Ogden JA, Utley T, Mee EW. Neurological and psychosocial outcome 4 to 7 years after subarachnoid hemorrhage. Neurosurgery 1997; 41:25–34.

108. Soelberg-Sørensen P, Marquardsen J, Pedersen H, Heltberg A, Munch O. Long-term prognosis and quality of life after reversible cerebral ischemic attacks. Acta Neurol Scand 1989; 79:204–213.

109. Scholte op Reimer WJ, de Haan RJ, Rijnders PT, Limburg M, van den Bos GA. The burden of caregiving in partners of long-term stroke survivors. Stroke 1998; 29:1605–1611.

110. Löfgren B, Gustafson Y, Nyberg L. Psychological well-being 3 years after severe stroke. Stroke 1999; 30:567–72.

111. Elmstahl S, Malmberg B, Annerstedt L. Caregiver's burden of patients 3 years after stroke assessed by a novel caregiver burden scale. Arch Phys Med Rehabil 1996; 77:177–182.

112. Kjendahl A, Sallstrom S, Osten PE, Stanghelle JK, Borchgevink CF. A one year follow-up study on the effects of acupuncture in the treatment of stroke patients in the subacute phase: a randomized controlled study. Clin Rehabil 1997; 11:192–200.

4

Prognosis After Stroke

Stroke Recurrence and Other Outcome Events

Jorge Moncayo-Gaete
Eugenio Espejo Hospital, Quito, Ecuador

Julien Bogousslavsky
University of Lausanne and Centre Hospitalier Universitaire Vaudois, Lausanne, Switzerland

I. INTRODUCTION

Stroke-related mortality has been on the decline in most Western and Asian countries in recent years. Currently, the main strategies used to prevent further strokes are antiplatelet and anticoagulant therapies, carotid endarterectomy, and control of vascular risk factors. A considerable number of stroke survivors, however, fail to receive any preventive therapy or fail to adhere to a regimen of preventive measures.

Stroke survivors are at high risk of experiencing a stroke recurrence. Of all well-established stroke risk factors, previous stroke is at the top of the list, with a risk seven times higher than that found in the general population. One-third of the approximately 730,000 strokes that occur in the United States every year are recurrences. Rates, predictors, patterns, and outcome after recurrence vary depending on stroke subtype. Therefore, the identification of subgroups of patients at high risk of recurrence after first-ever events has become a priority in order to target and optimize secondary stroke prevention.

This chapter examines the patterns, epidemiological aspects, and outcome of ischemic and hemorrhagic stroke recurrences, and their prevention according to different stroke subtypes.

II. EARLY ISCHEMIC-STROKE RECURRENCE

Over the past few years, the case-fatality rate at 28 days after stroke has fallen in most industrialized countries (1–5). Early case-fatality rates for ischemic stroke (IS) currently range from 5.8% to 20.4% (6–9). The result of this decline in the rate of short-term stroke mortality is the growing number of IS survivors at risk of developing a closely following further stroke, one of the most feared complications during the first days or weeks after the initial event.

Literature on this topic reflects the lack of a universally accepted definition of early IS recurrence. Differences exist as to the interval from index stroke to second event that qualifies as ''early'' recurrence. The first 14 days has sometimes been chosen as the boundary between early and long-term recurrences, particularly in studies assessing this matter in patients with brain infarction thought to derive from cardioembolic sources (10–12). Other series, on the other hand, have stretched the limit to 90 days after first IS (13–16). However, the first 30 days after index stroke is the cutoff point in most studies for speaking of short-term recurrence (17–19). The 1-month interval seems reasonable, since 30–60% of recurrences appear within the first 30 days after the initial event (16,18).

In most patients, the initial neurological condition after IS remains stable, but 25–30% of patients may experience deterioration during the first 96 h (20–23). The mechanisms responsible for initial neurological deterioration are not well understood (21,24,25) (Table 1). Criteria for early stroke recurrence should include a new neurological deficit of more than a 24-h duration (16,19,26,27) or a sudden worsening of a preexisting deficit (27,28). These circumstances should be attributable solely to the involvement of a different vascular territory or anatomical site and, finally, the recurring event should occur during the first 30 days after index stroke. Other neurological and systemic disorders may also worsen the initial neurological status and should be ruled out to avoid a misdiagnosis of stroke recurrence (29–35) (Table 1). In some instances, clinical worsening of an existing deficit is not easy to note, particularly in those infarcts involving the mainstem of the middle cerebral artery or the internal carotid artery (36).

A. Epidemiology and Predictors

Epidemiological data on early stroke recurrence have been strongly influenced by study design (retrospective vs. prospective), period of follow-up, type of treatment, and by whether studies are community- or population-based. Average rates of 3.4% (varying from 1.6% to 4.4%) have been found in hospital-based studies (17,20,37) while community-based studies have shown average rates of 3.18% (varying from 1.2% to 5.6%) (17,26,36,39,40). The immediate period (<7 days)

Table 1 Mechanisms and Causes
of Worsening After Ischemic Stroke

Mechanisms of worsening
  Thrombus propagation
  Progression of arterial stenosis
  Carotid siphon occlusion
  Poor collateral circulation
Neurological causes of worsening
  Stroke recurrence
  Increased intracranial pressure
  Obstructive hydrocephalus
  Focal seizures
Nonneurological causes
  Electrolyte and metabolic disturbances
  Pulmonary infections
  Coexisting cardiac disease
  Cardiac arrhythmia

after the index event carries the greatest risk of recurrence, with 50% of second
events falling within this interval (26,41,42).

The Stroke Data Bank investigators found that a diastolic blood pressure
>100 mmHg and a history of diabetes both increase the risk of early recurrence
by 5.2% and 4.9%, respectively (17). Moreover, patients with both hypertension
and an initial blood-sugar concentration higher than 200 mg/dL had a risk of
recurrence at 30 days of 4.9%, and this risk was twice as great when blood-
glucose concentration was over 300 mg/dL (17).

The risk of early stroke recurrence depends on the pathophysiological IS
subtype. Patients with infarcts due to large-vessel atherosclerosis possess a high
risk of early recurrence, estimated at 7.9% in the first 30 days (17). Microembolic
signals (MES) detected by transcranial Doppler (TCD) monitoring of patients
with IS of presumed arterial origin have been associated with a high probability
of ipsilateral early recurrence, regardless of the severity of carotid stenosis (43–
45)

Brain infarcts presumed to be of cardioembolic origin have been considered
to carry a higher risk of recurrence than other brain-infarct etiologies. In fact,
the Cerebral Embolism Task Force has estimated retrospectively that around 12%
of patients with cardioembolic stroke can be expected to experience a second
event within 2 weeks of an initial event (46). A much higher figure was found in
a study of 227 untreated patients with cardioembolic infarct (27% with rheumatic
valvular disease); one of every five patients developed a second ischemic event

within the first 14 days. Dehydration, low plasma levels of antithrombin III, rheumatic heart disease (RHD), prosthetic valves, and intracardiac thrombi were associated with these recurrences (41).

The embolism-recurrence rates at 30 days currently reported for patients with cardiac sources of embolism (CSE), which vary from 2.9% to 6.9%, are lower than those previously estimated (15,17,47,48). Rates of recurrence at 1 month after index IS in untreated patients with a CSE range from 10% to 17%, while in both treated (most with anticoagulant therapy) and untreated patients, the recurrence rates at 30 days range between 3% and 9% (49–51).

The rates of stroke recurrence at 30 days in community- and population-based studies for patients with nonvalvular atrial fibrillation (NVAF) vary from 1% to 6.2% (27,37,51–53). The contribution of NVAF to early stroke recurrence is still controversial, however. In the Framingham Study, AF was significantly associated with recurrence (54). In contrast, other series have not consistently found an elevated risk of early recurrence in such patients (27,55,56). In keeping with these last findings, one multicenter-based study, performed to evaluate the efficacy of early antithrombotic therapy in the acute phase of stroke, found that AF patients had stroke-recurrence rates of approximately 2% in the first month, similar to those of patients with sinus rhythm (55). In another community-based study, the risk rate was even lower: 1% for patients with AF versus 4% for patients with sinus rhythm (27).

The presence of a CSE has not by itself been found to constitute a strong predictor of early recurrence. The risk of recurrence increases when the cardiac source coexists with another risk factor or another cardiac disorder. Concurrent hypertension, valvular heart disease, and AF were found to promote recurrence, though none of these was a predictor when existing separately (42). It has long been suggested that RHD carries a high risk of early recurrent embolism. However, the risk of recurrence has not been strikingly different between patients with NVAF and those with RHD (13). In fact, RHD has been identified as an independent predictor of recurrence only when it coexists with congestive heart disease (15).

Scarcity of data has been a hindrance in establishing the rates of early stroke recurrence in other types of CSE. It has been found, however, that embolism rarely recurs in the setting of infective endocarditis, once antibiotic therapy has been started (57–59). No early stroke recurrences have been documented for patients with patent foramen ovale (PFO) and other interatrial septal abnormalities (60).

Lacunar infarcts have a favorable short-term prognosis and the lowest rates of early stroke recurrence among all other subtypes of brain infarcts (from 0% to 2.2% at 30 days) (17,36,61,62). Patients with brain infarcts of undetermined cause have a slightly higher risk of early recurrence (about 3%) than those with a definite lacunar etiology (17).

B. Prognosis

Prognosis is dismal for patients with early IS recurrence. These patients show a deterioration in motor deficit of approximately 60% (17). Early IS recurrence prolongs hospital stay by almost twice that of patients with no recurrence (17,42). In addition, case-fatality rates for patients with recurrent brain infarct are two or three times higher than for patients with first-ever IS (7,41,42). In the Stroke Data Bank the early case-fatality rate for patients with first-ever IS was 7.4%, and rose to 20% for patients with IS recurrence (17). In-hospital mortality was almost three times greater for patients with recurrent cardioembolic infarcts (70.8%) than for patients with no recurrence (24.4%) (42).

C. Prevention of Early Recurrence After Brain Infarct

Early anticoagulation to avoid stroke progression and recurrence after IS has been commonly prescribed in the acute phase. In two studies anticoagulation failed to prevent early recurrence in patients with noncardioembolic infarcts (63,64), but three recent randomized trials have suggested otherwise (55,65,66). However, the possible benefit appears to be offset by the risk of major bleeding episodes (Table 2).

Table 2 Ischemic Stroke Recurrence, Hemorrhagic Transformation, and Bleeding Complications with Heparin for Acute Stroke

Trial	No. of patients	Recurrence IS	Hemorrhagic transformation	Major extracranial bleeding
IST (55)				
Heparin[a]	4,855	2.9%[b]	1.2%	1.3%
Control	4,859	3.8%	0.4%	0.4%
TOAST (66)				
Danaparoid	638	1.56%[c]	1.72%[d]	5.01%
Placebo	628	1.75%	0.47%	1.59%
Low-molecular-weight heparin (65)				
Nadroparin	203	1.47%[e]	0.98%	0.49%
Control	105	0.95	0.95%	1.9%

IST: International Stroke Trial.
TOAST: Trial of ORG 10172 in Acute Stroke Treatment.
[a] Low and high doses of heparin.
[b] Stroke recurrence within 14 days.
[c] Stroke recurrence within 10 days.
[d] Symptomatic hemorrhagic transformation within 10 days.
[e] Stroke recurrence within 10 days.

Retrospective and nonrandomized studies have found that anticoagulation reduces by 60% the absolute risk of recurrence in the first month after a cardioembolic stroke (11,67,68). The recurrence rate was eight times higher within 21 days after IS in nonanticoagulated patients or those in whom anticoagulation was delayed (17.5%) compared with those early anticoagulated (2%) (69). Early anticoagulation with heparin was found to be relatively safe in 231 patients with cardioembolic strokes monitorized closely in a nonrandomized, noncontrolled observational study (70). The rate of in-hospital recurrence was 2.1% and the rate of major bleeding episodes was 3.4%; recurrences were significantly related to lower mean activated partial thromboplastin time (70). Anticoagulation has been common in NVAF-related strokes particularly in the absence of large infarcts or uncontrolled hypertension (11,71,72). Lower recurrence rates were observed in patients with NVAF (2.8%) than nonanticoagulated patients (4.9%), but the former group was more prone to develop hemorrhagic strokes (54).

Early anticoagulation in cardioembolic strokes has been considered potentially risky, because of the propensity for spontaneous brain hemorrhage conversion (73,74). In two studies immediate anticoagulation did not promote hemorrhagic transformation (11,75). In addition, neurological status can remain stable despite continuation of anticoagulation in the presence of hemorrhagic infarct (68,69,76,77).

Early anticoagulation in the acute phase of IS still remains controversial. Appropriateness of anticoagulation should be tailored to the individual patient weighing the risk-benefit ratio and taking into account the presence either of risk factors that might promote recurrence or hemorrhagic transformation.

Aspirin (ASA) has been found to prevent early recurrences to a slight extent at doses of between 160 and 300 mg/day administered within 48 hr after stroke (55,78). Recently, intravenous aspirin reduced MES in seven patients with recent brain infarct attributable to ipsilateral large-artery disease (79).

III. LONG-TERM STROKE RECURRENCE

There has been a trend toward improvement in long-term survival after initial stroke over time. Some evidence from population-based studies suggests that the risk of death 2 years after stroke in the 1990s was 40% lower than in the 1980s. Among all types of IS, atherothrombotic infarcts were found to have the best survival rates (3).

In spite of the benefits of secondary preventive measures after stroke (80–84), risk factors in patients with prior stroke remain to a large extent uncontrolled (85,86) or there are a considerable proportion of initial-stroke patients who lack treatment in the long term (87). Therefore, there exists a high risk of recurrence for a large proportion of those surviving at least 1 month after a first-ever stroke.

Recurring strokes may account for approximately 30% of all events (3,7,40,88–92). Despite a decline in stroke incidence during the 1980s, rates of stroke recurrence have not experienced a similar trend (93). Recently, however, a significant decline in recurrence rates was observed over a period of 4 years in Malmö, Sweden, most likely as the result of an improvement in secondary preventive measures (94).

Several studies record an annual incidence of symptomatic recurrence after IS of 4–14% (13,18,95–98). The risk of recurrence is especially great during the first year after IS. The Stroke Data Bank observed a rate of 9.3% in 1273 patients with IS during a mean follow-up of 1.1 years (18). From the second year on, it carries a risk of 5–8% per year (99). A rate of 14.1% at 2 years has been recorded (18), and other studies show rates ranging from 5% to 20% (100). A number of studies show a 5-year cumulative risk of recurrence of between 22% and 30% (26,39,90,96).

A. Predictors of Long-Term Stroke Recurrence

In most instances, determination of risk factors for stroke recurrence has yielded conflictive results (13,15,17,18,26,40,54,90,91,94,97,101,102,104–113) (Table 3). Some of these risk factors are linked to recurrence with particular stroke subtypes. Leonberg, Sobel, and, recently, Yamamoto provide highlights as to the importance of risk-factor profile in recurrence, stressing that the number of risk

Table 3 Predictors of Long-Term Ischemic Stroke Recurrence

Age (26,101,102)
Male gender (97)
Female sex (91)
Hypertension (17,18,40,97,102,104–107)
Diabetes (17,18,26,94,101,109)
Valvular heart disease (15)
Ischemic heart disease (15,97,101,102,104)
Congestive heart failure (15,97,101,102,104)
Atrial fibrillation (13,94,101,104)
Previous TIAs (94,104,105)
Ethanol abuse (40)
Current smoking (90)
Proximal aortic atheromas (plaques > 4 mm in thickness) (114,115)
Dementia following stroke (91)
Elevated fibrinogen-plasma levels (111)
High-serum lipoprotein (a) levels (111)
Positive anticardiolipin antibodies (112,113)

factors and their interaction play a substantial role in stroke recurrence (103,116,117).

IS is a heterogeneous disorder encompassing many pathophysiological mechanisms. Consequently, not all stroke patients are at similar risk of recurrence, the differences depending on stroke subtype, as well as the number of risk factors involved.

B. Atherothrombotic Infarcts

The medical treatment arms of two large carotid endarterectomy trials have provided data about the natural history of symptomatic extracranial carotid stenosis (83,84). Virtually 26% of patients with internal carotid stenosis greater than 70% experienced a new ipsilateral stroke within 2 years in the NASCET study (83), and the ECST study showed a figure of 22% at 3 years (84) (Table 4). In 1273 patients with IS, Hier et al. found a similar rate of recurrence at 2 years for patients with infarcts due to large-vessel atherosclerotic disease (18). In addition, recurrence rates rise in proportion to the number of risk factors present, being twice as high for patients with more than five stroke-risk factors (83).

Table 4 Rates of Ipsilateral Stroke in Patients with Stenosis or Occlusion in the Arteries of the Anterior and the Posterior Circulation

Artery	Rate of ipsilateral recurrence	Interval,[a] years
ICA stenosis > 70% (83)	26%	2
ICA stenosis > 70% (84)	22%	3
ICA stenosis 50–69% (120)	12.9%	2
ICA occlusion (122,123)	3%	Annual
Intracranial ICA stenosis 50–69% (130)	19.4%	3
Intracranial ICA stenosis > 85% (130)	45.7%	3
MCA stenosis (127,129)	7.8%	Annual
MCA occlusion (127,129)	7.1%	Annual
Intracranial vertebral stenosis 50%–99% (140)	7.8%	Annual
Intracranial basilar stenosis 50–99% (140)	13.7%	Annual
PICA (140)	6%	Annual
PCA (140)	6%	Annual

[a] Interval of ipsilateral stroke recurrence since first stroke.
ICA: internal carotid artery.
MCA: middle cerebral artery.
PICA: posterior-inferior cerebellar artery.
PCA: posterior cerebral artery.

The risk of ipsilateral stroke in subgroups of patients with symptomatic stenosis greater than 70% also correlates with the degree of stenosis. The rate of a further ipsilateral stroke at 1 year for patients with stenosis ranging between 70% and 79% was 12.8%, while it was three times higher for patients with stenosis ranging from 90% to 94% (118). In addition, the risk of ipsilateral stroke rises steeply in the presence of ulcerated plaques (defined by angiography) (119).

Patients with moderate internal carotid stenosis have a more benign course than those with severe stenosis. The rate of ipsilateral stroke at 2 years in 87 symptomatic patients with from 50% to 79% of internal carotid artery (ICA) stenosis was 12.9% (120). Progression of carotid stenosis, defined by color-flow duplex scanning, occurred in approximately 16% of these 87 patients during a mean follow-up period of 44 months, and their rate of ipsilateral stroke recurrence rose to 14.3% at 2 years (120). Occlusion of the internal carotid artery has been considered to have a prognosis similar to that of stenotic lesions (121), though some studies have yielded rates of ipsilateral stroke of about 3% per year (122,123).

The annual risk of ipsilateral stroke for patients with distal internal carotid stenosis or middle cerebral artery (MCA) stenosis runs from 4% to 12% (124–129). Intracranial ICA stenosis has been found to be an independent risk factor for ipsilateral stroke (130). For the patients included in the medical arm of the NASCET study, the estimated risk of ipsilateral stroke was 19.4% at 3 years in patients with intracranial ICA stenosis of between 50% and 69%, while for patients with an intracranial ICA stenosis of over 85% it rose to 45.7% (130).

Stenosis of the main branches of the ICA has received little attention. It occurs more often in African, African-American, and Asian subjects (131–136) than in Caucasian populations (137,138). Atherosclerotic stenosis of the MCA rarely causes brain infarctions in Western populations (136,139). There is relatively little information available concerning the prognosis of patients with atherosclerotic MCA disease, and most of it is usually derived from the EC/IC Bypass Study (127). The yearly rate of ipsilateral IS in the stenosis group was slightly higher than that of the occlusion group (7.8% and 7.1%, respectively) (127,129) (Table 4).

In a retrospective study of 68 patients with intracranial symptomatic stenosis ranging from 50% to 99% involving mainly the vertebral and basilar arteries, almost one-fourth developed further ischemic events, and two-thirds of these recurred in the same symptomatic territory over an average follow-up period of 13.8 months (140). For those patients having previous infarcts in the basilar and vertebral arteries, the annual rate of stroke recurrence in the same arterial territories was 10.7% and 7.8%, respectively (140) (Table 4). It was higher when all vascular territories were taken into account: 15% when first infarct was in the basilar-artery territory and 13.7% when it was in the vertebral-artery territory. Patients with initial infarcts in the posterior cerebral artery and in the posterior-inferior cerebral artery had lower rates of recurrence (about 6%). Rates of stroke recurrence involving the same territory as the first infarct were twice as high for patients treated with antiplatelet agents as for those who received warfarin therapy (140).

Recurrence of infarcts caused by large-vessel atherosclerotic disease most often happens in the same arterial territory as the first, particularly when the carotid circulation is involved (141,142). In addition, this kind of infarct often recurs as the same pathological type, with frequencies ranging between 64% and 82% (117,141). Cardioembolic and Lacunar infarct (LI) each account for approximately 15% of recurrences, while hemorrhagic strokes are less frequent (117).

C. Prevention of Long-Term Recurrence After Atherothrombotic Infarct

IS recurrence tends to be of the same pathological mechanism as the first event, but other mechanisms already present, though not etiologically related to the first stroke, may be responsible for further events. Consequently, extensive noninvasive investigations of the heart, aorta, and major craniocerebral arteries, as well as blood tests, should be performed on patients with first-ever stroke, even when there is a definite etiology for the current event, to identify all underlying pathological mechanisms that could contribute to a recurrence.

Medical options for secondary stroke prevention comprise antiplatelet aggregation, anticoagulation, and control of risk factors. Anticoagulation will be discussed in the section on secondary prevention of cardioembolic strokes. Aspirin, ticlopidine, dypiridamole, and, more recently, clopidogrel are the antiplatelet agents proven to be useful in secondary stroke prevention.

Aspirin was first demonstrated to be clinically efficacious in secondary stroke prevention some 25 years ago; 1300 mg/day of aspirin, alone or with sulfinpyrazone, significantly reduced the incidence of stroke or death by 31% among patients who had experienced a transient ischemic attack (TIA) 3 months previously (143).

Recently, pooled data from 145 trials of antiplatelet therapy, involving 70,000 subjects at high risk of cardiovascular events, have provided conclusive evidence that aspirin reduces the incidence of nonfatal stroke by 22% (80). Low doses of aspirin (50–325 mg/day) are currently recommended for the prevention of IS and TIA (144,145), and have the added benefit of reducing adverse effects, principally gastrointestinal toxicity (146–148).

Increased platelet aggregation lasting several months has been documented in patients with previous IS (149,150). Partial inhibition of platelet aggregation, either transient or permanent, may occur in 20–30% of patients with prior IS treated with aspirin (151). Moreover, initial total inhibition of platelet aggregation may be lost over time in one-third of patients treated with aspirin. Overall, 8%

of patients exhibit aspirin resistance, even at high doses (151). Therefore, stroke recurrence in some patients treated with aspirin may be due to an inadequate effect.

Two large multicenter trials have shown ticlopidine to be superior to both aspirin and placebo in reducing nonfatal or fatal strokes in patients with previous noncardioembolic strokes (81,152). Ticlopidine significantly reduced the risk of recurrence by 33% over placebo (81), while in the TASS Study, ticlopidine was 20% more effective than aspirin in reducing recurrences (152). Both trials established that such adverse effects as diarrhea, rash, and, most notably, neutropenia (severe in some instances) were more common in patients receiving ticlopidine than in those treated with aspirin (81,152).

The efficacy of clopidogrel in the prevention of cardiovascular events was established in a single multicenter study performed on 19,185 high-risk patients (with recent myocardial infarction, stroke, or significant peripheral arterial disease) (153). Patients were randomly allocated to either 325 mg/day of aspirin or 75 mg/day of clopidogrel, and were followed up over an average of 1.9 years. The relative risk reduction of cardiovascular events by clopidogrel was 8.7% over that of aspirin, but this finding was unfortunately statistically marginal (153). Analysis of the stroke subgroup showed a yearly rate of recurring stroke of 5.7% in patients on aspirin and 5.2% in those on clopidogrel, resulting in a nonsignificant risk reduction of about 7% (153).

Available evidence suggests that clopidogrel is safer than ticlopidine. Clopidogrel is devoid of the adverse hematological effects seen with ticlopidine; diarrhea and rash are also less frequent in patients on clopidogrel (153). On the other hand, analysis of cost-effectiveness favors aspirin over both clopidogrel and ticlopidine for the prevention of thromboembolic stroke recurrence (145).

Trials during the 1980s to evaluate the efficacy of dypiridamole in secondary stroke prevention, alone or in combination with aspirin, yielded inconclusive results (154–156). Not long ago an extended-release dypiridamole presentation was reassessed in a four-arm trial performed on 6602 patients with previous TIA or IS occurring no more than 3 months prior to randomization (157). Aspirin was tested at low doses (50 mg daily) and dypiridamole at high doses (400 mg daily). Aspirin and dypiridamole as sole therapy were both superior to placebo, and the combination of these two antiplatelet agents significantly reduced the risk of recurrence by 37% (157).

In light of the available evidence, aspirin so far constitutes the first-line therapy for a great proportion of patients with atherothrombotic infarcts. Clopidogrel may be chosen as a second-line treatment, particularly in instances where aspirin fails or is contraindicated.

Anticoagulation is often used in patients with brain infarcts and intracranial stenosis. In a nonrandomized retrospective study involving 151 patients with symptomatic, angiographically proven intracranial large-artery stenosis (>50%), warfarin prevented more annual stroke recurrences than aspirin (3.6/100 vs. 10.4/100 patients-years, respectively) (158). However, percutaneous transluminal angioplasty (PTA) and stenting may be alternative options in suitable patients. Both procedures are effective in the treatment of symptomatic extraintracranial carotid and vertebral atherosclerotic stenosis (159–161). Marks et al. reported that the annual rate of new ipsilateral ischemic events was 3.2% in the territory appropriate to the site of angioplasty in 23 patients with intracranial stenosis followed over 35 months (159). Other series of PTA have not reported stroke recurrences after angioplasty in patients with intracranial lesions in the anterior and posterior circulation (160,161). The experience is still limited, however, and requires further study (162–165). The only surgical option for secondary stroke prevention is carotid endarterectomy in extracranial symptomatic stenosis with a narrowing of carotid artery diameter of more than 70%, provided there is a low risk of perioperative morbidity and mortality (83,84).

Finally, any effort to reduce stroke recurrence should also include therapeutic interventions oriented toward controlling modifiable risk factors for stroke.

D. Long-Term Recurrence After Cardioembolic Infarct

Cardieombolism is the second most common cause of first IS, accounting for approximately 20–30% of all cases (20,166–171). Recurrence rates in the first year after cardioembolic stroke range from 5% to 12% (15,18,40,141). Cumulative rates of recurrence reach 32% at 5 years after index stroke (15,18,40,141). Recurrence rates depend on the specific underlying cardiac condition.

E. Atrial Fibrillation

Atrial fibrillation (AF) is by far the most common potential cardiac source of embolism (19,172,173). Currently, nonvalvular AF (NVAF) is much more frequent than rheumatic AF (173,174). Overall, one in six first ischemic strokes is related to NVAF (27,175,176), with frequencies increasing steeply with age (175). Patients older than 60 with NVAF have an overall rate of first-ever IS between 4.5% and 8% per year (69,177–179).

Age, diabetes, history of hypertension, and previous TIA or stroke are the risk factors that predict stroke in patients with NVAF (114). In the European Atrial Fibrillation Trial (EAFT), the predictors of recurrent vascular events were: a history of previous thromboembolism, ischemic heart disease, cardiothoracic ratio >50% on chest roentgenogram, systolic blood pressure greater than 160 mmHg at study entry, AF with a duration of more than 1 year prior to index stroke, and evidence of previous IS on computerized-tomography scan (180). One-third of the placebo-treated patients in the EAFT trial had three or more risk factors and a recurrence-hazard ratio of 3.9, compared to 1.9 in patients with only or two of the above-mentioned risk factors (180).

NVAF patients with previous stroke exhibit a yearly rate of further stroke twice as high (10–12%) as stroke-free AF patients (177,181,182). In the last few years, patients with NVAF have been categorized according to the presence of other risk factors in order to identify high-risk subgroups of systemic embolism (177,183–185). According to the Stroke Prevention Atrial Fibrillation (SPAF) I–III trials, AF patients at high risk of embolism include women older than 75, those over the age of 75 and with history of hypertension, or those of any age with a systolic blood pressure higher than 160 mmHg (186). The moderate-risk category comprises patients younger than 75 and patients with a history of hypertension or diabetes (186). Thus, patients in the high-risk group exhibited yearly rates of recurrence of 20%, whereas the rate decreased to 10% per year in the moderate-risk group. Low-risk patients had an annual recurrence rate of 5.9% (186).

In several studies, the risk of recurring stroke in AF patients was higher in the first year, with rates of approximately 10–15% (187,188), and especially high rates have been observed during the first quarter (27,82,189). One study obtained identical results for the first year, but found no decline over time, with rates in subsequent years remaining as high as in the first year after stroke recurrence (82).

Not all patients with AF share the same risk of first-ever stroke and recurrence. Lone AF mainly occurs in younger patients and carries an annual risk of first-ever stroke of less than 0.5% (190). Risk of recurrence remains low over time (<1/100 patient-years) (191).

F. Valvular Heart Disease

Valvular heart disease (VHD) accounts for 4–20% of potential cardiac sources of embolism (48,173). Mitral stenosis is responsible for most VHD (192). Approximately, 40% of patients with VHD also develop AF (193). Coexistent mitral stenosis and AF carries a high risk of embolism. The annual rate of systemic embolism ranges between 4% and 5%, with more than half of emboli lodging in cerebral vasculature (192,194). Recurring embolism seems to be high, with one- to two-thirds of cases occurring within the first year after initial event (192,195,196). The risk of recurring embolism is substantially reduced through long-term anticoagulation (192,196,197). Anticoagulated patients with mitral stenosis after brain infarct showed a 3.9% per year recurrence risk (198).

G. Interatrial Septal Abnormalities

Interatrial septal abnormalities (ISA), including patent foramen ovale (PFO) (199–203) and atrial septal aneurysms (ASA) (204–207), have been considered as possible CSE in patients with cryptogenic IS, particularly among younger subjects. Both these ISA are found to coexist in 30–40% of patients with IS (205,207,208).

Available information on recurrence of infarcts attributed to paradoxical embolism (PE) suggests that the risk is rather low. Hanna et al., in 15 patients with IS treated with aspirin, warfarin, or surgical closure of PFO, did not find any stroke recurrence during a mean follow-up of 28 months (208). Bogousslavsky et al. reported 140 patients with IS and PFO who were randomly allocated to antiplatelet aggregation, anticoagulation, or surgical closure. Stroke recurred in eight of these patients during a mean follow-up of 3 years, giving an estimated annual rate of recurrence of 1.9% per year (60). The predictors of stroke recurrence in this study were infarct involving the territory of the posterior cerebral artery, associated interatrial communication, a history of recent migraine, and coexisting cause of stroke, the latter found in 15% of patients (60). The French Study Group confirmed a low rate of stroke recurrence (1% per year) in patients with stroke and ISA. A higher rate of stroke recurrence occurred, however, in patients with coexisting PFO and ASA (4.4% per year), suggesting the existence of synergism between both abnormalities respecting risk of recurrence (209).

H. Patterns of Recurrence

In general, most recurrences in patients with first cardioembolic cerebral infarct are of the same etiology as the initial event (117). Large-artery disease with significant stenosis in the appropriate artery and small-vessel disease as a consequence of long-standing hypertension coexist in nearly 20% of all patients with IS and are a potential cardiac source of embolism (173,210–212). In accord with these findings, noncardiac non-LI and LI account for 20% and 5%, respectively, of recurrences in patients with first cardioembolic IS (117).

I. Prevention of Long-Term Recurrence After Cardioembolic Stroke

As in other subtypes of initial IS, the existence of a source of embolism from the heart does not preclude an extensive search for coexisting causes of stroke that may constitute alternative mechanisms for a recurrence, and such an investigation may allow for better secondary prevention.

The efficacy of anticoagulation in primary stroke prevention for patients with NVAF has been firmly substantiated by various placebo-controlled clinical trials (178,213–217). So far, the European Atrial Fibrillation Trial (EAFT) is the only major study devoted to this matter (82). This multicenter study was conducted on 1007 patients with NVAF and recent (<3 months) TIA or minor stroke. Patients were randomly allocated to either a warfarin-eligible group (open anticoagulation, or double-blind treatment with either aspirin at 300 mg/day or a placebo) or a warfarin-ineligible group (double-blind treatment with either aspirin or a placebo). The mean age of patients was 73 years, mean follow-up was 2.3 years, and the warfarin target was International Normalized Ratio (INR) 2.5–4.0 (84). Warfarin-treated patients had a hazard ratio of recurrence of 0.34, while patients receiving aspirin showed a hazard ratio of 0.86 (82). In absolute terms, anticoagulation prevented eight strokes per 100 patients annually, while aspirin avoided approximately two strokes per 100 patients annually. The rate of bleeding complications was 2.8% and 0.7% per year in the warfarin and nonanticoagulated groups, respectively (82). The issue of appropriate timing for starting anticoagulation after NVAF-related IS has not been addressed. In the EAFT study, anticoagulation was begun within 14 days after qualifying stroke in 46% of patients assigned to warfarin therapy (82). In a subsequent report of the EAFT Study Group, the optimal level of anticoagulation suggested for secondary prevention in patients with AF-related stroke ranges between INR 2.0 and 3.9, with a target INR of 3.0 (218). Low-intensity warfarin (INR 1.5–2.1) may be safer in older subjects (179,219). In consequence, warfarin anticoagulation with a target INR of 3.0 is the first choice for patients with AF, and aspirin is the alternative when warfarin is contraindicated.

Long-term anticoagulation is also the first choice for prevention of recurring strokes in patients after an ischemic event caused by rheumatic mitral stenosis, prosthetic heart valve, dilated cardiomiopathy, or left ventricular dyskinesia (220). The target INR should be between 2.0 and 3.0. If a recurrence occurs despite adequate treatment, the target therapeutic range can be increased to 3.5, or aspirin can be added (221). Anticoagulation with a target of INR 3.0–4.0 should be maintained in patients with mechanical prosthetic heart valves. In these patients, anticoagulation can be supplemented with aspirin if a new cardioembolic stroke occurs despite an INR within the therapeutic range at the time of event (222).

Antiplatelet therapy is the first line of treatment in patients with stroke and suspected Paradoxical Embolism (PE) (223). Surgical closure of PFO has been proposed for patients assumed to have a high risk of recurrence. Criteria for the latter approach include brain infarct with no other demonstrated cause along with at least two of the following: massive right-to-left shunt, recurring clinical brain infarcts or multiple silent ischemic lesions on brain magnetic resonance imaging (MRI) PFO associated with ASA, and Valsalva maneuver preceding onset of stroke (223). Long-term anticoagulation can be of benefit to surgical candidates who refuse the operation and to patients with no other demonstrated cause of brain infarct who have only one of the factors mentioned above (224).

J. Lacunar Infarcts

Lacunar infarcts (LI) make up 20–25% of all first IS (225–230). Survival rates for patients with LI are significantly better than for those with nonlacunar infarcts (61,227,231) and decrease approximately 5% per year after occurrence (110).

Thus, 80–90% of patients are still alive 2 years after LI, whereas 65–75% of patients survive 5 years after LI (110,225,226,229).

Of 172 patients with symptomatic LI as first-ever stroke (followed on average for 3 years), 16 patients (9%) suffered a further stroke (110). Higher frequencies (21%) were reported in 322 patients with minor stroke during a follow-up period of 10 years, but only one-third of these patients had LI (232).

The risk of recurrence in LI is higher in the first year after the qualifying event. At 1 year, the rate of recurrence ranges from 4.7% to 12% (141,225, 231,233). Hospital and population-based studies have estimated that the average annual rate of recurrence after the first year is 5–6% (225,227). In line with this finding, the cumulative rates of recurrence reported at 5 years and 7 years have been 26% (227) and 34%, respectively (225).

Most studies have not identified predictors of stroke recurrence in LI. Age, hypertension, heart disease, diabetes, cigarette smoking, and dyslipidemia have not been correlated with further strokes in patients with previous LI (108,110, 141,234). Only leukoaraiosis (LA) has been associated, by means of univariate analysis, with stroke recurrence in patients with LI as initial stroke (235), but this finding has not been corroborated in other studies (108,110,233). Recently, diabetes has been associated with stroke recurrence (117).

Most patients with LI as index stroke experience only one recurrence. However, 20% of patients may experience two or more ensuing strokes (110). The interval between the initial LI and a subsequent stroke is usually around twice as long as that observed for stroke recurrence of nonlacunar infarcts or hemorrhagic strokes. Yamamoto and Bogousslavsky found that the mean interval between the first and second events for 19 patients with initial LI was 68 months, whereas other types of stroke exhibited intervals ranging from 31 to 38 months (117).

Several patterns of recurrence have been identified in patients with first LI. Most series have shown that approximately 50% of patients with initial LI have a recurrence of the same type (108,117,141,233,236), though in a study reported by Boiten and Lodder a value of 85% was found (61). This frequency was lower in some other series, where only around 25% of patients with initial LI experienced a subsequent LI (110,225,227). The discrepancy among these series may support the fact that LI is not linked to a single pathological mechanism. In some instances, when recurrence of LI is in the same side as the qualifying event, it has likely not been considered as a recurring episode, but only a worsening of sequelae.

Recurrence may also manifest as nonlacunar IS. It should be kept in mind that at least one-third of first LI may also result from embolic or hemodynamic mechanisms in the appropriate penetrating artery territory, both in patients with and without classic risk factors for LI (237–241). Moreover, large-artery disease and cardiac source of embolism may coexist in patients with first-ever small deep infarct (242). Therefore, either of these etiologies could be the dominant factor in first LI, and it is reasonable to assume that one or both of them may also play a role in a subsequent stroke.

In keeping with these facts, the further ischemic event is of a nonlacunar nature in 15–45% of patients with first-ever LI (61,108,110,117,141,225,233,243). However, most of these series have made no distinction between ischemic recurrences resulting from large-artery disease and those arising from cardioembolic sources, or the latter have been excluded from the analysis. This distinction was established in one series, where it was found that approximately 15% of ischemic recurrences in patients with index LI resulted from heart-related embolus (117).

Asymptomatic ischemic recurrences in patients with initial LI have received little attention, although they may be at least as common as symptomatic recurrences. Out of 81 patients with symptomatic initial LI, MRI imaging identified asymptomatic recurrences in eight cases, and half of these showed a pattern of recurrence that was also LI (233).

Stroke-recurrence patterns for patients with minor stroke, including 30% with LI, resembled those where solely LI was involved (232). Half of all recurrences were also minor strokes, while the risk of a major infarct as recurrence was associated with either nonlacunar stroke, recurrent minor stroke, prior myocardial infarction or hypertension, or any combination thereof (232). Intracerebral hemorrhages,on the other hand, account for approximately 10–15% of recurrences in patients with initial LI resulting from the deleterious effects of hypertension on penetrating arteries (108,110,225,233).

Outcome is better for LI than for nonlacunar infarcts. Approximately 65–80% of patients are functionally independent 1 year after index stroke (110,141,231,233,244). These findings were corroborated in another study that included 102 patients with recurring strokes (117). Patients with first-ever LI exhibited significantly better functional outcomes than those with nonlacunar index stroke (117). After a subsequent stroke, and regardless of the pattern of recurrence, the initial difference in functional outcome observed among the various stroke types was lost (117). Nevertheless, functional outcome is more likely to be better in patients with first LI when the recurrent stroke is also LI (233).

K. Prevention of Long-Term Recurrence After LI

Most trials conducted to assess the efficacy of antiplatelet therapy in secondary stroke prevention have not specifically focused on this issue. In a retrospective analysis, aspirin (over 600 mg/day) and ticlopidine both prevented (though not significantly) more recurrent strokes in patients with LI than low doses of aspirin (325 mg/day) (245).

In the randomized AICLA trial, 16% of patients had presumed LI. In these patients, high doses of aspirin (1000 mg/day), administered both with and without 225 mg/day of dypiridamole, significantly reduced the incidence of recurring stroke by 62% (155). In effect, recurring-stroke incidence was 10% and 26% in the aspirin and placebo groups, respectively (155). A subgroup analysis of the TASS study showed that ticlopidine was slightly more effective than aspirin in reducing the risk of recurring stroke in patients with minor stroke (246).

L. Prognosis, Morbidity, and Mortality After Ischemic Stroke Recurrence

Hypertension, the most preventable risk factor, is associated with all stroke subtypes. The long-term effects of hypertension include coronary heart disease (CHD) and congestive heart failure (247). Thus, cardiac comorbidity is high in virtually all stroke types. The prevalence of CHD ranges from 28% to 41% in patients with TIA or cerebral infarction, although they do not usually have a history of CHD (248–250). Additionally, the prevalence of CHD correlates well with the severity of stenosis in the carotid arteries, being 17% in patients free of carotid stenosis and rising to 46% in those with stenosis over 75% (251). Patients who have had a stroke recurrence run a greater risk of myocardial infarction and vascular death than first-stroke sufferers (99). Patients with recurrent stroke have a higher mortality risk (1.8 times) than patients with first-ever stroke; mortality was higher in patients with contralateral recurrent stroke than patients with ipsilateral recurrence (234).

Recurring strokes are associated with a poor prognosis (252). Greater levels of disability are expected in patients with recurring stroke than in those with first-ever strokes. Survival at 2 years after stroke was higher for patients with a single episode (56.7%) than for patients with a recurrence (48%) (253).

M. Burden of Ischemic Stroke Recurrence

Stroke recurrence is important from the standpoint of public health, since the real burden of stroke is best expressed in terms of both first-ever and recurring-stroke rates (88). Recurring stroke imposes a significant economic and social burden. Available data on costs for patients with first and recurring IS comes from a sample of Medicare patients over the age of 65 (253). Costs of initial hospitalization and treatment costs for the first to the third month were not substantially different for patients with first strokes and for those with recurring events. However, total costs (including medication, doctors' fees, nursing-home bills, hospital and rehabilitation charges) were higher from the fourth to the twenty-fourth month for patients with recurring strokes, with an average per-patient difference of $375 per month, the difference being more pronounced in younger patients. Nursing-home and rehospitalization costs were responsible for the difference between first and recurring-stroke expense (253).

IV. LONG-TERM RECURRENCE AFTER INTRACEREBRAL HEMORRHAGES

Nontraumatic intracerebral hemorrhages (ICH) account for approximately 9–14% of all strokes in Western series (20,166,168,254–257). Frequency differs among racial groups, the highest incidence being found in Asian and Hispanic populations (258–263).

Traditional wisdom long maintained that hypertensive ICH would most likely occur only once in a lifetime (168,264–266). A number of recent studies suggest otherwise, however (263,267,268). Several factors may partially contribute to this trend. First, there has been an increase in the number of ICH survivors over time. In fact, most hospital-based series agree that the current early-case-fatality rate for ICH has fallen to 30–35% (265,269–272). Community-based studies show higher rates; the difference may be explained by the exclusion in hospital series of fatalities occurring before admission (255,256). Second, a large proportion of hypertensive patients remain uncontrolled after initial stroke (86,87). Finally, as life expectancy increases, it is to be expected that there will be a growing number of persons suffering from hypertension or other pathological processes common in the elderly, such as cerebral amyloid angiopathy (CAA).

Two European series in the 1980s failed to find ICH recurrence during a follow-up that lasted no longer than 29 months (264,265). Short and long-term follow-ups of Asian series have shown rates of rebleeding ranging from 1.8% to 5.9% in patients with first-ever primary ICH (273–277). A rate of recurrence between 2 and 2.4% per year was found in two studies of patients who survived to 30 days after ICH (278,279). Recently, both French and Mexican studies found, over a period of 10 years, a recurrence rate for primary ICH of 6.4% and 6%, respectively (263,268) (Table 5). Passero et al. have reported higher rates, however, with one-fourth of the patients in a group of 112 suffering at least one rebleeding during an average follow-up of 7 years after initial ICH (267). Although second or third rebleedings are considered uncommon, it has been found that anywhere from 6% to 25% of patients having a second ICH may also develop further episodes (268,277,280).

Commonly, recurrence after primary ICH happens soon after index stroke (281). Two-thirds of recurrences occur within 2 years of the first hemorrhage; of these recurrences, one-third to one-half are in the first year (263,267,277). Lower age (268), cirrhosis of the liver (282), and lobar location (267,268,278) have been associated with rebleeding. Moreover, patients receiving less than 3 months of antihypertensive therapy after first ICH and those with uncontrolled hypertension also face an increased risk of recurrence (277,283). Diastolic blood pressure (>90 mmHg) increases the risk of recurrence, with rates of 10% per year (279). Several case-control (284,285) and prospective studies (286,287) have demonstrated that alcohol consumption increases the risk of first hemorrhagic

Table 5 Rates of Recurrence of Intracerebral Hemorrhage and Predictors
of Recurrence

Author	Year	Rate of recurrence	Predictor
Lee (275)	1990	2.7%	Not described
Hirohata (273)	1991	1.8%	Not described
Chen (274)	1995	5.3%	Not described
Misra (280)	1995	4.7%	Not described
Passero (267)	1995	24%	Lobar location
Neau (268)	1997	6.4%	Younger age Lobar location
Gonzáles-Duarte (263)	1998	6.0%	Not described
Arakawa (279)	1998	2.0%	DBP > 90 mmHg
Bae (277)	1999	5.4%	Antihypertensive therapy < 3 months
Hill (278)	2000	2%	Lobar location

DBP: Diastolic blood pressure.

stroke in direct proportion to the amount consumed, but no studies have been made to assess the role of continued consumption in hemorrhagic recurrence (263,267,268,277).

Ganglionic hemorrhages usually predominate over lobar locations in patients with first-ever ICH, regardless of etiology (8,257,271,288,289). Most rebleeding occurs at locations different from the previous hemorrhage (268,274,275,280), although in one-third of all cases both the first and second hemorrhages are at the same site (267). "Lobar-lobar" and "ganglionic-ganglionic" are the most common patterns of recurrence. The former predominates in European series, showing up in 45–60% of cases (267,268,290), while the latter is more prevalent in Asian (273–276) and Hispano-American populations (263), where frequencies range from 50% to 85%. The difference is most likely due to the higher frequency of hypertension in patients with "ganglionic-ganglionic" recurrences (268).

Elderly patients usually show a "lobar-lobar" rather than a "ganglionic-ganglionic" pattern (267,268), most likely due to the contribution of CAA. Hemorrhages in the setting of CAA are usually lobar (291–293), and tend to recur sequentially over a period of months or years (294–300). Hypertension has been found in 25–65% of patients with recurring lobar hemorrhages (267,268,281). Thus, hypertension and CAA often coexist in the elderly and the former may contribute to both the first and the recurring CAA-related hemorrhage. Other patterns, such as ganglionic-thalamic, may occasionally predominate in certain series (277). Lobar-ganglionic or, vice versa, cerebellum-ganglionic and brain-stem-lobar patterns are uncommon (263,268).

Stroke recurrence in patients with initial ICH may also manifest as an ischemic event. Interestingly, the risk of cerebral infarct in survivors of first ICH has been estimated to be 3% per year (278). Cerebral infarcts accounted for 15–60% of all recurrences in patients with first ICH (117,281), and most were of noncardioembolic origin (117).

Recurrence of ICH worsens outcome (281). The worst prognosis of all is usually associated with ganglionic-ganglionic hemorrhages (263). Approximately 40% of patients have been reported to suffer severe disability after a second ICH (263,277), although 75% of the patients in the French study, in striking contrast, were able to walk with aids after a recurrence (268). Overall mortality after a second hemorrhage has been reported to be anywhere from 0% to 32% (263,274,275,277,280). Passero et al., however, have reported case fatalities reaching 70% (267).

A. Prevention of Long-Term Recurrence After Intracerebral Hemorrhage

Hypertension plays a paramount role in ganglionic hemorrhages, and probably lobar hemorrhages, as well. It also contributes greatly to IS caused by either large- or small-vessel disease. The present section therefore deals with the impact of high-blood-pressure treatment on stroke recurrence.

Treatment of high blood pressure in middle-aged and elderly hypertensive-free stroke subjects reduces the incidence of first-ever stroke by approximately 40% (301–304). Benefits of treatment may be age-related. In subjects younger than 65, reduction may reach 46%, whereas in patients over 65 years old it may be only 35% (305).

The possible advantage of treating high blood pressure to reduce stroke recurrence was suggested by two randomized clinical trials in the 1970s (306,307). The first trial included 50 patients allocated to antihypertensive treatment and 49 patients comprising a control group. Over a mean follow-up period of 3.6 years, the rate of stroke recurrence was twice as high in the control patients (306). In the second trial, 233 and 219 patients were assigned to treatment and control groups, respectively. Subjects were followed for 2.3 years and the rate of stroke recurrence was only slightly lower in the treatment group (307).

In the multicenter TEST (Tenormin after Stroke and TIA) study, no difference in the rate of recurrence was found between 372 patients with previous ischemic or hemorrhagic strokes who received 50 mg/day of atenolol and 348 patients given a placebo (308).

A relative risk reduction of approximately 30% in stroke recurrence was observed in 536 patients included in the INDANA database, but this finding was not significant (309). This database included patients from six different Western trials conducted to assess the efficacy of antihypertensive treatment in patients with and without a history of stroke (309). For the first time, results coming from the Post-stroke Antihypertensive Treatment Study (PATS) showed a significant reduction in relative risk of stroke recurrence on the order of 28% among subjects treated for hypertension (310). In this study, 2841 and 2824 Chinese patients with previous stroke were assigned to treatment and control groups, respectively. During a mean follow-up period of 1.8 years, rates of recurrence were 5.59% for the treatment group and 7.68% for the control group (310). In line with these findings, a recent meta-analysis of nine randomized clinical trials performed to evaluate the efficacy of antihypertensive treatment on main cardiovascular outcomes confirmed a significant relative reduction in stroke recurrence of 28% (311). However, most trials addressing efficacy in reducing stroke recurrence have not specifically compared the benefits of different antihypertensive drugs, nor have they taken into account the quality of blood pressure control.

Medical interventions to lower high blood pressure seem to be more efficacious in primary than in secondary stroke prevention. Bae et al. (277) have pointed out that treating hypertension is the most effective means to prevent recurring hemorrhage. Stroke recurrence may be the result of the effects of long-standing hypertension on the cerebral vasculature, the interaction of hypertension with other risk factors, or a consequence of other preexistent underlying mechanisms that are not modified by antihypertensive treatment. In all likelihood, any of these circumstances could explain the difference in the efficacy of antihypertensive treatment found between primary and secondary stroke prevention.

Currently, prevention of recurrence after CAA-related hemorrhages is mainly limited to the withdrawal of anticoagulant agents and control of hypertension, if present. Promising strategies may be based on restraining the mechanisms involved in amyloid production and its deposition in the vessel walls and those involved in the rupture of amyloid-laden vessels (312).

V. CONCLUSION

One-third of all strokes are recurrences. Rates of short- and long-term recurrence differ between first ischemic and first hemorrhagic strokes. For ischemic stroke, risk of recurrence depends on subtype and risk-factor profile. For hemorrhagic stroke, risk factors and patterns of recurrence are population related. In both cases, the etiology of recurrence is often of the same type as for the first event, although one-third of all recurrences are caused by different etiologies already present in the first stroke. Functional disability, morbidity, and mortality are higher after recurrence. The essential measures to prevent recurrence are the identification of all underlying potential mechanisms for stroke, vigorous control of risk factors, and optimal medical or surgical treatment after the first event.

ACKNOWLEDGMENT

The author wishes to thank Mr. Jeffrey Morrison for his help in editing and correcting the English text.

REFERENCES

1. Bonita R, Broad JB, Beaglehole R. Changes in stroke incidence and case-fatality in Auckland, New Zealand, 1981–91. Lancet 1993; 342:1470–1473.
2. Broderick JP. Stroke trends in Rochester Minnesota, during 1945 to 1984. Ann Epidemiol 1993; 3:476–479.
3. Shahar E, McGovern PG, Sprafka M, Pankow JS, Doliszny KM, Luepker RV, Blackburn H. Improved survival of stroke patients during the 1980s. The Minnesota Stroke Survey. Stroke. 1995, 26.1–6.
4. Barker WH, Mullooly JP. Stroke in a defined elderly population 1967–85. A less lethal and disabling but no less common disease. Stroke 1997; 28:284–290.
5. Immonen-Räihä P, Mähönen M, Tuomilehto M, Salomaa V, Kaarsalo E, Narva E, Salmi K, Sarti C, Sivenius J, Alhainen K, Torppa J. Trends in case-fatality of stroke in Finland during 1983 to 1992. Stroke 1997; 28:2493–2499.
6. Carolei A, Marini C, Di Napoli M, Di Gianfilippo G, Santalucia P, Baldassarre M, De Matteis G, Di Orio F. High stroke incidence in the prospective community-based L'Aquila Registry (1994–1998): first year results. Stroke 1997; 28:2500–2506.
7. Ellekjær H, Holmen J, Indredavik B, Terent A. Epidemiology of stroke in Innherred, Norway, 1994 to 1996. Incidence and 30-day case-fatality rate. Stroke. 1997; 28:2180–2184.
8. Kumral E, Özkaya B, Sagduyu A, Sirin H, Vardarli E, Pehlivan M. The Ege Stroke Registry: a hospital-based study in the Aegean Region, Izmir, Turkey. Analysis of 2,000 stroke patients. Cerebrovasc Dis 1998; 8:278–288.
9. Vemmos KN, Mots ML, Tsibouris PK, Zis VP, Grobbee DE, Stranjalis G, Stamatelopoulos S. Stroke incidence and case fatality in southern Greece. The Arcadia Stroke Registry. Stroke 1999; 30:363–370.
10. Hart RG, Coull BM, Hart D. Early recurrent embolism associated with non-valvular atrial fibrillation: a retrospective study. Stroke 1983; 14:688–693.
11. Cerebral Embolism Study Group. Immediate anticoagulation of embolic stroke: a randomized trial. Stroke. 1983; 14:668–676.
12. Sherman DG, Goldman L, Whiting RB, Jurgensen K, Kaste M, Easton JD. Thromboembolism in patients with atrial fibrillation, Arch Neurol 1984; 41:708–710.
13. Sage JI, Van Uitert RL. Risk of recurrent stroke in patients with atrial fibrillation and non-valvular heart disease. Stroke 1983; 14:537–540.

14. Goldstein LB, Perry A. Early recurrent ischemic stroke: a case-control study. Stroke 1992; 23:1010–1013.

15. Broderick JP, Phillips SJ, O'Fallon WM, Frye RL, Whisnant JP. Relationship of cardiac disease to stroke ocurrence, recurrence and mortality. Stroke 1992: 23: 1250–1256.

16. Moroney JT, Bagiella E, Paik MC, Sacco RL, Desmond DW. Risk factors for early recurrence after ischemic stroke. The role of stroke syndrome and subtype. Stroke 1998; 29:2118–2124.

17. Sacco RL, Foulkes MA, Mohr JP, Wolf PA, Hier DB, Price TR. Determinants of early recurrence of cerebral infarction: Stroke Data Bank. Stroke 1989; 20:983–989.

18. Hier DB, Foulkes MA, Swiontoniowski M, Sacco RL, Gorelick PB, Mohr JP. Stroke recurrence within two years after ischemic infarction. Stroke 1991; 22:155–161.

19. Sandercock P, Tangkanakul C. Very early prevention of stroke recurrence. Cerebrovasc Dis 1997; 7(suppl 1):10–15.

20. Bogousslavsky J, Van Melle G, Regli F. The Lausanne Stroke Registry: analysis of 1,000 consecutive patients with first stroke. Stroke 1988; 19:1083–1092.

21. Toni D, Fiorelli M, Gentile M, Bastianello S, Sacchetti ML, Argentin C, Pozzilli C, Fieschi C. Deteriorating neurological deficit secondary to acute ischemic stroke: a study of predictability, pathogenesis, and prognosis. Arch Neurol 1995; 52:670–675.

22. Yamamoto H, Bogousslavsky J, Van Melle G. Different predictors of neurological worsening in different causes of stroke. Arch Neurol 1998; 55:481–486.

23. DeGraba TJ, Hallenbeck JM, Pettigrew KD, Dutka AJ, Kelly BJ. Progression in acute stroke. Value of the initial NIH Stroke Scale Score on patient stratification in future trials. Stroke 1999; 30:1208–1212.

24. Irino T, Watanabe M, Nishide M, Gotoh M, Tsuchiya T. Angiographical analysis of acute cerebral infarction followed by "cascade" -like deterioration of minor neurological deficits: what is progressing stroke? Stroke 1983; 14:363–368.

25. Fisher M, Garcia JH. Evolving stroke and the ischemic penumbra. Neurology 1996; 47:884–888.

26. Petty GW, Brown RD, Whisnant JP, Sicks JD, O'Fallon WM, Wiebers DO. Survival and recurrence after first cerebral infarction. A population-based study in Rochester, Minnesota, 1975 trough 1989. Neurology. 1998; 50:208–216.

27. Sandercock P, Bamford J, Dennis M, Burn J, Slattery J, Jones L, Boonyakarnkul S, Warlow C. Atrial fibrillation and stroke: prevalence in different types of stroke and influence on early and long term prognosis (Oxfordshire community stroke project). Br Med J 1992; 305:1460–1465.

28. Horning CR, Dorndorf W. Early outcome and recurrences after cardiogenic brain embolism. Acta Neurol Scand 1993; 88:26–31.

29. Hacke W, Schwab S, Horn M, Spranger M, De Georgia M, von Kummer R. Malignant middle cerebral artery territory infarction: clinical course and prognostic signs. Arch Neurol 1996; 53:309–315.

30. Heinsius T, Bogousslavsky J, Van Melle G. Large infarcts in the middle cerebral artery territory: etiology and outcome patterns. Neurology 1998; 50:341–350.

31. Amarenco P, Hauw J-J. Infarctus cérébelleux œdémateux. Étude clinico-pathologique de 16 cas. Neurochirurgie 1990: 36:234–241.
32. Kilpatrick CJ, David SM, Hopper JL, Rossiter SC. Early seizures after acute stroke: risk of late seizures. Arch Neurol 1992: 49:509–511.
33. Lane RD, Walllace JD, Petrosky PP, Schwartz GE, Gradman AH. Supraventricular tachycardia in patients with right hemispheric strokes. Stroke 1992; 23:362–366.
34. Davenport RJ, Dennis MS, Wellwood I, Warlow CP. Complications following acute stroke. Stroke 1996; 27:415–420.
35. Johnston KC, Li JY, Lyden PD, Hanson SK, Feasby TE, Adams RJ, Faught E, Haley C, for the RANTTAS Investigators. Medical and neurological complications of ischemic stroke. Experience from the RANTTAS Trial. Stroke 1998; 29:447–453.
36. Bamford J, Sandercock P, Dennis M, Burn J, Warlow C. Classification and natural history of clinically identifiable subtypes of cerebral infarction. Lancet 1991; 337: 1521–1526.
37. Gustafsson C, Britton M. Pathogenetic mechanism of stroke in NVAF: follow up of stroke patients with and without AF. J Intern Med 1991; 230:11–16.
38. D'Alessandro G, Di Giovanni M, Roveyaz L, Iannizzi L, Compagnoni MP, Blanc S, Bottachi E. Incidence and prognosis of stroke in the Valle d'Aosta, Italy. First-year results of a community-based study. Stroke 1992; 23:1712–1715.
39. Lauria H, Gentile M, Fassetta G, Casetta I, Agnoli F, Andreotta G, Barp C, Caneve G, Cavallaro A, Cielo R, Mongillo D, Mosca M, Olivieri PG. Incidence and prognosis of stroke in the Belluno Province, Italy: first year results of a community-based study. Stroke 1995; 26:1787–1793.
40. Sacco RL, Shi T, Zamanillo MC, Kargman DE. Predictors of mortality and recurrence after hospitalized cerebral infarction in an urban community: the Northern Manhattan Stroke Study. Neurology 1994; 44:626–634.
41. Yasaka M, Yamaguchi T, Oita J, Sawada T, Sichiri M, Omae T. Clinical features of recurrent embolization in acute cardioembolic stroke. Stroke 1993; 24:1681–1685.
42. Arboix A, García-Eroles L, Oliveres M, Massons JB, Targa C. Clinical predictors of early embolic recurrence in presumed cardioembolic stroke. Cerebrovasc Dis 1998; 8:345–353.
43. Babikian VL, Wijman CAC, Hyde C, Cantelmo NL, Winter MR, Baker E, Pochay V. Cerebral microembolism and early recurrent cerebral or retinal ischemic events. Stroke 1997; 28:1314–1318.
44. Valton L, Larrue V, Pavy Le Traon A, Géraud G. Cerebral microembolism in patients with stroke or transient ischemic attack as a risk factor for early recurrence. J Neurol Neurosurg Psychiatry 1997; 63.784–787.
45. Valton L, Larrue V, Pavy Le Traon A, Massabuau P, Géraud G. Microembolic signals and risk of early recurrence in patients with stroke or transient ischemic attack. Stroke 1998; 29:2125–2128.
46. Cerebral Embolism Task Force. Cardiogenic brain embolism. Arch Neurol 1986; 43:71–84.
47. Hornig CR, Brainin M, Mast H. Cardioembolic stroke: results from three current stroke data banks. Neuroepidemiology 1994: 13:318–323.

48. Arboix A, Vericat MC, Pujades R, Massons J, García-Eroles L, Oliveres M. Cardi-oembolic infarction in the Sagrat Cor-Alianza Hospital of Barcelona Stroke Regis-try. Acta Neurol Scand 1997; 96:407–412.

49. Koller RL. Recurrent embolic cerebral infarction and anticoagulation. Neurology 1982; 32:283–285.

50. Bass E. Anticoagulation in cerebral embolism. Can J Neurol Sci 1983; 10:32–36.

51. Yasaka M, Yamaguchi T. Immediate anticoagulation for intracardiac thrombus in acute cardioembolic stroke. Angiology 1992; 43:886–892.

52. Yamanouchi H, Shimada H, Tomonaga M, Matsushita S. Recurrence of embolic stroke in non-valvular atrial fibrillation (NVAF). An autopsy study. Acta Neurol Scand 1989; 80:123–129.

53. Bogousslavsky J, Van Melle G, Regli F, Kappenberger L. Pathogenesis of anterior circulation stroke in patients with non-valvular atrial fibrillation: the Lausanne Stroke Registry. Neurology 1990; 40:1046–1050.

54. Lin HJ, Wolf PA, Kelly-Hayes M, Beiser AS, Kase CS, Benjamin EJ, D'Agostino RB. Stroke severity in atrial fibrillation: the Framingham Study. Stroke 1996; 27: 1760–1764.

55. International Stroke Trial Collaborative Group: The International Stroke Trial (IST): a randomised trial of aspirin, subcutaneous heparin, both or neither among 19435 patients with acute ischaemic stroke. Lancet 1997; 349:1569–1581.

56. Jorgensen HS, Nakayama H, Reith J, Raaschou HO, Olsen TS. Acute stroke with atrial fibrillation: the Copenhagen Stroke Study. Stroke 1996; 10:1765–1769.

57. Davenport J, Hart RG. Prosthetic valve endocarditis 1976–87. Antibiotics, antico-agulation, and stroke. Stroke 1990; 21:993–999.

58. Salgado AV, Furlan AJ, Keys TF, Nichols TR, Beck GJ. Neurological complica-tions of native and prosthetic valve endocarditis: a 12 year experience. Neurology. 1989; 30:173–178.

59. Hart RG, Foster JW, Luther MF, Kanter MC. Stroke in infective endocarditis. Stroke 1990; 21:695–700.

60. Bogousslavsky J, Garazi S, Jeanrenaud X, Aesbicher N, Van Melle G, for the Laus-sane Stroke with Paradoxical Embolism Study Group. Stroke recurrence in patients with patent foramen ovale: the Lausanne Study. Neurology 1996; 46:1301–1305.

61. Boiten J, Lodder J. Prognosis for survival, handicap and recurrence of stroke in lacunar and superficial infarction. Cerebrovasc Dis 1993; 3:221–226.

62. Samuelsson M, Lindell D, Norrving B. Presumed pathogenetic mechanisms of re-current stroke after lacunar infarction. Cerebrovasc Dis 1996; 6:128–136.

63. Marshall J, Shaw DA. Anticoagulant therapy in acute cerebrovascular accidents: a controlled trial. Lancet 1960; 1:995–998.

64. Turpie AG, Levine MN, Hirsh J, Carter CJ, Jay RM, Powers PJ, Andrew M, Mag-nani HN, Hull RD, Gent M. Double-blind randomised trial of Org 10172 low-molecular-weight heparinoid in prevention of deep-vein thrombosis in thrombotic stroke. Lancet 1987; 1:523–526.

65. Kay R, Wong KS, Yu YL, Chan YW, Tsoi TJ, Ahuja FL, Chan FL, Fong KY, Law CB, Wong A, Woo J. Low-molecular-weight heparin for the treatment of acute ischemic stroke. N Engl J Med 1995; 333:1588–1593.

66. The Publications Committee for the Trial of ORG 10172 in Acute Stroke Treatment

(TOAST) Investigators. Low molecular weight heparinoid, ORG 10172 (danaparoid), and outcome after acute ischemic stroke: a randomized controlled trial. JAMA 1998; 279:1265–1272.

67. Lodder J, Van der Lugt PJM. Evaluation of the risk of immediate anticoagulation treatment in patients with embolic stroke of cardiac origin. Stroke 1983; 14:42–46.

68. Cerebral Embolism Task Force. Cardiogenic brain embolism: second report of the Cerebral Embolism Task Force. Arch Neurol 1989; 46:727–741.

69. Pessin MS, Estol CJ, Lafranchise F, Caplan LR. Safety of anticoagulation after hemorrhagic infarction. Neurology 1993; 43:1298–1303.

70. Chamorro A, Vila N, Ascaso C, Blanc R. Heparin in acute stroke with atrial fibrillation. Arch Neurol 1999; 56:1098–1102.

71. Alberts MJ, Dawson DV, Massey EW. A follow-up survey of clinical practices for the use of heparin, warfarin, and aspirin. Neurology 1994; 44:618–621.

72. Mohr JP, Albers GW, Amarenco P, Babikian VL, Biller J, Brey RL, Coull B, Easton JD, Gomez CR, Helgason CM, Kase CS, Pullicino PM, Turpie AG. Etiology of stroke. Stroke 1997; 28:1506–1510.

73. Hart RG. Cardiogenic embolism to the brain. Lancet 1992; 339:589–594.

74. Caplan LR. Prevention of cardioembolic stroke. Heart Dis Stroke 1994; 3:297–303.

75. Rothrock JF; Dittrich HC, McAllen S, Taft BJ, Lyden PD. Acute anticoagulation following cardioembolic stroke. Stroke 1989; 20:730–734.

76. Furlan AJ, Cavalier SJ, Hobbs RE, Weinstein MA, Modic MT. Hemorrhage and anticoagulation after nonseptic embolic brain infarction. Neurology 1982; 32:280–282.

77. Ott BR, Zamani A, Kleefield J, Funkestein HH. The clinical spectrum of hemorrhagic infarction. Stroke 1986; 17:630–637.

78. Chinese Acute Stroke Trial (CAST) Collaborative Group. CAST: a randomised trial of early aspirin use in 20000 patients with acute ischemic stroke. Lancet 1997; 349:1569–1581.

79. Goertler M, Baeumer M, Kross R, Blaser T, Lutze G, Jost S, Wallesch CW. Rapid decline of cerebral microemboli of arterial origin after intravenous acetylsalicylic acid. Stroke 1999; 30:66–69.

80. Antiplatelet Trialists' Collaboration. Collaborative overview of randomized trials of antiplatelet treatment. Part I. Prevention of death, myocardial infarction and stroke by prolonged antiplatelet therapy in various categories of patients. Br Med J 1994; 308:81–106.

81. Gent M, Blakely JA, Easton JD, Ellis DJ, Hachinski VC, Harbison JW, Panak E, Roberts RS, Sicurella J, Turpie AGG. The Canadian American Ticlopidine Study (CATS) in thromboembolic stroke. Lancet 1989; 2:1215–1220.

82. European Atrial Fibrillation Trial Study Group. Secondary prevention of vascular events in patients with nonrheumatic atrial fibrillation and recent transient ischemic attack or minor ischemic stroke. Lancet 1993; 342:1255–1262.

83. North American Symptomatic Carotid Endarterectomy Trial Collaborators. Beneficial effect of carotid endarterectomy in symptomatic patients with high-grade carotid stenosis. N Engl J Med 1991; 325:445–453.

84. European Carotid Surgery Trialists' Collaborative Group. MRC European carotid surgery trial: interim results for symptomatic patients with severe (70–99%) or with mild (0–29%) carotid stenosis. Lancet 1991; 337:1235–1243.
85. Joseph LN, Babikian VL, Allen NC, Winter MR. Risk factor modification in stroke prevention. The experience of a stroke clinic. Stroke 1999; 30:16–20.
86. Klungel OH, Kaplan RC, Heckbert SR, Smith NL, Lemaitre RN, Longstreth Jr WT, Leufkens HGM, de Boer A, Psaty BM. Control of blood pressure and risk of stroke among pharmacologically treated hypertensive patients. Stroke 2000; 31: 420–424.
87. Hillen T, Dundas R, Lawrence E, Stewart JA, Rudd AG, Wolfe CD. Antithrombotic and antihypertensive management 3 months after ischemic stroke. A prospective study in an inner city population. Stroke 2000; 31:469–475.
88. Broderick J, Brott T, Kothari R, Miller R, Khoury J, Pancioli A, Gebel J, Mills D, Minneci L, Shukla R. The Greater Cincinatti/Northern Kentucky Stroke Study. Preliminary first-ever and total incidence rates of stroke among blacks. Stroke 1998; 29:415–421.
89. Lackland DT, Bachman DL, Carter TD, Barker DL, Timms S, Kohli H. The geographic variation in stroke incidence in two areas of the southeastern stroke belt. The Anderson and Pee Dee Stroke Study. Stroke 1998; 29:2061–2068.
90. Burn J, Dennis M, Bamford J, Sandercock P, Wade D, Warlow C. Long-term risk of recurrent stroke after a first-ever stroke: the Oxfordshire Community Stroke Project. Stroke 1994; 25:333–337.
91. Moroney JT, Bagiella E, Tatemichi TK, Paik MC, Stern Y, Desmond DW. Dementia after stroke increases the risk of long-term recurrence. Neurology 1997; 48: 1317–1325.
92. Jamrozik K, Broadhurst RJ, Lai N, Hankey GJ, Burvill PW, Anderson CS. Trends in the incidence, severity, and short-term outcome of stroke in Perth, Western Australia. Stroke 1999; 30:2105–2111.
93. Meissner I, Whisnant JP, Garraway WM. Hypertension management and stroke recurrence in a community (Rochester, Minnesota, 1950–1979). Stroke 1988; 19: 459–463.
94. Elneihoum AM, Göransson M, Falke P, Janzon L. Three-year survival and recurrence after stroke in Malmö, Sweden. An analysis of Stroke Registry Data. Stroke 1998; 29:2114–2117.
95. Scmidt EV, Smirnov VE, Ryabova VS. Results of the seven-year prospective study of stroke patients. Stroke 1988; 19:942–949.
96. Kannel WB, Dawber TR, Sorlie P, Wolf PA. Components of blood pressure and risk of atherothrombotic brain infarction: the Framingham Study. Stroke 1976; 7: 327–331.
97. Sacco RL, Wolf PA, Kannel WB, McNamara PM. Survival and recurrence following stroke: The Framingham Study. Stroke 1982; 13:290–295.
98. Feinberg WM. Primary and secondary stroke prevention. Curr Opin Neurol 1996; 9:46–52.
99. Easton JD. Epidemiology of stroke recurrence. Cerebrovasc Dis 1997; 7(suppl 1): 2–4.

100. Sacco RL. Identifying patient population at high risk for stroke. Neurology. 1998; 51(suppl 3):S27–S30.
101. Marquardsen J. The natural history of acute cerebrovascular disease. Acta Neurol Scand 1969; 45 (suppl)38:11.
102. Vitanen M, Eriksson S, Asplund K. Risk of recurrent stroke, myocardial infarction and epilepsy during long-term follow-up after stroke. Eur Neurol 1988; 28:227–231.
103. Sobel E, Alter M, Davanipour Z, Friday F, McCoy R, Levitt LP, Isack T. Stroke in the Leigh Valley: combined risk factors for recurrent ischemic stroke. Neurology 1989; 39:669–672.
104. Alter M, Sobel E, McCoy RL, Francis ME, Davanipour Z, Shofer F, Levitt LP, Meehan EF. Stroke in the Leigh Valley: risk factors for recurrent stroke. Neurology. 1987; 37:503–507.
105. Lai SM, Alter M, Friday G, Sobel E. A multifactorial analysis of risk factors for recurrence of ischemic stroke. Stroke 1994; 25:958–962.
106. Lai SM, Alter M, Friday G, Sobel E. Prognosis for survival after an initial stroke. Stroke 1995; 26:2011–2015.
107. Irie K, Yamaguchi T, Minematsu K, Omae T. The J-curve phenomenon in stroke recurrence. Stroke 1993; 24:1844–1849.
108. Salgado AV, Ferro JM, Gouveia-Oliveira A. Long-term prognosis of first-ever lacunar strokes: a hospital-based study. Stroke 1996; 27:661–666.
109. Alter M, Friday G, Lai SM, O'Connel J, Sobel E. Hypertension and risk of stroke recurrence. Stroke 1994; 25:1605–1610.
110. Clavier I, Hommel M, Besson G, Noèlle B, Ferjus Perret JE. Long-term prognosis of symptomatic lacunar infarcts: a hospital-based study. Stroke 1994; 25:2005–2009.
111. Tohgi H, Chiba K, Takahashi H, Tamura K, Sasaki K, Suzuki II. Comparison of symptomatic and asymptomatic reinfarctions after small subcortical stroke. Eur Neurol 1994; 34:140–146.
112. Levine SR, Brey RL, Joseph CLM, Havstad S. Antiphospholipid Antibodies in Stroke Study Group. Risk of recurrent thromboembolic events in patients with focal cerebral ischemia and antiphospholipid antibodies. Stroke 1992; 23 (suppl 1):29–32.
113. Tohgi H, Takahashi H, Kashiwata M, Watanabe K, Hayama K. The anticardiolipin antibody in elderly stroke patients: Its effects on stroke types, recurrence, and the coagulation fibrynolysis system. Acta Neurol Scand 1994; 90:86–90.
114. The French Study of Aortic Plaques in Stroke Group. Atherosclerotic disease of the aortic arch as a risk factor for recurrent ischemic stroke. N Engl J Med 1996; 334:1216–1221.
115. Tunick PA, Rosenzweig BP, Katz ES, Freedberg RS, Perez JL, Kronzon I. High risk for vascular events in patients with protruding aortic atheromas: a prospective study. J Am Coll Cardiol 1994; 23:1085–1090.
116. Leonberg SC, Elliott FA. Prevention of recurrent stroke. Stroke 1981; 12:731–735.
117. Yamamoto H, Bogousslavsky J. Mechanisms of second and further strokes. J Neurol Neurosurg Psychiatry 1998; 64:771–776.

118. Morgenstern LB, Fox AJ, Sharpe BL, Eliasziw M, Barnett HJ, Grotta JC, for the North American Symptomatic Carotid Endarterectomy Trial (NASCET) Group. The risks and benefits of carotid endarterectomy in patients with near occlusion of the carotid artery. Neurology 1997; 48:911–915.

119. Eliasziw M, Streifler JY, Fox AJ, Hachinski VC, Ferguson GG, Barnett HJ. Significance of plaque ulceration in symptomatic patients with high-grade carotid stenosis. North American Symptomatic Carotid Endarterectomy Trial. Stroke 1994; 25:304–308.

120. Mansour MA, Mattos MA, Faught WE, Hodgson KJ, Barkmeier LD, Ramsey DE, Summer DS. The natural history of moderate (50% to 79%) internal carotid artery stenosis in symptomatic, nonhemispheric, and asymptomatic patients. J Vasc Surg 1995; 21:346–357.

121. Bogousslavsky J, Regli F. Prognosis of symptomatic intracranial obstruction of internal carotid artery. Eur Neurol 1983; 22:351–358.

122. Furlan AJ, Whisnant JP, Baker HL Jr. Long-term prognosis after carotid artery occlusion. Neurology 1980; 30:986–988.

123. Cote R, Barnett HJM, Taylor DW. Internal carotid occlusion: a prospective study. Stroke 1983; 14:898–902.

124. Marzewski DJ, Furlan AJ, St Louis P, Little JR, Modic MT, Williams G. Intracranial internal carotid stenosis: long-term prognosis. Stroke 1982; 13:821–824.

125. Craig DR, Meguro K, Watridge C, Robertson JT, Barnett HJM, Fox AJ. Intracranial internal carotid artery stenosis. Stroke 1982; 13:825–828.

126. Borozan PG, Shuler JJ, LaRosa MP, Ware MS, Flanigan DP. The natural history of isolated carotid siphon stenosis. J Vasc Surg 1984; 1:744–749.

127. The EC/IC Bypass Study Group. Failure of extracranial-intracranial arterial bypass to reduce the risk of ischemic stroke: results of an international randomized trial. N Engl J Med. 1985; 313:1191–1200.

128. Wechsler LR, Kistler JP, Davis KR, Kaminski MJ. The prognosis of carotid siphon stenosis. Stroke 1986; 17:714–718.

129. Bogousslavksy J, Barnett HJM, Fox AJ, Hachinski VC, Taylor W, for the EC/IC Bypass Study Group. Atheroscleorotic disease of the middle cerebral artery. Stroke 1986; 17:1112–1120.

130. Kappelle LJ, Eliasziw M, Fox AJ, Sharpe BL, Barnett HJM, for the North American Symptomatic Carotid Endarterectomy Trial (NASCET) Group. Importance of intracranial atherosclerotic disease in patients with symptomatic stenosis of the internal carotid artery. Stroke 1999; 30:282–286.

131. Solberg LA, McGarry PA. Cerebral atherosclerosis in Negroes and Caucasians. Atherosclerosis 1972; 16:141–154.

132. Gorelick P, Caplan LR, Hier D, Parker S, Patel D. Racial differences in the distribution of anterior circulation occlusive disease. Neurology 1984; 34:54–59.

133. Feldmann E, Daneault N, Kwan E, Ho KJ, Pessin MS, Langenberg P, Caplan LR. Chinese-white differences in the distribution of occlusive cerebrovascular disease. Neurology 1990; 40:1541–1545.

134. Moosy J. Pathology of cerebral atherosclerosis: influence of age, race, and gender. Stroke 1993; 24 (suppl 1):1-22–1-23.

135. Leung SY, Ng THK, Yuen ST, Lauder IJ, Ho FCS. Pattern of cerebral atherosclero-

sis in Hong-Kong Chinese: severity in intracranial and extracranial vessels. Stroke 1993; 24:779–786.

136. Sacco RL, Kargman DE, Gu Q, Zamanillo MC. Race-ethnicity and determinants of intracranial atherosclerotic cerebral infarction: the Northern Manhattan Stroke Study. Stroke 1995; 26:14–20.

137. Hass WK, Fields WS, North RR, Kricheff II, Chase NE, Bauer RB. Joint study of extracranial artery occlusion. II. Arteriography, techniques, sites and complications. JAMA 1968; 203:959–968.

138. Hinton RC, Mohr JP, Ackerman RH, Adair LB, Fisher CM. Symptomatic middle cerebral artery stenosis. Ann Neurol 1979; 5:152–157.

139. Caplan L, Babikian V, Helgason C, Hier DB, De Witt D, Patel D, Stein R. Occlusive disease of the middle cerebral artery. Neurology 1985; 35:975–982.

140. The Warfarin-Aspirin Symptomatic Intracranial Disease (WASID) Study Group. Prognosis of patients with symptomatic vertebral or basilar artery stenosis. Stroke 1998; 29:1389–1392.

141. Nadeau SE, Jordan JE, Mishra SK, Haerer AF. Stroke rates in patients with lacunar and large vessel cerebral infarctions. J Neurol Sci 1993; 114:128–137.

142. Cillessen JPM, Kapelle LJ, van Swieten JC, Algra A, van Gijn J. Does cerebral infarction after a previous warning occur in the same vascular territory? Stroke 1993; 24:351–354.

143. The Canadian Cooperative Study Group. A randomized trial of aspirin and sufinpyrazone in threatened stroke. N Engl J Med 1978; 299:53–59.

144. Hankey GJ, Warlow CP. Treatment and secondary prevention of stroke: evidence, costs, and effects on individuals and populations. Lancet 1999; 354:1457–1463.

145. Gorelick PB, Born GV, D'Agostino RB, Hanley DF Jr, Moye L, Pepine CJ. Therapeutic benefit. Aspirin revisited in light of the introduction of clopidogrel. Stroke 1999; 30:1716–1721.

146. UK-TIA Study Group. The United Kingdom transient ischemic attack (UK-TIA) aspirin trial: final results. J Neurol Neurosurg Psychiatry 1991; 54:1044–1054.

147. Dutch TIA Trial Study Group. A comparison of two doses of aspirin (30 mg vs 283 mg a day) in patients after transient ischemic attack or minor ischemic stroke. N Engl J Med 1991; 325:1261–1266.

148. Patrono C, Collor BS, Dalen JE, Fuster V, Gent M, Harker LA, Hirsh J, Roth G. Platelet-active drugs: the relationships among dose, effectiveness, and side effects. Chest 1998; 114 (suppl 5):470S–488S.

149. Iwamoto T, Kubo H, Takasaki M. Platelet activation in the cerebral circulation in different subtypes of ischemic stroke and Binswanger's disease. Stroke 1995; 26: 52–57.

150. Van Kooten F, Ciabattoni G, Koudstaal PJ, Dippel DWJ, Patrono C. Increased platelet activation in the chronic phase after cerebral ischemia and intracerebral hemorrhage. Stroke 1999; 30:546–549.

151. Helgason CM, Bolin KM, Hoff JA, Winkler SR, Mangat A, Tortorice KL, Brace LD. Development of aspirin resistance in persons with previous ischemic stroke. Stroke 1994; 25:2331–2336.

152. Hass WK, Easton JD, Adams HP Jr, Pryse-Phillips W, Molony BA, Anderson S, Kamm B. A randomized trial comparing ticlopidine hydrochloride with aspirin for

the prevention of stroke in high-risk patients. Ticlopidine Aspirin Stroke Study Group. N Engl J Med 1989; 321:501–507.

153. CAPRIE Steering Committee A randomised blinded, trial of clopidogrel versus aspirin in patients at risk of ischaemic events (CAPRIE). Lancet 1996; 348:1329–1339.

154. Guiraud-Chaumeil B, Rascol A, David J, Boneu B, Clantet M, Bierme R. Prévention des récidives des accidents vasculaires cérébraux ischémiques par les anti-agrégants plaquettaires. Rev Neurol (Paris) 1982; 138:367–385.

155. Bousser MG, Eschwege E, Haguenau M, Lefaucconnier JM, Thibult N, Touboul D, Touboul PJ. "AICLA" controlled trial of aspirin and dypiridamole in the secondary prevention of atherothrombotic cerebral ischemia. Stroke 1983; 14:5–14.

156. The American-Canadian Co-operative Study Group. Persantine aspirin trial in cerebral ischemia. Part II. Endpoint results. Stroke 1985:16:406–415.

157. Diener HC, Cumha L, Forbes C, Sivenius J, Smets P, Lowenthal A. European Stroke Prevention Study 2: dypiridamole and acetylsalicylic acid in the secondary prevention of stroke. J Neurol Sci 1996; 143:1–13.

158. Chimowitz MI, Kokkinos J, Strong J, Brown MB, Levine SR, Silliman S, Pessin MS, Weichel E, Sila CA, Furlan AJ, Kargmann DE, Sacco RL, Wityk RJ, Ford G, Fayad PB, for the Warfarin-Aspirin Symptomatic Intracranial Disease Study Group. The Warfarin-Aspirin Symptomatic Intracranial Disease Study. Neurology. 1995; 45:1488–1493.

159. Marks MP, Marcellus M, Norbash AM, Steinberg GK, Tong D, Albers GW. Outcome of angioplasty for atherosclerotic intracranial stenosis. Stroke 1999; 30:1065–1069.

160. Clark WM, Barnwell SL, Nesbit G, O'Neill OR, Wynn ML, Coull BM. Safety and efficacy of percutaneous transluminal angioplasty for intracranial atherosclerototic stenosis. Stroke 1995; 26:1200–1204.

161. Takis C, Kwan ES, Pessin MS, Jacobs DH, Caplan LR. Intracranial angioplasty: experience and complications. Am J Neuroradiol 1997; 18:1661–1668.

162. Yadav JS, Roubin GS, Iyer S, Vitek J, King P, Jordan WD. Elective stenting of the extracranial carotid arteries. Circulation 1997; 95:376–381.

163. Al-Mubarak N, Gomez CR, Vitek JJ, Roubin GS. Stenting of symptomatic intracranial internal carotid artery stenosis: a case report. Am J Neuroradiol 1998; 19:1949–1951.

164. Mori T, Kazita K, Mori K. Cerebral angioplasty and stenting for intracranial vertebral atherosclerotic stenosis. Am J Neuroradiol 1999; 20:787–789.

165. Gomez CR, Misra VK, Liu MW, Wadlington WR, Terry JB, Tulyapronchote R, Campbell MS. Elective stenting of symptomatic basilar artery stenosis. Stroke 2000; 31:95–99.

166. Foulkes MA, Wolf PA, Price TR, Mohr JP, Hier DB. The Stroke Data Bank: design, methods, and baseline characteristics. Stroke 1988; 19:547–554.

167. Norrving B, Löwenhielm P. Epidemiology of stroke in Lund-Orup, Sweden, 1983–85. Incidence of first stroke and aged-related changes in subtypes. Acta Neurol Scand 1988; 78:408–413.

168. Mohr JP, Caplan LR, Melski JW, Goldstein RJ, Duncan GW, Kistler JP, Pessin

MS, Bleich HL: The Harvard Cooperative Stroke Registry: a prospective registry. Neurology 1978; 28:754–762.

169. Sacco RL, Ellenberg JH, Mohr JP, Tatemichi TK, Hier DB, Price TR, Wolf PA. Infarcts of undetermined cause: the NINCDS Stroke Data Bank. Ann Neurol 1989; 25:382–390.

170. Lindgren A, Roijer A, Norrving B, Wallin L, Eskilsson J, Johansson BB. Carotid artery and heart disease in subtypes of cerebral infarction. Stroke 1994; 25:2536–2562.

171. Rothrock JF, Lyden PD, Brody ML, Taft-Alvarez B, Kelly N, Mayer J, Wiederholt WC. An analysis of ischemic stroke in an urban southern California population. The University of California, San Diego, Stroke Data Bank. Arch Intern Med 1993; 153:619–624.

172. Ramirez-Lassepas M, Cipolle RJ, Bjork RJ, Kowitz J, Snyder BD, Weber JC, Stein SD. Can embolic stroke be diagnosed on the basis of neurologic clinical criteria? Arch Neurol 1987; 44:87–89.

173. Bogousslavsky J, Cachin C, Regli F, Despland PA, Van Melle G, Kappenberger L (for the Lausanne Stroke Registry Group). Cardiac sources of embolism and cerebral infarction—clinical consequences and vascular concomitants: the Lausanne Stroke Registry Group. Neurology 1991; 41:855–859.

174. Kittner SJ, Sharkness CM, Sloan MA, Price TR, Dambrosia JM, Tuhrim S, Wolf PA, Mohr JP, Hier DB, Caplan LR. Infarcts with a cardiac source of embolism in the NINDS Stroke Data Bank: neurologic examination. Neurology 1992; 42:299–302.

175. Wolf PA, Abott RD, Kannel WB. Atrial fibrillation: a major contributor to stroke in the elderly. The Framingham study. Arch Intern Med 1987; 147:1561–1564.

176. Boysen G, Nyboe J, Appleyard M, Sorensen PS, Boas J, Somnier F, Jensen G, Schnohr P. Stroke incidence and risk factors for stroke in Copenhagen, Denmark. Stroke 1988; 19:1345–1353.

177. Atrial Fibrillation Investigators: Atrial Fibrillation, Aspirin, Anticoagulation Study; Boston Area Anticoagulation Trial for Atrial Fibrillation Study; Canadian Atrial Fibrillation Anticoagulation Study; Stroke Prevention in Atrial Fibrillation Study; Veterans Affairs Stroke Prevention in Nonrheumatic Atrial Fibrillation Study. Risk factors for stroke and efficacy of antithrombotic therapy in atrial fibrillation. Arch Intern Med 1994; 154:1449–1457.

178. Stroke Prevention in Atrial Fibrillation Investigators. Stroke Prevention in Atrial Fibrillation Study. Final Results. Circulation 1991; 84:527–539.

179. Hart RG. Sherman DG, Easton JD, Cairns JA. Prevention of stroke in patients with nonvalvular atrial fibrillation. Neurology 1998; 51:674–681.

180. Van Latum JC, Koudstaal PJ, Venables GS, Van Gijn J, Kapelle LJ, Algra A, for the European Atrial Fibrillation Trial (EAFT) Study Group. Predictors of major vascular events in patients with a transient ischemic attack or minor ischemic stroke and with nonrheumatic atrial fibrillation. Stroke 1995; 16:801–806.

181. Feinberg WM. Anticoagulation for prevention of stroke. Neurology 1998; 51 (suppl 3):S20–S22.

182. Lip GY, Lowe GD. Antithrombotic treatment for atrial fibrillation. Br Med J 1996; 312:45–49.

183. Laupacis A, Albers GW, Dalen JE, Dunn MI, Feinberg W, Jacobson AK. Antithrombotic therapy in atrial fibrillation. Chest 1995; 108(suppl 4):352S–359S.
184. Stroke Prevention in Atrial Fibrillation Investigators. Risk factors for thromboembolism during aspirin therapy in atrial fibrillation. Cerebrovasc Dis 1995; 5:147–157.
185. Stroke Prevention in Atrial Fibrillation Investigators. Patients with nonvalvular atrial fibrillation at low risk of stroke during treatment with aspirin. JAMA 1998; 279:1273–1277.
186. Hart RG, Pearce LA, McBride R, Rothbart RM, Asinger RW; on behalf of the Stroke Prevention in Atrial Fibrillation (SPAF) Investigators. Factors associated with ischemic stroke during aspirin therapy in atrial fibrillation. Analysis of 2012 participants in the SPAF I–III clinical trials. Stroke 1999; 30:1223–1229.
187. Sherman DG, Hart RG, Easton JD. The secondary prevention of stroke in patients with atrial fibrillation. Arch Neurol 1986; 43:68–70.
188. Lodder J, Dennis MS, Van Raak L, Jones LN, Warlow CP. Cooperative study on the value of long term anticoagulation in patients with stroke and non-rheumatic atrial fibrillation. Br Med J (Clin Rev Ed) 1988; 296:1435–1438.
189. Diener HC, Forbes C, Riekkinin PJ, Sivenius J, Smets P, Lowenthal A. European Stroke Prevention Study II. Efficacy and safety data. J Neurol Sci 1997; 151:S13–S17.
190. Kopecky SL, Gersh BJ, McGoon MD, Whisnant JP, Holmes DR Jr, Ilstrup DM, Frye RL. The natural history of lone atrial fibrillation. A population-based study over three decades. N Engl J Med 1987; 317:669–674.
191. Bogousslavsky J, Adnet-Bonte C, Regli F, Van Melle G, Kappenberger L. Lone atrial fibrillation and stroke. Acta Neurol Scand 1990; 82:143–146.
192. Szekely P. Systemic embolism and anticoagulant prophylaxis in rheumatic heart disease. Br Med J 1964; 1:1209–1212.
193. Diker E, Aydogdu S, Ozdemir M, Kural T, Polat K, Cehreli S, Erdogan A, Goksel S. Prevalence and predictors of atrial fibrillation in rheumatic valvular heart disease. Am J Cardiol 1996; 77:96–98.
194. Wolf PA, Dawber TR, Thomas HE Jr, Kannel WB. Epidemiologic assessment of chronic atrial fibrillation and risk of stroke: the Framingham study. Neurology 1978; 28:973–977.
195. Daley R, Mattingly TW, Holt CL. Systemic arterial embolism in rheumatic heart disease. Am Heart J 1951; 42:566.
196. Levine HJ, Pauker SG, Salzman EW. Antithrombotic therapy in valvular heart disease. Chest 1989; 95 (suppl):98S–106S.
197. Coulshed N, Epstein EJ, McKendrick CS, Galloway RW, Walker E. Systemic embolism in mitral valve disease. Br Heart J 1970; 32:26–34.
198. Seigel R, Tresch DD, Keelan MH, Brooks HL. Effects of anticoagulation on recurrent systemic emboli in mitral stenosis. Am J Cardiol 1987; 60:1191–1192.
199. Lechat P, Mas JL, Lascault G, Loron P, Theard M, Klimczac M, Drobinski G, Thomas D, Grosgogeat Y. Prevalence of patent foramen ovale in patients with stroke. N Engl J Med 1988; 318:1148–1152.
200. Webster MWI, Chancellor AM, Smith HJ, Swift DL, Sharpe DN, Bass NM, Glasgow GL. Patent foramen ovale in young stroke patients. Lancet 1988; 2:11–12.

201. Jeanrenaud X, Bogousslavsky J, Payot M, Regli F, Kapenberger L. Foramen ovale perméable et infarctus cérébral du sujet jeune. Schweiz Med Wochenschr 1990; 120:823–829.
202. Gautier JC, Dürr A, Koussa S, Lascault G, Grosgogeat Y. Paradoxical cerebral embolism with a patent foramen ovale. Cerebrovasc Dis 1991; 1:193–202.
203. Di Tullio M, Sacco RL, Gopal A, Mohr JP, Homma S. Patent foramen ovale as a risk factor for cryptgenic stroke. Ann Intern Med 1992; 117:461–465.
204. Nater B, Bogousslavsky J, Regli F, Stauffer JC. Stroke patterns with atrial septal aneurysm. Cerebrovasc Dis 1992; 2:342–346.
205. Cabanes L, Mas JL, Cohen A, Amarenco P, Cabanes PA, Oubary P, Chedru F, Guérin F, Bousser MG, de Recondo J. Atrial septal aneurysm and patent foramen ovale as risk factors for cryptogenic stroke in patients less than 55 years of age. A study using transesophageal echocardiography. Stroke 1993; 24:1865–1873.
206. Lucas C, Goullard L, Marchau M Jr, Godefroy O, Rondepierre Ph, Chamas E, Mounier-Vehier F, Leys D, Higher prevalence of atrial septal aneurysms in patients with ischemic stroke of unknown cause. Acta Neurol Scand 1994; 89:210–213.
207. Mügge A, Daniel WG, Angermann Ch, Spes Ch, Khandheria BK, Kronzon I, Freedberg RS, Keren A, Dennig K, Engberding R, Sutherland GR, Vered Z, Erbel R, Visser CA, Lindert O, Haussmann D, Wenzlaff P. Atrial septal aneurysm in adult patients. A multicenter study using transthoracic and transesophageal echocardiography. Circulation 1995; 91:2785–2792.
208. Hanna JP, Ping Sung J, Furlan AJ, Stewart WJ, Sila CA, Tan M. Patent foramen ovale and brain infarct. Echocardiographic predictors, recurrence, and prevention. Stroke 1994; 25:782–786.
209. Mas JL, Zuber M. Recurrent cerebrovascular events in patients with patent foramen ovale, atrial septal aneurysm or both and cryptogenic stroke or transient ischemic attack. French Study Group on Patent Foramen Ovale and Atrial Septal Aneurysm. Am Heart J 1995; 130:1083–1088.
210. Gagliardi R, Benvenuti L, Frosini F, Ammannati F, Barletta GA, Fantini F. Frequency of echocardiographic abnormalities in patients with ischemia of the carotid territory—a preliminary report. Stroke 1985; 16:118–120.
211. Olsen TS, Skriver EB, Herning M. Cause of cerebral infarction in the carotid territory: its relation to the size and the location of the infarct and to the underlying vascular lesion. Stroke 1985; 16:459–466.
212. Albers GW, Comess KA, DeRook FA, Bracci P, Atwood JE, Bolger A, Hotson J. Transesophageal echocardiographic findings in stroke subtypes. Stroke 1994; 25:232–238.
213. Petersen P, Boysen G, Godtfredsen J, Andersen ED, Anderson B. Placebo-controlled, randomised trial of warfarin and aspirin for prevention of thromboembolic complications in chronic atrial fibrillation. The Copenhagen AFASAK study. Lancet 1989; 1:175–179.
214. The Boston Area Anticoagulation Trial for Atrial Fibrillation Investigators. The effect of low-dose warfarin on the risk of stroke in patients with nonrheumatic atrial fibrillation. N Engl J Med 1990; 323:1505–1511.
215. Stroke Prevention in Atrial Fibrillation Investigators. Warfarin versus aspirin for

prevention of thromboembolism in atrial fibrillation: Stroke Prevention in Atrial Fibrillation II Study. Lancet 1994; 343:687–691.

216. Connolly SJ, Laupacis A, Gent M, Roberts RS, Cairns JA, Joyner C. Canadian Atrial Fibrillation Anticoagulation (CAFA) study. J Am Coll Cardiol 1991; 18: 349–355.

217. Ezekowitz MD, Bridgers SL, James KE, Carlinger NH, Colling CL, Gornick CC, Krause-Steinrauf H, Kurtzke JF, Nazarian SM, Radford MJ. Warfarin in the prevention of stroke associated with nonrheumatic atrial fibrillation. N Engl J Med 1992; 327:1406–1412.

218. The European Atrial Fibrillation Trial Study Group. Optimal oral anticoagulant therapy in patients with nonrheumatic atrial fibrillation and recent cerebral ischemia. N Engl J Med 1995; 333:5–10.

219. Yamaguchi T, for Japanese Nonvalvular Atrial Fibrillation-Embolism Secondary Prevention Cooperative Study Group. Opitimal intensity of warfarin therapy for secondary prevention of stroke in patients with nonvalvular atrial fibrillation. A multicenter, prospective, randomized trial. Stroke 2000; 31:817–821.

220. Poole RM, Chimowitz MI. Cardiac sources of embolism: diagnosis, management and prevention. In: Batjer HH, Caplan RL, Friberg L, Greenlee RG Jr, Kopitnik TA Jr, Young WL, eds. Cerebrovascular Disease. Philadelphia: Lippincott-Raven, 1997, pp 377–383.

221. Hirsh J, Fuster V. Guide to anticoagulant therapy. Part 2. Oral anticoagulation. Circulation 1994; 89:1469–1480.

222. Turpie AG, Gent M, Laupacis A, Latour Y, Gunstensen J, Basile F, Klimek M, Hirsh J. A comparison of aspirin with placebo in patients treated with warfarin after heart-valve replacement. N Engl J Med 1993; 329:524–529.

223. Devuyst G, Bogousslavsky J, Ruchat P, Jeanrenaud X, Despland PA, Regli F, Aebischer N, Karpuz HM, Castillo V, Guffi M, Sadeghi H. Prognosis after stroke followed by surgical closure of patent foramen ovale: a prospective follow-up study with brain MRI and simultaneous transesophageal and transcranial Doppler ultrasound. Neurology 1996; 47:1162–1166.

224. Devuyst G, Bogousslavsky J. Status of patent foramen ovale, atrial septal aneurysm, atrial septal defect and aortic arch atheroma as risk factors for stroke. Neuroepidemiology 1997; 16:217–223.

225. Gandolfo C, Moretti C, Dall Agata D, Primavera A, Brusa G, Loeb C. Long-term prognosis of patients with lacunar syndromes. Acta Neurol Scand 1986; 74:224–229.

226. Arboix A, Marti-Vilalta JL, Garcia JH. Clinical study of 227 patients with lacunar infarcts. Stroke 1990; 21:842–847.

227. Sacco SE, Whisnant JP, Broderick JP, Phillips SJ, O'Fallon WM. Epidemiological characteristics of lacunar infarction in a population. Stroke 1991; 22:1236–1241.

228. Chamorro A, Sacco RL, Mohr JP, Foulkes MA, Kase CS, Tatemichi TK, Wolf PA, Price TR, Hier DB. Clinical-computed tomographic correlations of lacunar infarction in the Stroke Data Bank. Stroke 1991; 22:175–181.

229. Giroud M, Gras P, Milan C, Arveux P, Beuriat P, Vion PH, Dumas R. Histoire naturelle des syndromes lacunaires: apport du registre dijonnais des accidents vasculaires cérébraux. Rev Neurol 1991; 147:566–572.

230. Bogousslavsky J, Regli F, Maeder Ph. Intracranial large-artery disease and "lacunar" infarction. Cerebrovasc Dis 1991; 1:154–159.

231. Bamford J, Sandercock P, Jones L, Warlow C. The natural history of lacunar infarction: the Oxfordshire Community Project. Stroke 1987; 18:554–551.

232. Prencipe M, Culasso F, Rasura M, Anzini A, Beccia M, Cao M, Giubilei F, Fieschi C. Long-term prognosis after a minor stroke. 10-year mortality and major stroke recurrence rates in a Hospital-Based cohort. Stroke 1998; 29:126–132.

233. Samuelsson M, Lindell D, Olsson G-B. Lacunar infarcts a 1-year clinical and MRI follow-up study. Cerebrovasc Dis 1994; 4:265–272.

234. Jørgensen HS, Nakayama H, Reith J, Raaschou HO, Olsen TS. Stroke recurrence: predictors, severity, and prognosis. The Copenhagen Stroke Study. Neurology 1997; 48:891–895.

235. Miyao S, Takano A, Teramoto J, Takahashi A. Leukoaraiosis in relation to prognosis for patients with lacunar infarction. Stroke 1992; 23:1434–1438.

236. Samuelsson M, Soderfeldt B, Olsson GB. Functional outcome in patients with lacunar infarction. Stroke 1996; 27:842–846.

237. Pullicino P, Nelson RF, Kendal BE, Marshall J. Small deep infarcts diagnosed on computed tomography. Neurology 1980; 30:1090–1096.

238. Guika J, Bogousslavsky J, Regli F. Infarcts in the territory of the deep perforators from the carotid system. Neurology 1989; 39:507–512.

239. Horowitz DR, Tuhrim S, Weinberg JM, Rudolph SH. Mechanisms in lacunar infarction. Stroke 1992; 23:325–327.

240. Waterston JA, Brown MM, Butler P, Swash M. Small deep cerebral infarcts associated with occlusive internal carotid artery disease. Arch Neurol 1990; 47:953–957.

241. Mast H, Nüssel F, Vogel H-P, Heinsius T, Dissmann R, Völler H, Marx P. Cranial computerized tomography stroke patterns in patients with cardiac sources of embolism, extracranial large-artery disease or no extracranial source. Cerebrovasc Dis 1994; 4:20–25.

242. Moncayo J, Devuyst G, Van Melle G, Bogousslavsky J. Coexisting causes of ischemic stroke. Arch Neurol 2000, 57:1139–1144.

243. Kapelle LJ, van Latum JC, Algra A, Koudstaal PJ, Van Gijn J. Dutch TIA Trial Study Group. Recurrent stroke after transient ischemic attack or minor ischemic stroke: does the distinction between small and large vessel disease remain true to type?. J Neurol Neurosurg Psychiatry 1995; 59:127–131.

244. Landi G, Cella E, Bocardi E, Mussico M. Lacunar versus non-lacunar infarcts: pathogenetic and prognostic differences. J Neurol Neurosurg Psychiatry 1992; 55: 441–445.

245. Weisberg LA. Lacunar infarcts. Clinical and computed tomographic correlates. Arch Neurol 1982; 39:37–40.

246. Harbinson JW. Ticlopidine versus aspirin for the prevention of recurrent stroke: analysis of patients with minor stroke from the Ticlopidine Aspirin Stroke Study. Stroke 1992; 23:1723–1727.

247. Kannel WB. Hypertension as a risk factor for cardiac events—epidemiologic results of long-term studies. J Cardiovasc Pharmacol 1993; 21(suppl 2):S27–37.

248. Rokey R, Rolak R, Harati T, Kutka N, Verani MS. Coronary artery disease in

patients with cerebrovascular disease: a prospective study. Ann Neurol 1984; 16: 50–53.

249. Di Pasquale GD, Andreoli A, Pinelli G, Grazi P, Manini G, Tognetti F, Testa C. Cerebral ischemic and asymptomatic coronary artery disease: a prospective study of 83 patients. Stroke 1986; 17:1098–1101.

250. Love BB, Grover-Mckay M, Biller J, Rezai K, McKay CR. Coronary artery disease and cardiac events with asymptomatic and symptomatic cerebrovascular disease. Stroke 1992; 23:939–945.

251. O'Leary DH, Polak JF, Kronmal RA, Kittner SJ, Bond MG, Wolfson SK, Bommer W, Price TR, Gardin JM, Savage PJ. Distribution and correlates of sonographically detected carotid artery disease in the Cardiovascular Health Study. Stroke 1992; 23:1752–1760.

252. May DS, Caspar ML, Croft JB, Giles WH. Trends in survival after stroke among Medicare beneficiaries. Stroke 1994; 25:1617–1622.

253. Samsa GP, Bian J, Lipscomb J, Matchar DB. Epidemiology of recurrent cerebral infarction. A Medicare claims-based comparison of first and recurrent stroke on 2-year survival and cost. Stroke 1999; 30:338–349.

254. Caplan LR, Hier DB, D'Cruz I. Cerebral embolism in the Michael Reese Stroke Registry. Stroke 1983; 14:530–536.

255. Bamford J, Sandercock P, Dennis M, Burn J, Warlow C. A prospective study of acute cerebrovascular disease in the community: the Oxfordshire Community Stroke Project—1981–86. 2. Incidence, case fatality rates and overall outcome at one year of cerebral infarction, primary intracerebral and subarachnoid haemorrhage. J Neurol Neurosurg Psychiatry 1990; 53:16–22.

256. Giroud M, Gras P, Chadan N, Beuriat P, Milan C, Arveux P, Dumas R. Cerebral haemorrhage in a French prospective population study. J Neurol Neurosurg Psychiatry 1991; 54:595–598.

257. Moulin Th, Tatu L, Crépin-Leblond Th, Chavot D, Bergès S, Rumbach L. The Besançon Stroke Registry: an acute stroke registry of 2,500 consecutive patients. Eur Neurol 1997; 38:10–20.

258. Tanaka H, Ueda Y, Date C, Baba T, Yamashita H, Hayashi M, Shoji H, Owada K, Baba Kl, Shibuya M, Kon T, Detels R. Incidence of stroke in Shibata, Japan: 1976–1978. Stroke 1981; 12:460–466.

259. Suzuki K, Kutsuzawsa T, Takita K, Ito M, Sakamoto T, Hirayama A, Ito T, Ooishi H, Kawakami K, Hirota K, Ogasawara T, Yoshida J, Tamura T, Hattori S, Iwabuchi S, Karouji Y, Waga T, Oosato Y, Yazaki K, Saito T, Oouchi T, Kojima S. Clinico-epidemiologic study of stroke in Akita Japan. Stroke 1987; 18:402–406.

260. Shi F, Hart RG, Shermann DG, Tegeler CH. Stroke in the People's Republic of China. Stroke 1989; 20:577–582.

261. Yano K, Reed DM, MacLean CJ. Serum cholesterol and hemorrhagic stroke in the Honolulu Heart Program. Stroke 1989; 20:1460–1465.

262. Del Brutto OH, Mosquera A, Sanchez X, Santos J, Noboa CA. Stroke subtypes among Hispanics living in Guayaquil, Ecuador: Results from the Luis Vernaza Hospital Stroke Registry. Stroke 1993; 24:1833–1836.

263. Gonzáles-Duarte A, Cantú C, Ruíz-Sandoval JL, Barinagarrementeria F. Recurrent

primary cerebral hemorrhage. Frequency, mechanisms, and prognosis. Stroke 1998; 29:1802–1805.

264. Douglas MA, Haerer AF. Long-term prognosis of hypertensive intracerebral hemorrhage. Stroke 1982; 3:488–491.

265. Fieschi C, Carolei A, Fiorelli M, Argentino C, Bozzao L, Fazio C, Salvetti M, Bastianello S. Changing prognosis of primary intracerebral hemorrhage: results of a clinical and computed tomographic follow-up study of 104 patients. Stroke 1988; 19:192–195.

266. Trouillat R, Bogousslavsky J, Regli F, Uske A. Hémorragies intracérébrales supratentorielles. Schweiz Med Wochenschr 1990; 120:1056–1063.

267. Passero S, Burgalassi L, D'Andrea P, Battistini N. Recurrence of bleeding in patients with primary intracerebral hemorrhage. Stroke 1995; 26:1189–1192.

268. Neau JP, Ingrand P, Couderq C, Rosier M-P, Bailbe M, Dumas P, Vandermarcq P, Gil R. Recurrent intracerebral hemorrhage. Neurology 1997; 49:106–113.

269. Tuhrim S, Dambrosia JM, Price TR, Mohr JP, Wolf PA, Hier DB, Kase CS. Intracerebral hemorrhage: external validation and extension of a model for prediction of 30-day survival. Ann Neurol 1991; 29:658–663.

270. Schütz H, Bödeker R-H, Damian M, Krack P, Dorndorf W. Age-related spontaneous intracerebral hematoma in a German community. Stroke 1990; 21:1412–1418.

271. Anderson CS, Chakera TM, Stewart-Wynne EG, Jamrozik KD. Spectrum of primary intracerebral hemorrhage in Perth, Western Australia, 1989–90: incidence and outcome. J Neurol Neurosurg Psychiatry 1994; 57:936–940.

272. Dandapani BK, Suzuki S, Kelley RE, Reyes-Iglesias Y, Duncan RC. Relation between blood pressure and outcome in intracerebral hemorrhage. Stroke 1995; 26: 21–24.

273. Hirohata T, Sasaki U, Uozumi T, Ohta M, Shinohara S, Takeda T, Murakami Y, Matsui S, Zenke K, Ueda T. Study on recurrence of hypertensive intracerebral hemorrhage. Neurol Med Chir (Tokyo) 1991; 31:887–891.

274. Chen ST, Chiang CY, Hsu CY, Lee TH, Tang LM. Recurrent hypertensive intracerebral hemorrhage. Acta Neurol Scand 1995; 91:128–132.

275. Lee KS, Bae HG, Yung IG. Recurrent intracerebral hemorrhage due to hypertension. Neurosurgery 1990; 26:586–590.

276. Maruishi M, Shima T, Okada T, Nishida M, Yamane K, Okita S. Clinical findings in patients with recurrent intracerebral hemorrhage. Surg Neurol 1995; 44:444–449.

277. Bae HG, Jeong DS, Doh JW, Lee KS, Yun IG. Recurrence of bleeding in patients with hypertensive intracerebral hemorrhage. Cerebrovasc Dis 1999; 9:102–108.

278. Hill MD, Silver FL, Austin PC, Tu JV. Rate of stroke recurrence in patients with primary intracerebral hemorrhage. Stroke 2000; 31:123–127.

279. Arakawa S, Saku Y, Ibayashi S, Nagao T, Fujishima M. Blood pressure control and recurrence of hypertensive brain hemorrhage. Stroke 1998; 29:1806–1809.

280. Misra UK, Kalita J. Recurrent hypertensive intracerebral hemorrhage. Case report. Am J Med Sci 1995; 310:156–157.

281. Counsell C, Boonyakarnkul S, Dennis M, Sandercock P, Bamford J, Burn J, Warlow C. Primary intracerebral hemorrhage in the Oxfordshire Community Stroke Project. 2. Prognosis. Cerebrovasc Dis 1995; 5:26–34.

282. Boudouresques G, Hauw JJ, Meininger V, Escourolle R, Pertuiset B, Buge A, Lhermitte F, Castaigne P. Etude neuropathologique des hemorrhagies intracraniennes de l'adulte. Rev Neurol 1979; 135:197–210.

283. Ruíz-Sandoval JL, Cantú C, Barrinagarrementeria F. Intracerebral hemorrhage in young people. Analysis of risk factors, location, causes and prognosis. Stroke 1999; 30:537–541.

284. Petitti DB, Wingerd J, Pellegrin F, Ramcharan S. Risk of vascular disease in women: smoking, oral contraceptives, noncontraceptive estrogens, and other factors. JAMA 1979; 242:1150–1154.

285. Stemmerman GN, Hayashi T, Resch JA, et al. Risk factors related to ischemic and hemorrhagic cerebrovascular disease at autopsy: the Honolulu Heart Study. Stroke 1984; 15:23–28.

286. Donahue RP, Abbott RD, Reed DM, Yano K. Alcohol and hemorrhagic stroke: the Honolulu Heart Study. JAMA 1986; 255:2311–2314.

287. Stampfer MJ, Colditz GA, Willett WA, Speizer FE, Hennekens CH. A prospective study of moderate alcohol consumption and the risk of coronary disease and stroke in women. N Engl J Med 1988; 319:267–273.

288. Kase CS. Intracerebral hemorrhage: non-hypertensive causes. Stroke 1986; 17: 590–595.

289. Awada A, Russell N, Al Rajeh S, Omojola M. Non-traumatic cerebral hemorrhage in Saudi Arabs: a hospital-based study of 243 cases. J Neurol Sci 1996; 144:198–203.

290. Gras P, Arveux P, Giroud M, Sautreaux JL, Aube H, Blettery B, Dumas R. Les hémorragies intracérébrales spontanées du sujuet jeune: étude de 33 cas. Rev Neurol 1991; 147:653–657.

291. Cosgrove GR, Leblanc R, Meagher-Villemure K, Ethier R. Cerebral amyloid angiopathy. Neurology 1985; 35:625–631.

292. Jellinger K. Cerebrovascular amyloidosis with cerebral hemorrhage. J Neurol 1977; 214:195–206.

293. Okazaki H, Reegan TH, Campbell RJ. Clinicopathologic studies of primary intracerebral amyloid angiopathy. Mayo Clin Proc 1979; 54:22–31.

294. Kase CS, Vonsattel JP, Richardson EP. Case records of the Massachussets General Hospital (Case 10-1988). N Engl J Med 1988; 318:623–631.

295. Ackerman RH, Richardson EP, Heros RC. Case records of the Massachusetts General Hospital (Case 49-1982). N Engl J Med 1982; 307:1507–1514.

296. Finelli PF, Kessimian N, Bernstein PW. Cerebral amyloid angiopathy manifesting as recurrent intracerebral hemorrhage. Arch Neurol 1984; 41:330–333.

297. Patel DV, Hier DB, Thomas CM, Hemmati M. Intracerebral hemorrhage secondary to cerebral amyloid angiopathy. Radiology 1984; 151:397–400.

298. Gilles C, Brucher JM, Khoubesserian P, Vanderhaeghen JJ. Cerebral amyloid angiopathy as a cause of multiple intracerebral hemorrhages. Neurology 1984; 34:730–735.

299. Roosen N, Martin JJ, De la Porte C, van Vyve M. Intracerebral hemorrhage due to cerebral amyloid angiopathy: case report. J Neurosurg 1985; 63:965–969.

300. Brown RT, Coates RK, Gilbert JJ. Radiographic-pathologic correlation in cerebral amyloid angiopathy. J Can Assoc Radiol 1985; 36:308–311.

301. Hypertension Detection and Follow-Up Program Cooperative Group. Five-year findings of the Hypertension Detection and Follow-Up Program III. Reduction in stroke incidence among persons with high blood pressure. JAMA 1982; 247:633–638.

302. Collins R, Peto R, MacMahon S, Hebert P, Fiebach NH, Eberlein KA, Godwin J, Qizilbash N, Taylor JO. Hennekens CH. Blood pressure, stroke, and coronary heart disease. Part 2. Short-term reductions in blood pressure: overview of randomised drug trials in their epidemiological context. Lancet 1990; 335:827–838.

303. SHEP Cooperative Research Group. Prevention of stroke by antihipertensive drug treatment in older persons with isolated systolic hypertension: final results of the Systolic Hypertension in the Elderly Program (SHEP). JAMA 1991; 265:3255–3264.

304. Staessen JA, Fagard R, Thijs L, Celis H, Arabidze GG, Birkenhager WH, Bulpitt CJ, de Leeuw PW, Dollery CT. Fletcher AE, Forette F, Leonetti G, Nachev C, O'Brien ET, Rosenfeld J, Rodiccio JL, Tuomilehto J, Zanchetti A. Randomized double-blind comparison of placebo and active treatment for older patients with isolated systolic hypertension: the Systolic Hypertension in Europe (Sys-Eur) Trial Investigators. Lancet 1997; 350:757–764.

305. Lièvre M, Leizorovicz A. Treatment of high blood pressure in patients aged over 60 years: lessons from randomized clinical trials. Cardiol Elderly 1995; 3:217–222.

306. Carter AB. Hypotensive therapy in stroke survivors. Lancet 1970; 1:485–489.

307. Hypertension Stroke Co-operative Study Group. Effect of antihypertensive treatment on stroke recurrence. JAMA 1974; 229:409–418.

308. Eriksson S, Olofsson BO, Wester PO for the TEST Study Group. Atenolol in secondary prevention of stroke. Cerebrovasc Dis 1995; 5:21–25.

309. Gueyffier F, Boutitie F, Boissel JP, Coope J, Cutler J, Ekbom T, Fagard R, Friedman L, Perry HM, Pocock S, Prineas R, Schron E. INDANA: a meta-analysis on individual patient data in hypertension. Protocol and preliminary results. Thérapie 1995; 50:353–362

310. PATS Collaborating Group. Post-stroke Antihypertensive Treatment Study. A preliminary result. Chin Med J 1995; 108:710–717.

311. The INDANA (INdividual Data ANalysis of Antihypertensive intervention trials) Project Collaborators. Gueyffier F, Boissel JP, Boutitie F, Pocock S, Coope J, Cutler J, Ekbom T, Fagard R, Friedman L, Kerlikowske K, Perry M, Prineas R, Schron E. Effect of antihypertensive treatment in patients having already suffered from stroke. Gathering the evidence. Stroke 1997; 28:2557–2562.

312. Greenberg SM, Vonsattel JP, Segal AZ, Chiu RI, Clatworthy AE, Liao A, Hyman BT, Rebeck GW. Association of apolipoprotein E E2 and vasculopathy in cerebral amyloid angiopathy. Neurology 1998; 50:961–965.

5
Mortality in Patients with Stroke

Philip A. Wolf
Boston University School of Medicine, Boston, Massachusetts

I. INTRODUCTION

The diagnostic category *stroke*, defined as brain injury resulting from disease of
the blood vessels, is obviously a heterogeneous group with different pathological
bases and varying clinical outcomes. In general, prognosis, including mortality,
after stroke is largely determined by the mechanissm or type of stroke. Hemorrhage is considerably more likely to be lethal than infarction; however, even
within these two major categories, mortality is related to the specific stroke subtype. Stroke mortality is generally divided into *acute*, usually within 30 days
following stroke—the 30-day case fatality rate (CFR), and *long-term*, 1–5 years
poststroke. Factors mediating acute mortality are generally a reflection of the
severity of the initial insult while age and comorbid disease play a greater role
in late deaths. Vital statistics, usually based on death certificate data, often lack
the specificity to distinguish hemorrhage from ischemic stroke. Clinical series of
well-studied stroke patients generally achieve this distinction with ease provided
a computed tomography scan of the brain (CT-brain) is made soon after stroke
onset.

It is usually possible to separate hemorrhage and ischemic stroke subtypes
into distinct pathophysiological categories. In these studies, the severity of the
deficit, recurrence rates, and mortality are closely related to the specific stroke
subtype. For hemorrhage, the clinical features as well as the outcomes differ
in patients with subarachnoid hemorrhage from aneurysm and those with intracerebral hemorrhage resulting from hypertensive arteriolar disease. Other, less
common varieties include intraparenchymatous bleeding from vascular malformations, amyloid angiopathy, and bleeding diatheses. Among ischemic stroke

subtypes, lacunar infarcts have the lowest CFR, infarction secondary to large-artery atherothrombosis or occlusion is next, and cerebral embolism from a cardiac source has the highest CFR. Thus, the 30-day CFR reflects the severity of the acute stroke insult and modifying factors including comorbidity. Death usually results from mass effect or from complications (aspiration, urinary sepsis, pulmonary embolism) following the acute stroke. Late (1–5 year) mortality, on the other hand, is more often due to recurrent stroke or other coexisting diseases, particularly cardiac diseases. In addition, specific stroke types, e.g., cardiogenic embolism in persons with atrial fibrillation (AF), are more likely to have a stroke recurrence during the 30 days following initial stroke. Survivors of the acute stroke have considerably greater risk of stroke recurrence during the subsequent months and years.

II. GEOGRAPHIC VARIATION IN STROKE MORTALITY

Death rates for stroke vary widely in different geographic locales probably reflecting powerful environmental influences (Fig. 1). Death rates are highest in Asia and Eastern Europe presumably reflecting the influence of poverty, poor sanitation and nutrition, and suboptimal health practices. These wide variations in death rates, presumably an indication of variations in stroke incidence, reflect the considerable importance of environmental factors on stroke occurrence. However, even within the United States, the geographic distribution of stroke deaths varies from 20–24 deaths/100,000 population in the Southwest to 29–42/100,000

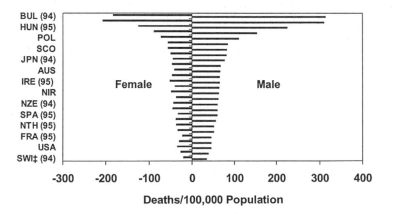

Fig. 1   Age-adjusted death rates for stroke by country and sex, age 35–74, 1996. (From: National Institutes of Health: Morbidity and Mortality: 1996 Chartbook on Cardiovascular, Lung, and Blood Diseases. Bethesda, MD: NIH, 1996.)

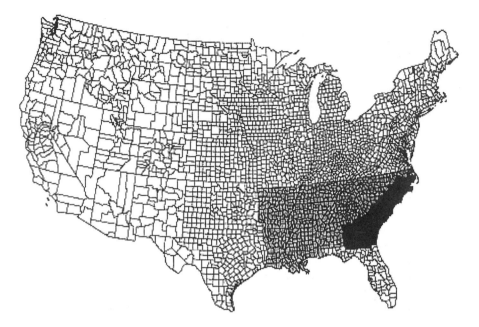

Fig. 2 The stroke belt. Map of U.S. countries showing the stroke buckle (dark shading), stroke belt (light shading), and the remainder of the United States (not shaded). Note that Alaska and Hawaii are included in the remainder of the United States but are not shown in the map. (From: Evaluation of Social Status as a Contributing Factor to the Stroke Belt Region of the United States, George Howard, DrPH; Roger Anderson, PhD; Norman J. Johnson, PhD; Paul Sorlie, PhD; Gregory Russell, MS; Virginia J. Howard, MSPH. Stroke 1997; 28:936–940.)

population in the Southeast, a region designated the *stroke belt* (Fig. 2). These high death rates from stroke in the coastal plains of North and South Carolina and Georgia occur in whites as well as African-Americans, and in both sexes. The basis for these geographic variations generally and for the 40% excess in stroke deaths in the stroke belt remains unexplained (1,2).

III. SECULAR TRENDS IN STROKE MORTALITY

During the past three decades, total stroke mortality rates have fallen more than 60% (figure from ASA). This decline has occurred in both men and women, in whites and nonwhites, throughout North America, Japan, Western Europe, and in most industrialized nations (3). These declines in deaths have taken place in the absence of clear or uniform evidence of a decline in overall stroke *incidence* and may reflect improved survival either from better medical management or as a reflection of decreased stroke *severity*. In turn, the apparent reduction in stroke severity may be a result of a decrease in the proportion of strokes due to large *intracerebral hemorrhages* (IH) or from an overall reduction in *severity* of strokes, both infarcts and hemorrhages. Regarding the change in the "case mix," there clearly appears to be a smaller proportion of stroke secondary to *fatal* IH. This apparent diminution in IH may reflect the routine use of CT or MRI imaging and the attendant capacity to detect smaller and less lethal hemorrhages (4). In addition, declining *incidence* of IH has been noted for more than 30 years (5,6). In a recent report from the Canadian Collaborative Study Group of Stroke Hospitalizations, a decline in 30-day CFR for cerebral infarction was noted. There was an even greater decline in 30-day CFR for intracerebral hemorrhage during the two time periods 1982–1983 and 1991–1992 (7) (Table 1). The analyses were based on large numbers: a total of 335,283 discharges for stroke over the 10-year period (309,631 cerebral infarctions and 25,652 intracerebral hemorrhages) from Canada's 10 provinces. The age-specific decline in 30-day CFR varied from 11% following cerebral infarction for men and women aged 15–54 and ≥85 years with a fall of 23% for the age group 65–74. For intracerebral hemorrhage, even more striking declines in 30-day CFR were seen. Decreases were three- to fourfold greater than for cerebral infarction and ranged from 38% to 51% (7).

Table 1 Age-Specific, 30-Day, In-Hospital Case-Fatality Rates in Canada in 1982–1983 and 1991–1992 and Estimated Change[a] over This Period (Rate, %)

Age group, years	1982–1983	1991–1992	% Change (95% CI)
Cerebral infarction			
15–54	5.5	6.9	−11 (−28 to 11)
55–64	9.7	7.5	−17 (−27 to −7)
65–74	13.2	11.3	−23 (−28 to −17)
75–84	19.6	16.3	−18 (−22 to −13)
≥85	29.8	27.3	−11 (−17 to −5)
Intracerebral hemorrhage			
15–54	36.2	29.3	−46 (−56 to −33)
55–64	55.5	37.1	−40 (−51 to −26)
65–74	48.8	40.9	−38 (−48 to −27)
75–84	65.7	44.7	−51 (−59 to −41)
≥85	71.9	58.8	−48 (−62 to −28)

[a] Sex-adjusted; excludes data from British Columbia (1982) and Alberta (1989, 1990, and 1991). From Mayo N, Neville D, Kirkland S, Ostbye T, Mustard CA, Reeder B, Joffres M, Brauer G, Levy AR. Hospitalization and case-fatality rates for stroke in Canada from 1982 through 1991. Stroke 1996; 27:1215–1220.

This improvement in survival following acute stroke is quite remarkable particularly since there was no specific therapeutic tool or strategy for treatment of stroke during the decade under study. Unfortunately, no revolutionary therapy exists even now.

A. Intracerebral Hemorrhage

In rural Japan during the years following World War II, massive intraparenchymatous hemorrhage accounted for a large proportion of stroke. This was attributed to high-salt, low-animal-protein and low-fat diet, and high levels of uncontrolled hypertension (8–10). Improvements in nutrition, sanitation, and public health generally have been associated with a marked decline in IH incidence and mortality.

B. Subarachnoid Hemorrhage

Recent data from New Zealand continue to show a decline in mortality and suggest a decline in incidence rates of SH (11). However, no change in CFRs was seen despite substantial improvements in critical care during the past 20 years (11,12). By contrast, in the Rochester, Minnesota, population, 30-day survival was 71% during 1985–1994, compared with 40% for 1955–1964 (p = 0.006) (13). Previous analyses disclosed no change in incidence but this most recent time period showed a trend toward a reduction in incidence in the most recent 10-year period (12,14).

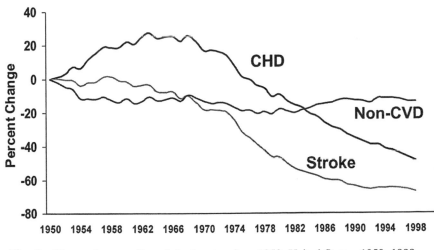

Fig. 3   Change in age-adjusted death rates since 1950, United States, 1950–1998.

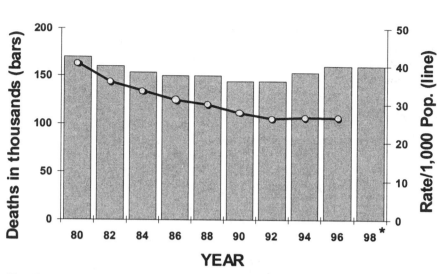

*Preliminary

Fig. 4 Mortality from stroke in the United States, 1980–1998. (Data from: Vital Statistics of U.S., NCHS.)

C. Ischemic Stroke

Since 1960 death rates for stroke have declined more than 60% (Fig. 3). Evidence for a decreased incidence is scanty while improved survival has been documented in many studies (7,11,15–19). As noted previously, the decline in severity of hospitalized stroke patients and the improved detection of smaller, milder strokes by modern techniques are both probable contributors to this pattern. The decline in stroke mortality seems to have reached a plateau with rates leveling off in the 1990s (20) (Fig. 4). With an increasing proportion of the population surviving to ages where stroke incidence is high, it is quite likely stroke will continue to grow as a cause of death in the years to come.

IV. ACUTE MORTALITY FOLLOWING STROKE

A. Hemorrhage

1. Subarachnoid Hemorrhage (SAH)

Aneurysm rupture accounts for most cases of subarachnoid hemorrhage. The 28-day (or 30-day) CFRs do not increase with increasing age below 65 years since the severity of the brain injury (as attested to by the presence of coma or diminished level of consciousness) rather than comorbid diseases is determinative. However, SAH in persons above age 65 years is higher and approaches 80% (11). Overall, 28-day CFR ranges from 25% to 55% (11,15,22–24). In Framingham, CFR with coma at onset of hemorrhage was 83% (21). For those with focal deficits CFR was 56% and in persons free of coma or focal deficits it was 13% (21). A clear correlation to the Hunt and Hess Grade of Glascow Coma Scale (GCS) has also been noted. In Rochester, Minnesota, the 30-day CFR ranged from 30% in Grade 1–2 patients (asymptomatic but for headache, neck rigidity, and no focal deficit but for cranial nerve palsy), 65% in Grade 3 (drowsy, confused, or mild focal neurological deficit), to 85% in Grade 4–5 (stupor to coma, moderate to severe hemiparesis, decerebrate rigidity) (12). Rebleeding risk may be as high as 50% in the 60 days following the initial hemorrhage and carries additional risk of mortality (12).

2. Intracerebral Hemorrhage

Spontaneous bleeding into the brain, commonly referred to as "hypertensive" intracerebral hemorrhage (ICH), has the highest 30-day CFR of all stroke subtypes. These deep hemorrhages, principally a consequence of uncontrolled hypertension, commonly occur in specific sites: basal ganglia, thalamus, cerebellum, or pons. The other principal type, *lobar* hemorrhage, largely due to amyloid angioplasty, is becoming more prevalent with the aging of the population. In the pre-CT era, where decrease in level of consciousness was a key indicator leading to the ICH diagnosis, the 30-day CFR was approximately 90% (21,25). In modern CT-based studies, CFR ranges from a mean of 35% for hospital-based studies to 48% in community-based studies. Most of these studies occur within 2 days of onset and are the direct result of the brain injury by the expanding hematoma. Volume of hemorrhage, pulse pressure, and level of consciousness as assessed by means of the GCS measured on admission were the key indicators of outcome in the NINDS Stroke Data Bank series (26). Thirty-day survival was far greater and reached 98% in patients with smaller hematomas (small), GCS $\geq$ 9, and pulse pressure $\leq$ 40 mmHg. By contrast, when the hematoma was *large*, the GCS $\leq$ 8, and the pulse pressure $>$ 65 mmHg, survival at 30 days was 8%. This estimation of acute survival was based on an algorithm derived from 94 systemically studied acute intracerebral hemorrhages in the Stroke Data Bank (27). Much of the improvement in 30-day CFR in recent years is more likely due to improved detection of smaller, less lethal, hemorrhages by means of imaging than from specific improvement in the treatment of patients with ICH (25).

3. Cerebral Infarction

Ischemic infarction accounts for approximately 85% of all stroke events with hemorrhage making up the balance. Using data obtained from communities or

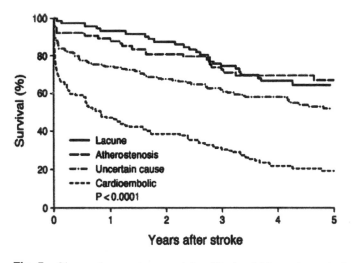

Fig. 5 Observed percentage surviving (Kaplan-Meier estimates) after incident ischemic stroke among 442 residents of Rochester, Minnesota, 1985–1989, with common ischemic stroke subtypes. (From Ref. 35.)

general population samples, a less distorted picture is obtained than from hospital or referral-based data. In Rochester, Minnesota, the overall 30-day CFR for cerebral infarction was 13.9% (20). In the Framingham Study, 30-day CFR following atherothrombotic brain infarction was 15%. A recent report from Rochester, Minnesota, population, for the years 1985–1989, disclosed wide variation in 30-day CFR depending upon the specific ischemic stroke subtype (20). Case-fatality rates at 30 days ranged from 1.4% following lacunar infarction, to 8.1% following stroke related to large artery stenosis, to 14.0% for infarct of uncertain cause, to 30.3% following cardioembolic stroke (Fig. 5). Similarly, acute mortality from cardioembolic stroke, particularly in subjects with atrial fibrillation, was four times greater than in patients with stroke due to large artery atherosclerosis (20). Increasing age, stroke severity, and congestive heart failure also had an adverse influence on 30-day CFR. Similarly, in the Framingham study, among ischemic strokes, the 30-day CFR of 25% was greatest for cardioembolic stroke in persons with atrial fibrillation (28). Uniformly, lacunar infarction has an extremely low 30-day CFR; in the Rochester, Minnesota, study it was 1.4% (20).

B. Late Mortality

1. Hemorrhage

There are few reports of long-term outcome, including recurrence, among survivors of major intracerebral hemorrhage secondary to hypertensive small vessel disease. Following rupture of an aneurysm arising from the circle of Willis, recurrence of subarachnoid hemorrhage is common, often within days or weeks of the initial bleed, and contributes to acute and subacute mortality from the condition. Owing to the high acute mortality, follow-up data are sparse.

2. Lobar Hemorrhage

Cerebral amyloid angioplasty is thought to underlie lobar intracerebral hemorrhage in the elderly—usually above the age of 60 years—and accounts for approximately one-third of all cases of intracerebral hemorrhage (29). Lobar hemorrhage is less likely to be fatal than the "hypertensive" variety and has a tendency to recur (30). Recurrence, in fact, is one of the hallmarks of this condition, occurring in 19 of 71 lobar hemorrhage survivors, a cumulative rate of recurrence of 21% during a mean follow-up period of 23.9 ± 14.8 months (31). Recurrence appears to be related to apolipoprotein E genotype with either the ε2 or ε4 allele predisposing to recurrent hemorrhage (31). Cerebral amyloid angiopathy is thought to be more frequent in persons with memory loss and these congophilic changes in the walls of cerebral arteries are often present in Alzheimer's disease brains. With an increasing population of elderly it is likely this variety of cerebral hemorrhage and recurrent hemorrhage will account for increasing morbidity and mortality from stroke.

3. Cerebral Infarction

While ischemic stroke subtype is strongly related to 30-day CFR and stroke severity, 1- and 5-year mortality is more often related to age and comorbid disease. Rates vary widely by the age of the population, calendar year, and between different case series in different geographic settings. During the 30-year period between 1955–1959 and 1985–1989 1-year survival following cerebral infarction rose from 75% to 79% for men (mean age 68 and 70 years, respectively) and from 62% to 64% for women (mean age 74 and 79 years, respectively). However, a Cox proportional hazards model showed 1-year survival to be strongly dependent upon age and calendar year (both $p < 0.0001$). The gender difference was no longer significant after this statistical analysis took the older ages of the women in the population into account (32). Extensive physical and lifestyle data were available on the participants of the Cardiovascular Health Study of 5201 men and women, aged 65–84 years at entry. After 7 years of follow-up there was a total of 455 *incident* strokes, 101 of which were fatal. As noted in other studies, hemorrhage was more likely to be lethal than infarction and cardiogenic embolism more deadly than other ischemic stroke subtypes. However, no specific analyses of determinants of late mortality (as compared with 30-day CFR) were reported. In all, 11% of persons with incident ischemic stroke died during the follow-up period. Of those subjects with incident strokes who died, 51.3% died of stroke. These stroke deaths were attributed to either the index event, late effects of the stroke, or a recurrent stroke event. Only 16.2% died of coronary heart disease and 4.6% from other atherosclerotic or cardiovascular diseases. Independent determinants of fatality were: age; stroke type (hemorrhage vs. ischemic stroke); taking longer to perform a timed walk prior to stroke onset. Other variables analyzed that did not reach statistical significance were: stroke location, gender, race, education, smoking status, alcohol use, income, clinic site, blocks walked in the previous week, previous transient ischemic attack, previous myocardial infarction, previous angina pectoris, previous congestive heart failure, previous atrial fibrillation, self-reported diabetes, self-reported hypertension, use of aspirin two or more times in the last 2 weeks, use of any antihypertensive medication, use of any diuretic, height, weight in quartiles, systolic and diastolic blood pressure as continuous variables and in quartiles, kcal expended per week, grip strength, modified Mini-Mental State Examination score, Digit Symbol Substitution score, depression score, Activities of Daily Living, Instrumental Activities of Daily Living, potassium, creatinine, hematocrit, factor VII, fibrinogen, C-reactive protein, forced expiratory volume in 1 sec, forced vital capacity, maximum wall thickness of internal carotid artery, maximum wall thickness of common carotid artery, and procedure-related stroke (33). Small case series report, in addition to age and initial stroke severity, that congestive heart failure and diabetes (or elevated blood sugar at the time of stroke) are significant factors in long-term mortality (34).

REFERENCES

1. Howard G, Anderson R, Johnson NJ, Sorlie P, Russell G, Howard VJ. Evaluation of social status as a contributing factor to the stroke belt region of the United States. Stroke 1997; 28(5):936–940.
2. Howard G, Evans GW, Pearce K, Howard VJ, Bell RA, Mayer EJ, Burke GL. Is the stroke belt disappearing? An analysis of racial, temporal, and age effects. Stroke 1995; 26:1153–1158.
3. Thom TJ. Stroke mortality trends. An international perspective. Ann Epidemiol 1993; 3:509–518.
4. Garraway WM, Whisnant JP, Drury I. The changing pattern of survival following stroke. Stroke 1983; 14:699–703.
5. Aurell M, Hood B. Cerebral hemorrhage in a population after a decade of active antihypertensive treatment. Acta Med Scand 1964; 176:377–383.
6. Shimamoto T, Komachi Y, Inada H, Doi M, Iso H, Sato S, Kitamura A, Iida M, Konishi M, Nakanishi N. Trends for coronary heart disease and stroke and their risk factors in Japan. Circulation 1989; 79:503–515.
7. Mayo NE, Neville D, Kirkland S, Ostbye T, Mustard CA, Reeder B, Joffres M, Brauer G, Levy AR. Hospitalization and case-fatality rates for stroke in Canada from 1982 through 1991. The Canadian Collaborative Study Group of Stroke Hospitalizations. Stroke 1996; 27(7):1215–1220.

8. Ueda K, Omae T, Hiroda Y, Takeshita M, Katsuki S, Tanaka K, Enjoji M. Decreasing trend in incidence and mortality from stroke in Hisayama residents, Japan. Stroke 1981; 12:154–160.

9. Ueda K, Hasuo Y, Kiyohara Y, Wada J, Kawano H, Kato I, Fujii I, Yanai T, Omae T, Fujishima M. Intracerebral hemorrhage in a Japanese community. Hisayama: incidence, changing pattern during long-term follow-up, and related factors. Stroke 1988; 19:48–52.

10. Tanaka H, Ueda Y, Hayashi M, Date C, Baba T, Yamashita H, Shoji H, Tanaka Y, Owada K, Detels R. Risk factors for cerebral hemorrhage and cerebral infarction in a Japanese rural community. Stroke 1982; 13:62–73.

11. Truelsen T, Bonita R, Duncan J, Anderson NE, Mee E. Changes in subarachnoid hemorrhage mortality, incidence, and case fatality in New Zealand between 1981–1983 and 1991–1993. Stroke 1998; 29(11):2298–2303.

12. Phillips LH, Whisnant JP, O'Fallon WM, Sundt TM, Jr. The unchanging pattern of subarachnoid hemorrhage in a community. Neurology 1980; 30:1034–1040.

13. Brown RD, Whisnant JP, Sicks J, O'Fallon WM, Petty GW, Wiebers, DO. Subarachnoid hemorrhage and intracerebral hemorrhage: trends in incidence and survival in a population-based study. Neurology 2001; 56(Suppl 3):A86–A87.

14. Ingall TJ, Whisnant JP, Wiebers DO, OFallon WM. Has there been a decline in subarachnoid hemorrhoid mortality? Stroke 1989; 20:718–724.

15. Kolominsky-Rabas PL, Sarti C, Heuschmann PU, Graf C, Siemonsen S, Neundoerfer B, Katalinic A, Lang E, Gassmann KG, von Stockert TR. A prospective community-based study of stroke in Germany—the Erlangen Sroke Project (ESPro): incidence and case fatality at 1, 3, and 12 months. Stroke 1998; 29(12):2501–2506.

16. McGovern PG, Burke GL, Sprafka JM, Xue S, Folsom AR, Blackburn H. Trends in mortality, morbidity, and risk factor levels for stroke from 1960 through 1990. The Minnesota Heart Survey. JAMA 1992; 268(6):753–759.

17. Chang CC, Chen CJ. Secular trend of mortality from cerebral infarction and cerebral hemorrhage in Taiwan, 1974–1988. Stroke 1993; 24(2):212–218.

18. Howard G, Craven TE, Sanders L, Evans GW. Relationship of hospitalized stroke rate and in-hospital mortality to the decline in US stroke mortality. Neuroepidemiology 1991; 10(5–6):251–259.

19. Bonita R, Beaglehole R. The enigma of the decline in stroke deaths in the United States: the search for an explanation. Stroke 1996; 27(3):370–372.

20. Petty GW, Brown RD, Jr., Whisnant JP, Sicks JD, O'Fallon WM, Wiebers DO. Survival and recurrence after first cerebral infarction: a population-based study in Rochester, Minnesota, 1975 through 1989. Neurology 1998; 50(1):208–216.

21. Sacco RL, Wolf PA, Bharucha NE, Meeks SL, Kannel WB, Charette LJ, McNamara PM, Palmer EP, D'Agostino R. Subarachnoid and intracerebral hemorrhage: natural history, prognosis, and precursive factors in the Framingham Study. Neurology 1984; 34:847–854.

22. Anderson CS, Jamrozik KD, Broadhurst RJ, Stewart-Wynne EG. Predicting survival for 1 year among different subtypes of stroke. Results from the Perth Community Stroke Study. Stroke 1994; 25(10):1935–1944.

23. Bamford J, Sandercock P, Dennis M, Burn J, Warlow C. A prospective study of acute cerebrovascular disease in the community: the Oxfordshire Community Stroke

Project—1981–86. 2. Incidence, case fatality rates and overall outcome at one year of cerebral infarction, primary intracerebral and subarachnoid haemorrhage. J Neurol Neurosurg Psychiatry 1990; 53(1):16–22.

24. Giroud M, Milan C, Beuriat P, Gras P, Essayagh E, Arveux P, Dumas R. Incidence and survival rates during a two-year period of intracerebral and subarachnoid haemorrhages, cortical infarcts, lacunes and transient ischaemic attacks. The Stroke Registry of Dijon: 1985–1989. Int J Epidemiol 1991; 20(4):892–899.

25. Drury I, Whisnant JP, Garraway WM. Primary intracerebral hemorrhage: impact of CT on incidence. Neurology 1984; 34:653–657.

26. Tuhrim S, Dambrosia JM, Price TR, Mohr JP, Wolf PA, Heyman A, Kase CS. Prediction of intracerebral hemorrhage survival. Ann Neurol 1988; 24:258–263.

27. Tuhrim S, Dambrosia JM, Price TR, Mohr JP, Wolf PA, Hier DB, Kase CS. Intracerebral hemorrhage: external validation and extension of a model for prediction of 30-day survival. Ann Neurol 1991; 29:658–663.

28. Lin HJ, Wolf PA, Kelly-Hayes M, Beiser AS, Kase CS, Benjamin EJ, D'Agostino RB. Stroke severity in atrial fibrillation: the Framingham Study. Stroke 1996; 27(1): 1760–1764.

29. Sacco RL. Lobar intracerebral hemorrhage. N Engl J Med 2000; 342(4):276–279.

30. Vinters HV. Cerebral amyloid angiopathy. In: HJM barnett, JP Mohr, BM Stein, FM Yatsu, editors. Stroke: Pathophysiology, Diagnosis, and Management. Philadelphia: Churchill Livingstone, 1998, pp 945–962.

31. O'Donnell HC, Rosand J, Knudsen KA, Furie KL, Segal AZ, Chiu RI, Ikeda D, Greenberg SM. Apolipoprotein E genotype and the risk of recurrent lobar intracerebral hemorrhage. N Engl J Med 2000; 342(4):240–245.

32. Brown RD, Jr., Petty GW, O'Fallon WM, Wiebers DO, Whisnant JP. Incidence of transient ischemic attack in Rochester, Minnesota, 1985–1989. Stroke 1998; 29(10): 2109–2113.

33. Longstreth WT, Jr., Bernick C, Fitzpatrick A, Cushman M, Knepper L, Lima J, Furberg CD. Frequency and predictors of stroke death in 5,888 participants in the Cardiovascular Health Study. Neurology 2001; 56(3):368–375.

34. Sacco RL, Shi T, Zamanillo MC, Kargman DE. Predictors of mortality and recurrence after hospitalized cerebral infarction in an urban community: the Northern Manhattan Stroke Study. Neurology 1994; 44:626–634.

35. Petty GW, Brown RD, Whisnant JP, Sicks JD, O'Fallon WM, Wiebers DO. Ischemic Stroke Subtypes. A Population-based Study of Functional Outcome, Survival, and Recurrence. Stroke 2000; 31:1062–1069.

6

Motor Dysfunction and Recovery

Rüdiger J. Seitz and Hans-Joachim Freund
University Hospital Düsseldorf, Düsseldorf, Germany

Ferdinand Binkofski
University Hospital Lübeck, Lübeck, Germany

I. INTRODUCTION

The challenging aspect in each stroke patient is the question to what degree he or she will recover from his or her neurological deficit. Studies on large clinical cohorts showed that approximately half of the patients with completed stroke have persistent hemiparesis (1). Most recovery occurs during the first weeks following stroke (2,3). Stroke can interfere with virtually every single capacity of the human brain. The resulting deficits can either be assessed in global terms such as the disability level of daily activities or scored for specific neurological impairments (4). The adequate assessment of the functional state has become increasingly important, as the correlation with the tissue perfusion state and with the recruitment of perilesional areas during functional activation provides the ground for evaluation of the efficacy of new therapeutic interventions that have recently come into clinical use. Since most of the recovery takes place early after stroke, a major question regarding the underlying mechanisms is how far the restoration of tissue function contributes to the reorganization of the remaining network.

These processes will be discussed in this chapter with reference to the clinical predictors, lesion patterns, electrophysiological data, and evidence from neuroimaging.

II. CLINICAL PREDICTORS

The severity and resolution of hemiparesis after brain infarction vary between patients. This variability has turned out to be one of the major problems of assessing stroke recovery (5). Many patients experience transient deficits that disappear within 24 hr (6) or suffer from slight or moderate hemiparesis that regresses completely within a couple of days (2,7). Of the patients with severe completed stroke approximately 50% recover from hemiparesis (1,8). In most of these patients recovery takes place within 4 weeks after infarction usually starting with shoulder and synergistic arm-hand movements (2,3,9). In subcortical infarctions, functional restoration may be slower, continuing over several years (10,11). This suggests that a variety of mechanisms are involved in the restoration of executive functions after brain infarction. Also, hitherto-undetected white matter changes and the large prevalence of silent stroke lesions in patients presenting with the clinical symptoms of acute infarction affect the cognitive and attentional state of the patients and their capacity to recover (12–14).

In a prospective study of patients admitted to our neurology service we found that patients with hemiparetic stroke fell into three groups, when a score designed to measure motor impairment, including paresis, apraxia, and motor neglect, was applied (15). Patients could be assigned to these three groups on the basis of their different degree of motor recovery (Fig. 1). Patients were separated by a critical score value defining a group with a severe acute motor deficit and poor recovery, another group with a severe initial deficit and moderate to good recovery, and a third group with a slight initial deficit and excellent recovery. Patients with a score value below 16 recovered completely within 4 weeks, while more severely affected patients showed a protracted recovery course.

These results imply that postlesional recovery is strongly influenced by a critical residual spared function that appears to determine whether a given system can undergo recovery or not. Furthermore, these data accord with multivariate analyses indicating that the severity of the initial motor deficit and clinical state after 1 week are reliable predictors for stroke outcome (16,17). Prolonged flaccidity of the affected half of the body after stroke has been found to indicate poor motor recovery (18–20). Furthermore, younger age allows for better functional recovery than advanced age (16,20–22). Nevertheless, young stroke victims face an increased mortality risk compared with the general population as found by a prospective follow-up over 8 years (23).

The differences in functional restoration among patients make it likely that apart from the cortical output system, feedback provided by the use of a partly compromised limb may play a major role for the reshaping of the remaining circuits. This is best illustrated by the inability of deafferented patients to learn new movement patterns. The situation in a paralyzed limb is similar, because the lack of active limb use precludes any motor-related feedback (24). The hypothesis that a critical minimum of residual executive capacity is a necessary condition for tuning the remaining network into function holds promise for new approaches to rehabilitative strategies (25,26). Feedback can even be provided by the visual domain. For example, visual neglect compromises recovery from hemiparesis

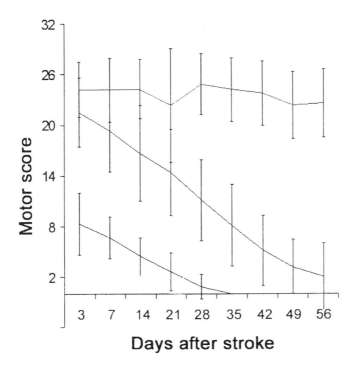

Fig. 1 Analysis of poststroke recovery shows three different groups irrespective of cortical and subcortical lesion location. Less severely affected patients with initial motor scores below 16 recovered within 30 days ($n = 17$). Severely affected patients with initial motor scores greater than 16 showed negligible recovery ($n = 19$) or recovered well in a longer time course ($n = 16$). (From Ref. 46.)

(20,27). Conversely, neuroimaging data provided evidence that patients who have recovered from hemiparesis employ the visual system in relation to the execution of finger movements (28).

Epidemiological studies showed that early physiotherapy and patient mobilization after stroke is beneficial (29). It is unclear at present how these data obtained in humans can be reconciled with observations in animal experiments showing that training during the first days aggravates postischemic brain lesions (30,31). In the early chronic phase, the intensity of repetitive training has been shown to fascilitate motor recovery (32–35). Even rhythmic movement fascilitation as well as robot training appear to be beneficial for motor recovery (36–38). Repetitive training and voluntary contraction of affected muscles fascilitate motor cortical activity as shown by transcranial magnetic stimulation (37,39). These data correspond to evidence from animal experiments showing an enlarge-

ment of the motor cortical representation in monkeys that were subjected to rehabilitative training after experimental stroke in motor cortex (Fig. 2). Furthermore,
it was shown by functional neuroimaging that the supplementary motor area that
plays a prominent role in movement initiation is activated in patients who have
recovered from hemiparetic infarction in the area of the middle cerebral artery
(40,41).

Apart from the affected side, also the body half ipsilateral to the brain
infarction is compromised after brain infarction. In the acute stage after hemiplegic stroke the ipsilesional arm moves less and can exert only reduced grip force
(42). However, even at a chronic stage ipsilateral deficits in fine motor control
have been shown to persist (43). This may be related to simultaneous affection

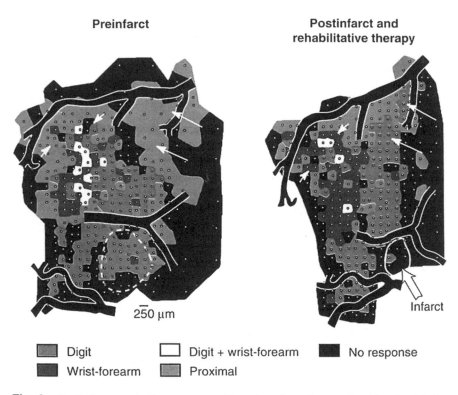

Fig. 2 Cortical reorganization as assessed by microelectrode mapping after focal ischemic lesion (dashed circle) in the monkey motor cortex. The long white arrows show the
expansion of the partially lesioned digit representation into the adjacent cortical representation of the proximal arm following some 4 weeks of dedicated rehabilitative training. Note
also, the expanded wrist-forearm representation (short white arrows). (From Ref. 145.)

of ispilateral corticospinal projections (44,45), or to transcallosal diaschisis (28). Moreover, left-hemisphere damage resulting in apraxia induces bilateral long-standing deficits in hand use (46–48).

III. LESION SIZE AND LOCATION

Lesion volume of infarction does not predict recovery except for very large lesions that do not allow for recovery (49–51). Accordingly, the motor score and lesion size were not correlated (Fig. 3). In contrast, lesion location within the affected hemisphere as well as in right versus left hemisphere as assessed with CT or MRI is an important determinant for recovery (47,52–54). Measurements of cerebral oxygen extraction (50) and diffusion weighted MR imaging (55–58)

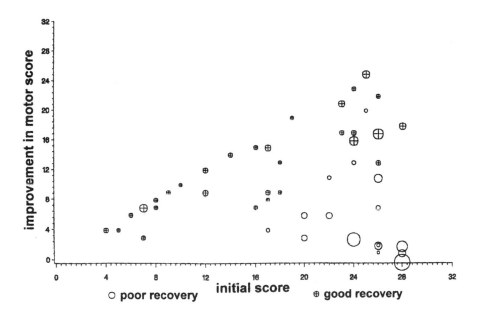

Fig. 3 The relation of postischemic recovery and stroke lesion volume for the individual patients shown in Fig. 1. Note that the improvement in motor score approximates the initial impairment in the majority of patients. Some patients with more severe initial hemiparesis and score values greater than 16 did not recover irrespective of lesion volume. While the smaller lesion occurred in either cortical or subcortical location, the very large lesions involved both cortical and subcortical structures including the basal ganglia and thalamus. Lesion volume is coded by circle diameter. (From ref. 46 with permission.)

showed a tendency for large infarctions to be associated with little recovery. However, this relation did not hold for less than very large infarctions (Fig. 3). One possible explanation of the poor recovery in the cases with quasi sensorimotor hemispherectomies is that the candidate structures for the mediation of functional substitution are destroyed altogether: primary sensorimotor cortex, premotor, and parietal areas. This view is supported by findings showing that in addition to corticospinal tract damage, thalamic affection contributes to poor outcome (10,49). Moreover, multivariate analyses of neuroimaging data showed that distributed cortical networks affect also other brain areas and functional systems in remote locations that normally subserve hand function (28,40). Finally, a particular mortality risk in stroke is the involvement of the insular cortex causing sudden death probably due to affection of autonomic functions (59).

One of the most important factors influencing motor recovery appears to be the integrity of the pyramidal motor output system. It has been well documented that extensive brain lesions in the area of the cortical motor representations along the precentral gyrus induce a contralateral hemiparesis in animals and humans with permanent loss of prehension or locomotor movements (49,60–64). However, subcortical lesions involving the pyramidal tract can also cause severe contralateral hemiparesis that may not or only slowly resolve over time. Owing to the convergence of nerve fibers from the motor cortex as they approach the internal capsule and the resulting increase in nerve fiber density, a small lesion in the pyramidal tract at the level of the internal capsule is comparable to a larger cortical lesion in terms of the amount of affected axons (49).

IV. ELECTROPHYSIOLOGICAL PREDICTORS

Physiological evidence of the importance of the pyramidal output system for motor recovery in humans has been obtained from transcranial magnetic stimulation, which showed that in the acute stage after stroke, but also after 2 months, absence of magnetic evoked motor potentials (MEPs) and somatosensory evoked potentials (SSEPs) was related to poor motor recovery after stroke (65–68). Specifically, it was shown that the reduction of corticospinal tract affection during the first 4 weeks after stroke was related to an increase of the MEP amplitudes and to clinical motor recovery in a quantitative manner (49). The MEPs first reoccurred in the proximal muscles and later in the distal hand muscles in parallel to the clinical pattern of recovery (42) when recovered amplitude and central conduction times approached normal values.

Fractionated finger movements, as opposed to leg and arm muscle activity, usually remain severely impaired when the corticospinal output system is extensively damaged at whatever level. This was demonstrated in monkeys with cortical and brainstem lesions (60,69–71) and in patients with hemispheric brain infarctions (49) and brainstem lesions (72,73). In these studies it was estimated that approximately 20% of corticospinal tract fibers must be spared to ensure restitution of fractionated finger movements. Phylogenetic comparisons and onto-genetic data in the monkey revealed that the development of fractionated finger movements was parallelled by an extension of cortical projections and probably by direct synaptic connections to the motor neurons at the lower cervical levels of the spinal cord (74–77). This point is well illustrated by the famous case reported by Foerster (78). This patient underwent ablation of the motor cortex for intractable focal epilepsy and later, at autopsy, showed complete unilateral pyramidal tract degeneration. He had regained the capacity to lift his arm straight over his head and to hold a pen. However, his fractionated finger movements remained severely handicapped. Further evidence for the role of the pyramidal tract was obtained from morphometric measurements that revealed a good corre-lation of neurological impairment and tract affection as well as from MR diffusion tensor imaging (79–81).

Owing to the multifold affection of the cortex by ischemia, enhanced in-hibition and disinhibition have been shown to develop in a spatially distinct manner and with a defined time course (82). In humans enhanced inhibition was shown by transcranial magnetic stimulation to occur after extensive isch-emia of premotor or parietal cortex resulting in hemiparesis (83,84). This inhi-bition regressed in parallel to clinical recovery (Fig. 4). These observations are supported by experimental studies in rats showing that cortical ischemia impairs synaptic transmission, while the direct wave of motor evoked potentials and the early potential of the somatosensory evoked potentials promptly recovered (85). In contrast, disinhibition occurs after circumscribed infarction of motor cortex as can be demonstrated by a shortened silent period after transcranial magnetic stimulation (86,87). In such patients, paired transcranial magnetic stimulation revealed disinhibition of the cerebral cortex being associated with rapid clinical recovery (88).

V. THE ROLE OF NEUROIMAGING FOR PREDICTION OF STROKE RECOVERY

In the patients who recover from stroke, recovery was attributed to reorganization within the remaining functional network. However, in patients with transient functional impairment in the sense of transient ischemic attack, recovery may result from restitution of tissue function after transient ischemia. These mecha-nisms can now be studied in humans with the new imaging techniques. Perfusion and diffusion weighted imaging (PI, DWI) with magnetic resonance imaging (MRI) and MR angiography provide information on the hemodynamic status of ischemic brain areas and about irreversible brain damage as well as about the

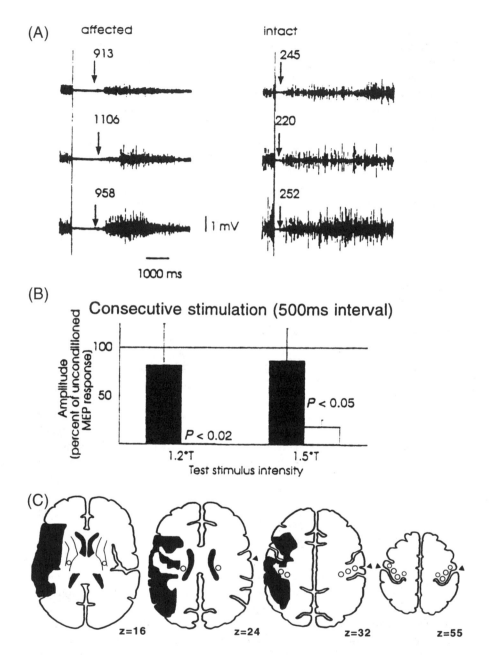

(A) affected

913
1106
958

intact

245
220
252

|1 mV

1000 ms

(B)

Consecutive stimulation (500ms interval)

Amplitude
(percent of unconditioned
MEP response)

100

50

$P < 0.02$

$P < 0.05$

1.2°T   1.5°T
Test stimulus intensity

(C)

z=16   z=24   z=32   z=55

major brain-supplying arteries. These techniques have significantly improved the accuracy of early stroke diagnosis (89). They further allow measurement of the apparent diffusion coefficient providing quantitative information about the functional state of brain tissue after ischemic brain injury (90).

A. Stroke Imaging

Interruption of circulation due to cerebral artery occlusion induces immediate changes in cerebral electrical activity with peri-infarct depolarization resulting in repeated episodes of metabolic stress and growth of the infarction from 4 to 24 hr postocclusion and characteristic lesion patterns (89,91–94). Clinically, middle cerebral artery (MCA) occlusion is manifest by apoplectiform contralateral hemiplegia within 60 sec (95). Usually, recanalization of the occluded cerebral artery with partial restoration of perfusion occurs within 24 hr (96,97). Early recanalization of MCA occlusion within 8 hr and good leptomeningeal collaterals critically increase the chances of functional restitution with favorable clinical outcome (98–100). This is probably also the mode of action in acute thrombolysis as evident from functional imaging (101,102) and monitoring with MRI and transcranial Doppler sonography (103). Figure 5 illustrates a patient with a severe perfusion deficit due to acute thrombembolic occlusion of the distal MCA in the presence of a small manifest infarct lesion as evident from DWI. After restoration of brain perfusion, the patient had a remarkable clinical recovery.

Mounting evidence shows that secondary inflammatory and apoptotic processes ensue in the subacute ischemic state leading to augmentation of infarct volume following reperfusion (104–106). Furthermore, arteriosclerotic lesions in the extracranial arteries are prone to augmentation by inflammatory changes that lead to placque destabilization and the occurrence of microemboli (107,108). These microemboli are predictive of the occurrence of subsequent brain infarction adding to preexisting ischemic lesions. The inflammatory leukocytic invasion into tissue can be visualized in humans by imaging with GABA-A receptor ligand PK11195 (109). Conversely, hyperperfusion of the infarcted brain tissue is not

---

Fig. 4 Exaggerated silent period in hemiparesis. (A) Prolonged and variable silent period in the affected arm about 20 days after middle cerebral artery infarction. (B) Double stimulation revealed the enhanced suppression of the second stimulus at two different stimulation strengths. The regression of the duration and variability of the silent period correlated with the clinical recovery. (C) Chronic infarct lesion in one of the patients with an exaggerated silent period as plotted onto axial brain slices of standard anatomy (252). The infarct lesion involved the premotor, parietal, and peri-insular cortex, while the dorsal part of the motor cortex including the representation of the hand were spared. Dots indicate location of motor cortex and corticospinal tract. [From Classen et al. (83) with permission.]

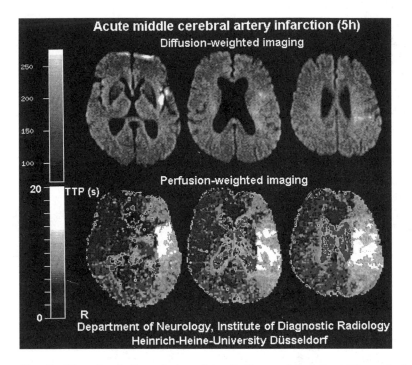

Fig. 5 Thrombembolic occlusion of the distal part of the left middle cerebral artery on the basis of an acute occlusion of the left internal carotid artery in a 65-year-old patient. Note the extensive area of severely impaired perfusion in the presence of a small infarct lesion in the left insula as evident from diffusion-weighted imaging.

a factor contributing to aggravation of infarction (110). The therapeutically important aspect of acute stroke is that the secondary events after ischemia are possibly at least partially reversible by the inhibition of caspases (111).

During ischemia the thresholds for selective neuronal and tissue necrosis are a function of rCBF (90). In patients with early recanalization and effective leptomeningeal collaterals, the amount of brain tissue subjected to necrosis is, therefore, smaller than in those with prolonged MCA occlusion and poor leptomeningeal collaterals. Consequently, persisting metabolic abnormalities around the necrotic core of brain infarction within the affected perfusion area are probably the result of selective ischemic nerve cell damage in the presence of viable glia (91,112). These data indicate that recovery of function in brain infarction is critically determined by the spatial extent and duration of severe ischemia. Hemiplegia and depression of rCBF produced by temporary carotid artery balloon occlusion have been shown to normalize completely with 15 min (95). This implies that a chronic structural brain lesion as evident in CT and MRI reflects only a portion of the total amount of brain tissue affected at the acute stage of brain infarction. Accordingly, the neuronal loss after transient ischemia significantly exceeds the area showing a DWI abnormality (94).

As evident from PI and DWI imaging, during stroke evolution the hypoperfused area is typically larger then the DWI lesion resulting in a prominent PI-DWI mismatch (Fig. 6). The PI abnormalities correlate better with the initial neurological deficit (58,113–115) than the DWI lesions (56,58,113), rendering perfusion imaging an important diagnostic tool for acute stroke. While the PI deficit closely reflects the functional effect of ischemia, the so called PI-DWI mismatch region reflects tissue at risk that can be recruited into the ischemic infarct during the subsequent hours. Experimentally, it has been shown that the flow thresholds for irreversible structural damage and functional disturbances are different (90). The PI method is sensitive enough to detect perfusion deficits in mild hypoperfusion states that are below the threshold for function but above the threshold for structural damage. Identification and follow-up of these areas has

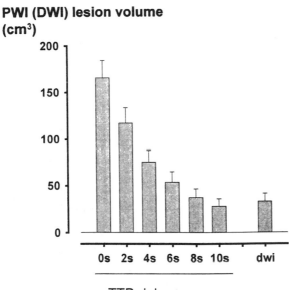

PWI (DWI) lesion volume (cm³)

TTP-delay ≥x sec.

Fig. 6 Quantitation of the perfusion-diffusion mismatch in acute stroke. Quantitative assessment showed that a delay of perfusion of 6 sec in the infarct compared to the nonaffected hemisphere was predictive for the ischemic lesion as indicated by the lesion in the diffusion-weighted MR-image. Further details in Neumann-Haefelin et al. (113).

provided new ground for our thinking about structure function relationships during stroke evolution. This is illustrated in Fig. 7, which shows that the initial PI-DWI mismatch is followed by a subsequent increase of the DWI lesion, which returns to the lesion size of the initial perfusion defect after 30 days. It should be noted, however, that the first MR scan was done after treatment initiation on average more than 5 hr after stroke onset (116). DWI lesions more than 5 hr of age readily predict the infarct lesion as measured with T2-weighted MR at 7 days (115,117).

Figure 8 shows the example of such a mismatch between PI and DWI areas in a transient ischemic attack 2 hr after onset. A subsequent scan 24 hr later demonstrated that the hypoperfused area diminished in size, whereas infarct size only marginally increased. This is the typical event after TIA, showing that TIAs may result in small lacunar infarct lesions. The same dynamics of PI and DWI evolution were observed with a more protracted time course also after completed infarction in the majority of our patients (115). These observations contradict experimental results indicating that the PI area is invariably recruited into the infarct.

A second insight that was learned from early stroke imaging was that the hypoperfused state could be maintained much longer than formerly thought. In

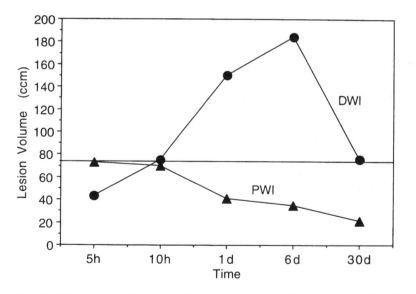

Fig. 7 Time course of lesion evolution after treatment initiation in the first 30 days after stroke. The perfusion deficit at 5 hr predicted the final infarct lesion as evident in diffusion-weighted imaging. While the perfusion deficit decreased over time, the diffusion lesion culminated at day 6. [From Beaulieu et al. (116).]

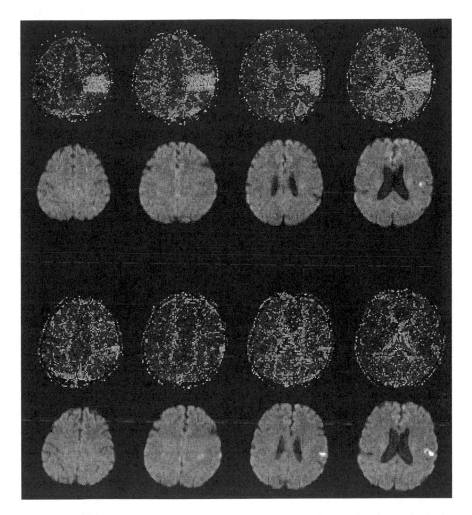

Fig. 8 Perfusion and diffusion-weighted imaging of a transitory ischemic attack. At the time of MR scanning the initial hemiparesis and motor aphasia had already nearly completely resolved. Note the severe initial perfusion-diffusion mismatch (upper two rows). One day later, when the patient was normal again, virtually no perfusion deficit was detectable, while there were small infarct lesions along the central sulcus (lower two rows).

hemodynamically relevant carotid artery stenosis, DWI shows only a small infarct whereas PI shows a relatively large hypoperfused area (118). That is, in acute stroke the total PI-DWI mismatch is often larger in those with ipsilateral carotid stenosis > 70% than in patients without carotid stenosis (118). In these cases, hypoperfusion clears as soon as such a patient is operated on for the carotid artery stenosis or acute occlusion (Fig. 9). Such findings indicate that most of the total mismatch in these patients is not necessarily at high risk of irreversible tissue damage. Between the acute and the follow-up MR study after 7 days in the stenosis group only 7% of the total PI-DWI mismatch became recruited into the infarct, as compared to 40% of the patients without carotid artery stenosis (118). This was probably due to the fact that the severity of the perfusion deficit in the periphery of the mismatch was relatively mild in most patients with carotid stenosis. While previous studies found that a positive PI-DWI mismatch was associated with subsequent lesion enlargement (57,116,119), apparently a considerably smaller percentage of the total PI-DWI mismatch is at risk of becoming recruited into the infarct in patients with severe carotid stenosis than in those without carotid stenosis (118). Although these observations need to be corroborated by further investigations, the evidence from early stroke imaging indicates that partial hypoperfusion can persist longer than previously thought. Consequently its resolution can underlie functional improvement in terms not only of

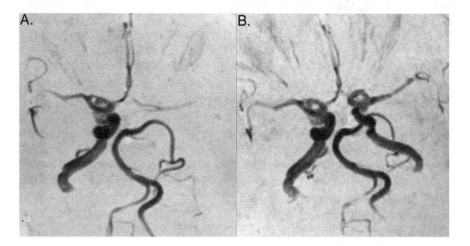

Fig. 9 Effect of acute carotid endarterectomy as demonstrated by time-of-flight magnetic resonance angiography in the patient shown in Fig. 5. Note the lack of signal in the left internal carotid artery and the reduced signal in the left middle cerebral artery about 3 hr after stroke onset (A). Restoration of the intra-arterial perfusion signal occurred after carotid endarterectomy performed 8 hr after stroke onset (B).

hours but probably also of a couple of days. How many patients maintain such hypoperfused stage for how long is still unclear. Nevertheless, these observations suggest that recovery may well be the consequence of the resolution of partially hypoperfused states.

In acute stroke patients with extracranial severe carotid artery disease, PI abnormalities may be due to blood flow obstruction at the level of the stenosis or to emboli lodging in downstream intracranial cerebral vessels. These emboli severely alter the perfusion pattern in the stroke area as was demonstrated in experimental ischemia (120). Furthermore, the ischemic abnormalities grow from the center to the periphery of the infarctions at later stages. Collateral flow, mainly via the circle of Willis, can partially compensate for the local flow obstruction such that CBF is often only moderately reduced in patients with severe carotid disease without prior stroke (121). Evidence from multitracer imaging with positron emission tomography shows that the perfusion deficit pattern does not correlate with the angiographic studies in such patients with severe occlusive artery disease (122,123). Collateral blood flow by small vessels below the resolution capacity of intraarterial angiography, therefore, seems to play an important role in the compensation of locally reduced cerebral perfusion. Likewise, good CBF has been shown to reduce the risk of stroke or TIA in association with carotid artery surgery and on a long-term scale (124).

Currently, it is a matter of debate which perfusion parameters—time-to-peak (TTP), regional mean transit time (rMTT), regional cerebral blood flow (rCBF) or regional cerebral blood volume (rCBV)—are optimal for differentiating critical from only moderate perfusion abnormalities. TTP maps obtained after an intravenous Gd-DTPA bolus are relatively easy to generate and perfusion deficits are easily visualized. Quantification of the TTP delay may be used to semiquantitatively assess the severity of the perfusion deficit in the PI-DWI mismatch (Fig. 6) and is clearly superior to purely qualitative forms of evaluation (125). But TTP is only an indirect measure of tissue perfusion. Absolute quantification of CBF, CBV, and MTT, on the other hand, has been shown to be possible in healthy volunteers using deconvolution methods that require determination of an arterial input function (126,127). However, although absolute flow quantification would be ideal for defining tissue at risk, it is currently unknown how accurate these methods will be when applied to acute stroke patients.

Most investigators using relative rMTT, rCBF, or rCBV maps measured total lesion volumes, but did not attempt to quantify the severity of the perfusion deficit. Recently, however, Schlaug et al. (128) determined rCBF and rCBV values in comparison to unaffected contralateral tissue in the DWI lesion and in the "penumbra," which was operationally defined as tissue that became recruited into the infarct lesion. Among other parameters, rCBF values of 0.12 and 0.37 were reported for the ischemic core and the "penumbra," respectively. However, normal rCBF is almost three times higher in gray than in white matter, indicating that ideally gray and white matter should be evaluated separately to assess the degree of cerebral ischemia.

In addition to the acute changes of perfusion and oxidative metabolism following stroke (91), there are also topographically specific, chronic changes in perilesional and remote locations reflecting the damage of the brain induced by the infarct (129–132). Specifically, categorical comparisons with healthy controls showed that in patients with hemiplegic infarction, rCBF and the cerebral metabolism were reduced in the affected motor cortex, the adjacent premotor and parietal cortex, the basal ganglia, the thalamus, and the contralesional cerebellum (130,131). Application of a principal component analysis (PCA) revealed an abnormally configured network in such stroke patients that reflected the topographic extent of lesion-related abnormalities affecting the damaged cerebral hemisphere and also the unaffected contralesional hemisphere, and subcortical structures such as the basal ganglia and the thalamus (Fig. 10). Spectral EEG analysis provided supporting evidence for transhemispheric diaschisis (133). Figure 11 shows the bilateral suppression of EEG activity after a severe MCA infarction. It is evident that the contralateral EEG recovered in a protracted manner in parallel to some degree of clinical recovery. These findings are consistent with recent descriptions of contralateral abnormalities in electroencephalographic and magnetoencephalographic recordings of spontaneous and movement-related brain activity after hemiparetic stroke (134,135). Also, in accordance with earlier observations in patients with suprathalamic infarctions in the middle cerebral territory (130), no lesion-related abnormalities were observed in the contralesional cerebellum. Interestingly, stroke patients retain subtle motor and cognitive deficits that are most likely reflected by deficient cortical activation patterns even after clinical motor

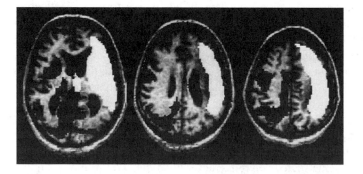

Fig. 10 Lesion-related abnormalities of the regional cerebral blood flow in patients with infarctions of the middle cerebral artery territory as visualized by a network analysis. The white areas indicate the perilesional zone, while the gray areas indicate the remote abnormalities in the contralesional hemisphere. (From ref. 28.)

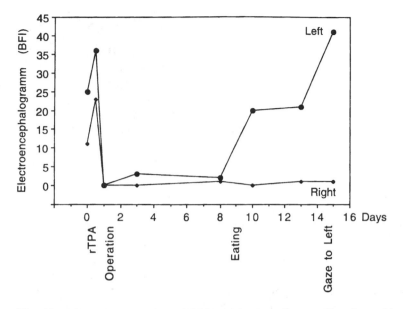

Fig. 11 Bilateral suppression of EEG activity in a 49-year-old patient with malignant right hemispheric brain infarction 24 hr after thrombolysis with rtPA. Eight days after craniectomy the patient's state improved, which was paralleled by reoccurrence of EEG activity in the contralesional cerebral hemisphere. For methodological details see Siebler et al. (135).

recovery (136,138). Such deficits may be augmented by changes related to a vascular encephalopathy (139,140).

B. Functional Imaging

Functional activation studies with PET and fMRI make it possible to map the cerebral structures that participate in the execution of an experimental task or a certain function. While heavily employed for studying normal brain function (see ref. 141), they more recently have also been used for studying the reorganization of functional representations in the human brain related to disease and functional recovery in a number of cerebral disorders including brain ischemia. Similar to other disease conditions, such as psychosis, it is important to study stroke patients with tasks they can perform (142), since the activation patterns are heavily influenced by the disease and disease-related functional changes that affect the brain activation patterns obscuring the task-specific activation patterns. This work led to new insights into the capacity of the human brain to reorganize. In this section mechanisms for such a reorganization will be discussed.

1. Reorganization

Since the pioneering work of Merzenich and Sameshima (143) it is known that functional reorganization can take place in the adult nervous system. The classic experiments were first shown for input manipulation where the overuse or disuse of particular inputs led to an increase or decrease of the corresponding cortical representation areas. The pivotal question for restorative neurology was whether such plasticity also operates after cortical damage. Ablation of areas 1, 2, and 3 in the hand area of the primary somatosensory cortex of the monkey (SI) led to an immediate unresponsiveness on the hand representation in SII, the second somatosensory cortex, a functionally related but distinct cooperative area (144). Twenty-four hours later the formally unresponsive hand area was then occupied by a foot representation. Nudo et al. (145) observed that the cortical finger representations adjacent to partly damaged finger representations became enlarged in relation to rehabilitative treatment, while they remained unchanged in the monkeys not subjected to rehabilitative treatment (Fig. 2). This and other experiments of this kind showed that reorganization occurs in the adult nervous system also after focal brain damage. It shows further that this reorganization operates rapidly, as in the case of input manipulation. The time course of this functional reorganization clearly exceeds the more protracted recovery curves seen in stroke patients in Fig. 1. It follows that for many patients, in particular those with partial or mild initial deficits, these reorganization processes could fully account for the observed recovery. On the other hand, tissue-born recovery could contribute in a similar way, so that the two processes might overlap and both underlie early recovery. At present it is impossible to single out the contribution of either mechanism to recovery in the individual patient.

Imaging studies in patients who had recovered from their first hemiparetic stroke involving the internal capsule and the basal ganglia consistently showed enlarged areas of activation in the cortical areas ipsilateral to the infarction during movement activity of the affected hand (146–148). However, the magnitude of the rCBF increases in the motor cortex was unrelated to the local remote decrease in rCBF, being as high as normal and probably corresponding to the normal MEPs of the affected hand (138,149). Thus, there are good reasons to believe that the motor cortex of the affected hemisphere was actively involved in task performance. In contrast, movement imagery does not induce rCBF increases in the motor cortex (150–152). Individual data analysis in recovering patients demonstrated that additional rCBF increases occurred, in particular in premoter and frontomesial cortical areas of both cerebral hemispheres, suggesting parallel involvement of a number of cortical areas in motor restitution (149,153,154).

In contrast, after recovery from hemiparetic stroke in the MCA territory with predominantly cortical involvement there was a lack of activation in motor cortex and SI, although the corticospinal tract was functional as assessed by motor evoked potentials and metabolic studies (41,52). This is illustrated for the chronic state in Fig. 12. While in the chronic stage no rCBF changes were observed in sensorimotor cortex adjacent to the stroke lesion, in the subacute stage after stroke activation of sensorimotor cortex close to the lesion has been well demonstrated (Fig. 13). These data showed lateral displacement of the activation area as also present in brain tumors (155,156). The data suggest a local reorganization employing the plastic capacity of the underlying neural machinery (157). Moreover, the patterns and cerebral locations of the most effective stimulation sites of MEPs in patients who have recovered from cortical infarction were not distinguishable from those in recovered patients with subcortical infarction (158). This suggests that in both subcortical and cortical brain infarctions motor cortex was most likely active during finger movement performance. Nevertheless, diminished rCBF increases due to sensorimotor stimulation have been reported after transient ischemic attacks and subcortical stroke (138,159). Possibly these observations indicate an uncoupling of rCBF (no response) and rCMRGlu (persistent response) after pharmacological inhibition of the neuronal nitric oxide synthetase (160).

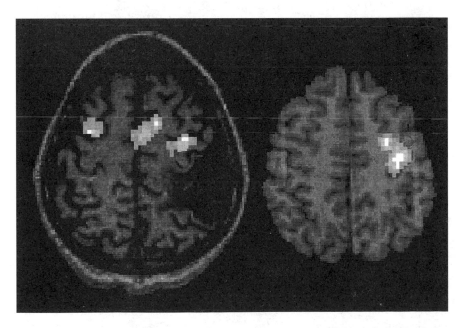

Fig. 12 Abnormal activations in patients who have recovered from their first brain infarction involving the middle cerebral artery territory as demonstrated with PET. While healthy controls (right) performing the same finger sequence task showed a significant rCBF increase in the motor and premotor cortex, the patients (left) had activations of bilateral premotor cortex and of the supplementary motor area. Further details in ref. 41.

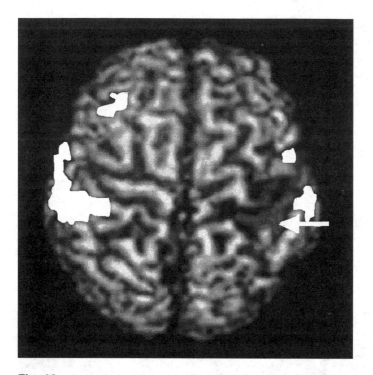

Fig. 13 Activation pattern in left sensorimotor cortex infarction (arrow) during tactile exploration of a complex geometrical object with the affected, partially recovered right hand as demonstrated with functional MRI. Note the lateral displacement of the postcentral activation and the extensive activation of the homolog area in the contralesional hemisphere. Related to the task demand, there were also activations in left premotor and right prefrontal cortex.

    An important mechanism for recovery-related reorganization is the possibility that projection systems of the homolog system in the contralateral cerebral hemisphere can become engaged in the restoration of executive functions. We observed that in MCA infarction involving the anterior parietal lobule, somatosensory discrimination of macrogeometric objects induced rCBF increases in contralesional parietal cortical regions (41). They occurred in an area that in normal subjects seems to participate in voluntary controlled movement (152,161). In this connection, it is noteworthy that the rCBF in the supplementary motor area and in parietal cortex was shown to be related to the exertion of force (162). Nevertheless, the parietal activation probably reflected a large-scale reorganization of the sensorimotor system to meet the task demands of the sensorimotor activation paradigm. Indeed, there is kinematic evidence showing that patients with parietal cortex lesions retain abnormal fingers movements when required to explore macrogeometric objects after recovery from hermisparesis (46). In addition, there is abnormal prefrontal cortex activation suggesting enhanced cognitive control for a task that is relatively difficult for patients as compared with healthy subjects (41).

Interestingly, there was relatively little activation in the frontomesial cortex including the SMA in the patients who had recovered from striatocapsular infarction (149,163) in contrast to the patients who had recovered from MCA infarction. Activation of the SMA probably corresponds to the initiative role of the SMA in movement control (164,165). The lack of SMA activation in the striatocapsular infarctions is probably due to damage of the corticospinal projection from the SMA to the basal ganglia by the stroke lesion. Thus, these patients appeared to activate instead the contralesional premotor cortex. Also, the lateral promoter cortex was activated in both hemispheres in the patients with MCA infarction. Conversely, stroke patients with involvement of premotor cortex exhibit an additional motor deficit that counteracts recovery (64,166). Nevertheless, during somatosensory activation, both, patients with subcortical and cortical stroke showed parietal lobe activation (Fig. 13). The parietal cortex subserves sensorimotor integration being heavily interwoven with executive functions mediated in the frontal motor cortical areas (149).

There is convincing clinical evidence showing that the motor system in the contralesional hemisphere plays an important role for deficit compensation by postischemic reorganization (167). The first to show this in brain lesions acquired in adulthood using PET were Chollet et al. (146). Later it was replicated by Cao et al. (168) using fMRI. However, it was noted that those patients who exhibited significant rCBF increases in motor cortex contralateral to the cerebral infarction had associated movements of the nonaffected hand (153). Obviously, this corresponded to electromyographic findings in healthy subjects in whom effort, force, and activity with the nondominant hand were accompanied by increased muscle activity in the homologe muscles contralateral to the moving hand (169,170). The associated rCBF increases in the motor cortex of the nonaffected hemisphere occurred in those patients with limited recovery (149,153). They probably corresponded to the presence of ipsilateral MEPs in such patients (171,172) reflecting an unmasking of ipsilateral corticospinal projections in relation to heightened effort and action with the affected hand. That associated finger movements can occur in hemiparesis has long been known (173). Typically, their onset is significantly shorter than those evoked by high effort of the normal hand (174). It could be that these movements are mediated by exposure of the zone in the motor cortex, which has been shown in the monkey to be involved in bilateral hand movements (175). However, fMRI showed that the ipsilateral activation does not occur in a homolog location compared with the contralateral motor cortical representation (176). Similarly, the recovery may be brought about by recruitment of ipsilateral corticospinal projections as evident from patients with congenital brain lesions (44,45,177,178). Usually, this leads to initial reoccurrence of proximal movements compared to the later recovery of distal movements (42,179). This hypothesis is corroborated by the ipsilateral impairment of forearm function in the acute stage after stroke (180). Remarkably, the more asymmetrical the activations, the worse the clinical outcome (181).

It is important to realize that involvement of homolog areas including the premoter cortical areas contralateral to a stroke lesion has repeatedly been reported as a mechanism for recovery that applies also for aphasia (182–184). Most comspiciously, recovery from hemiplegia may be connected also with activation of the lower premotor cortex including the inferior frontal cortex ipsilateral to the moving hand during execution of fast and sequential finger movements with the recovered hand (41,153). These areas are also activated in healthy subjects during learning of finger movement sequences (185,186) but not after skill acquisition (187).

The situation is different in congenital hemispheric brain lesions involving the pre- and postcentral gyrus. In these patients motor function in the contralateral hand may be remarkable and even allow independent finger movements (188,189). Sabatini et al. (189) reported a case presenting 19 years after a large porencephalic lesion in the area of the right middle cerebral artery, in whom rCBF increases were confined to the motor cortex of the nonaffected hemisphere during finger movements of either hand. Electrophysiological support for such findings has been obtained in patients with congenital hemiplegic palsy and hemispherectomy, showing unmasking of ipsilateral corticospinal motor projections that are usually not excitable in healthy people (44,45,177). It should be stressed that these observations were obtained many years after birth and hemispherectomy, respectively. One can, therefore, postulate that in these patients the cortical reorganization mediating recovery of motor functions had occurred very early in life having had sufficient time to take place. It appears likely that the capacity for cerebral reorganization of the focally damaged brain, as for instance after stroke, is less extensive in the adult brain.

2. The Role of Reafferent Feedback

It appears from Fig. 1 that most patients recover well and early. One group who were severely impaired initially recovered in contrast to other severely affected patients who did not recover at all. It is likely that the decisive distinctive feature is the absence of residual function in the nonrecovering patients. Evidence from combined clinical and electrophysiological studies suggests that in addition to the motor score the presence of SSEPs indicates good recovery (190). Furthermore, illusory arm movements have been reported to activate beyond motor areas also the somatosensory cortex (191). It may therefore be assumed that the absence of residual function over a critical time span prevents functional restitution. Conversely, animal experiments show an enlargement of the somatosensory representations during skill recovery after focal lesions of the primary somatosensory cortex (192). Further, deafferented monkeys who were not using the affected limb many weeks after injury failed to recover (193). From these observations the concept was derived that the animals learned not to use the affected limb because of discomfort, stress, the frustration when doing so, but rather used the intact arm. This concept of "learned nonuse" laid the ground for subsequent therapy studies in severely impaired chronic human stroke victims. This concept imposed constraints on the unaffected limb because it has to be worn in a cast for many hours a day forcing the subject to use the minimal residual functions of the affected arm for whatever purpose. This so-called "constrained induced" therapy has now been shown to be very successful even when applied in the chronic state for severely affected patients (193,194). Thus, there is good evidence to support the view that reafferent somatosensory information from the partly compromised limb is critically required for tuning the remaining network into function as may be evident from scanning passive movements (195). These data are corroborated further by the observation that there is a posterior shift of the sensorimotor area in patients with sensorimotor strokes (134).

Another modality that seems to play an important role in postischemic recovery is the visual system. Monkeys with focal ischemic lesions in motor cortex visually inspect their hand when retrieving objects with the affected hand (196). In humans, it was observed that patients who had recovered from ischemic stroke differed significantly from healthy controls by the recruitment of a predominantly contralesional network, involving visual cortical areas, prefrontal cortex, thalamus, hippocampus, and cerebellum during the blindfolded performance of sequential finger movements (28). Greater expression of this cortical-subcortical network correlated with a more severe sensorimotor deficit in the acute stage after stroke, reflecting its role for poststroke recovery. Thus, a visuomotor brain system appeared to compensate for a sensorimotor deficit in patients who had recovered from hemiparetic stroke. This observation corresponds to animal models of focal brain lesions and to the developing human visual and auditory systems (197–200), suggesting that postlesional reorganization involves a network usually not active in sensorimotor activity.

In addition, it was shown that the lesion-affected and the recovery-related network in stroke patients shared the same structures in the contralesional thalamus and bilateral in visual association areas (28). Thus, these sharing structures accommodated simultaneously passive lesion effects and active recovery-related changes in locations remote from the site of the brain infarction. This observation corresponds to the original conception of diaschisis as a restorative mechanism in functional recovery. That is, recovery is mediated by areas that have regained activity after initial inhibition by a distant brain lesion (201). Thus, postlesional reorganization appeared as a task-related rewiring of intrinsic cerebral networks. While such a reorganization was shown to be effective in the perilesional vicinity (157), there seems to be also large-scale interregional reorganization. These affected regions did not show metabolic depressions in categorical comparisons with healthy subjects, which therefore did not seem to be a prerequisite for diaschisis. The type of activation-related interregional interactions suggests a task-related engagement of preexisting, hitherto latent pathways. Accordingly, when the functional changes as evident from brain imaging correlate with neurological deficits or with neurological recovery, they may be referred to as instances of diaschisis and the regression of diaschisis. Similar conclusions were also proposed recently for psychologically impaired patients (142).

As evidenced by PET activation studies in patients recovered from hemiplegic stroke, such unused, but functionally related pathways take on backup or facilitatory functions (146,147,149,153). They may become engaged as alternative neural routes in patients with congenital or developmental brain diseases (44,45,177,189). From a phenomenological point of view, these cases represent temporary loss of function and its reappearance after a shorter or longer period of time. Disturbances of complex motor behavior like neglect and limb kinetic apraxia also tend to disappear with time (166,202). Nevertheless, ideomotor apraxia, visuomotor ataxia, and motor aphasia may be sufficiently stable in some patients or detectable by adequate neuropsychological testing (203–205). As in the case of simple motor functions, the clinical presentation and resolution of these complex cerebral dysfunctions appear to be determined by the localization and size of the underlying brain lesion (206–211). In aphasia, however, the location of the original lesion appears to vary more widely between subjects, reflecting the great variability of language localization (212,213). Also, there is some evidence that larger lesions in the frontal operculum induce a more severe aphasia (214).

An alternative hypothesis is that recovering patients select an alternative strategy to compensate for their neurological deficit as was shown in monkeys (215). A simple approach is that patients employ more extended finger movements for object exploration than they usually would (216). In contrast to the hand representation in motor cortex (217–219), there is no overlapping somatotopy of digit representation in the somatosensory cortex (220). Thus, a spatially enhanced input is processed in a large portion of the sensorimotor cortex in these patients. Similarly, there is evidence suggesting that patients with hemianopia can learn to exaggerate saccadic eye movements to compensate for their visual field defect (221,222). Likewise, hemiparetic patients may engage muscles for moving a paretic limb that are usually only used for auxillatory actions or reserved for high levels of exertion. This compensatory behavior is most prominent in patients with dystrophic muscle diseases, for instance while they are standing up or lifting a limb (223), but probably also holds for brain lesions. Finally, patients with Parkinson's disease sometimes employ sensory cues to initiate locomotion (224–226). Clearly, these altered actions rely on abnormal sensorimotor or visuomotor information processing and are most likely to produce abnormal cortical activation patterns.

3. The Role of the Perilesional Area

There is plenty of evidence from experimental studies that the perilesional zone after focal ischemia is grossly abnormal. This does not refer to the concept of penumbra, which has been defined for tissue at risk during the first minutes and hours after the insult. Rather the perilesional zone accommodates persistent and severe changes in tissue function in a surprisingly large area surrounding a lesion as demonstrated experimentally (82). In the thrombosis model of the rat, small focal cortical lesions lead to changes that can be revealed by electrophysiological, anatomical, and audioradiographic methods. Specifically, intracortical excitability is increased, intracortical inhibition decreased, and spontaneous activity and stimulus response characteristics are distinctly altered. Figure 14 shows that intracortical inhibition is severely changed in area up to 6 mm from the border of a 2-mm stroke lesion. In close accordance, audioradiography revealed a decreased inhibition as it shows down-regulation of GABA α and β receptors (227,228). In addition, there was an increase in glutamate receptor densities. These changes persist over many weeks. The implication of these prolonged changes for functional restoration and the cooperation of these perilesional areas with the remaining network are as yet unknown. Moreover, the perilesional area can be visualized microscipically by different staining methods in the histological pictures but cannot be properly recognized even at high field (7 Tesla) MRI, although its electrophysiological, audioradiographic, and metabolic patterns are clearly defined (229). Rather, neuroimaging in baboons and humans suggests that decreased labeling of the GABA-B receptor indicated irreversibly damaged brain tissue (109,230–233).

For the clinician this means that we do not see the remote changes. This is similar to the fact that we do not see relevant pathophysiology in basal ganglia, such as increased, spontaneous activity, abnormal synchronization, and the like, by imaging methods. Nevertheless, we must assume that this perilesional area is of considerable influence for the postischemic neurological deficit and the pattern of functional restoration. The structural and the functional component of reafferent feedback emphasize that the old mechanistic view that the size of a destructed

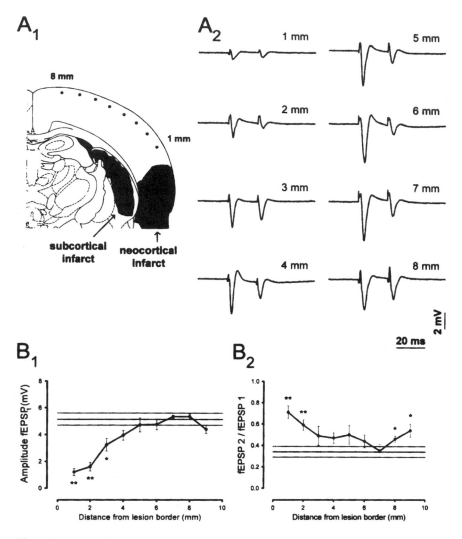

Fig. 14 Excitability changes in the cerebral cortex 7 days after 1-hr occlusion of the middle cerebral artery. (A$_1$) Schematic diagram of the microelectrode recording sites in rat cortex. (A$_2$) Field potentials of the excitatory postsynaptic potentials (fEPSP) obtained at the recording sites illustrated in A1. (B$_1$) Note the severe suppression of the first fEPSP in the vicinity of the lesion border, which gradually normalizes in relation to an increasing distance to the lesion border suggesting perilesional decreased activity. (B$_2$) Close to the lesion and remote from the lesion the ratio of the first and second fEPSP was significantly greater than in control animals as indicated by the horizontal lines. At day 27 the first to second fEPSP ratio had normalized in the perilesional area but remained abnormal in remote location allowing for locally enhanced excitability. [From Neuman-Haefelin and Witte (251).]

area is the major determinant for the resulting functional impairment is certainly too simplistic.

VI. PERSPECTIVES

Motor activity represents relatively well-defined brain functions, whereas higher cortical functions like neglect, apraxia, and aphasia are more difficult to study as they are composed of a number of different subfunctions. Initial activation studies in stroke patients suggest comparable determinants for recovery. In higher cortical functions the mechanisms include the critical preservation of the circuits normally subserving attention or language production and frustrane activation of the contralateral homolog areas in poor recovery (234–238). However, these studies point to the importance of brain-mapping studies for a better understanding of recovery from brain lesion and the development of neurobiologically based therapeutic regimens.

Motor functions represent good models for studying modulating actions of neurotransmitters and pharmaceuticals. There is evidence from animal experiments for the importance of the widely projecting, adrenergic and cholinergic neurons for brain function (239–241). These neurons become retrogradely affected by the ischemic tissue lesion and their damage has been related to the manifestation of diaschisis (242). Likewise, adrenergic mediators have been shown to promote recovery in animals, while adrenergic receptor blockers and related drugs are found to impair it (243–247). Randomized and double-blind studies in humans are still lacking, but retrospective analysis of large groups of patients recovering from stroke seem to corroborate the animal data (248). Recently, it was reported that epinephrine and fluoxetin augmented electromyographic activity in leg muscles in paraplegia during aided walking as well as brain activity related to movement (249,250). Thus, functional recovery may be enhanced also by drug action.

Finally, on the horizon of today's knowledge, there is the possibility of using molecular approaches for regeneration of nervous tissue such as gene transfer and stem cell engineering. If shown operational, they will open new perspectives of research on the prognosis of functional restoration after stroke.

REFERENCES

1. Gresham GE, Kelly-Hayes M, Wolf PA, Beiser AS, Kase CS, D'Agostino RB. Survival and functional status 20 or more years after first stroke: the Framingham Study. Stroke 1998; 29(4):793–797.
2. Duncan PW, Goldstein LB, Matchar D, Divine GW, Feussner J. Measurement of

motor recovery after stroke. Outcome assessment and sample size requirements. Stroke 1992; 23(8):1084–1089.

3. Donnan GA, Bladin PF, Berkovic SF, Longley WA, Saling MM. The stroke syndrome of striatocapsular infarction. Brain 1991; 114(Pt 1A):51–70.

4. Duncan PW, Lai SM, Keighley J. Defining post-stroke recovery: implications for design and interpretation of drug trials. Neuropharmacology 2000; 39(5):835–841.

5. Kwakkel G, Wagenaar RC, Kollen BJ, Lankhorst GJ. Predicting disability in stroke—a critical review of the literature. Age Ageing 1996; 25(6):479–489.

6. Hennerici M, Aulich A, Freund H-J. Carotid artery syndromes. In: Vinken PJ, Bruyn GW, Klawans HL, Toole JF, eds. Handbook of Neurology. Amsterdam: Elsevier, 1988, pp 291–337.

7. Gray CS, French JM, Bates D, Cartlidge NE, James OF, Venables G. Motor recovery following acute stroke. Age Ageing 1990; 19(3):179–184.

8. Heinemann AW, Roth EJ, Cichowski K, Betts HB. Multivariate analysis of improvement and outcome following stroke rehabilitation [see comments]. Arch Neurol 1987; 44(11):1167–1172.

9. Katrak P, Bowring G, Conroy P, Chilvers M, Poulos R, McNeil D. Predicting upper limb recovery after stroke: the place of early shoulder and hand movement. Arch Phys Med Rehabil 1998; 79(7):758–761.

10. Fries W, Danek A, Scheidtmann K, Hamburger C. Motor recovery following capsular stroke. Role of descending pathways from multiple motor areas. Brain 1993; 116(Pt 2):369–382.

11. Manto M, Jacquy J, Hildebrand J, Godaux E. Recovery of hypermetria after a cerebellar stroke occurs as a multistage process. Ann Neurol 1995; 38(3):437–445.

12. Kase CS, Wolf PA, Chodosh EH, Zacker HB, Kelly-Hayes M, Kannel WB, et al. Prevalence of silent stroke in patients presenting with initial stroke: the Framingham Study. Stroke 1989; 20(7):850–852.

13. Sultzer DL, Mahler ME, Cummings JL, Van Gorp WG, Hinkin CH, Brown C. Cortical abnormalities associated with subcortical lesions in vascular dementia. Clinical and position emission tomographic findings. Arch Neurol 1995; 52(8): 773–780.

14. van Zagten M, Boiten J, Kessels F, Lodder J. Significant progression of white matter lesions and small deep (lacunar) infarcts in patients with stroke. Arch Neurol 1996; 53(7):650–655.

15. Kunesch E, Binkofski F, Steinmetz H, Freund HJ. The pattern of motor deficits in relation to the site of stroke lesions. Eur Neurol 1995; 35(1):20–26.

16. Wozniak MA, Kittner SJ, Price TR, Hebel JR, Sloan MA, Gardner JF. Stroke location is not associated with return to work after first ischemic stroke. Stroke 1999; 30(12):2568–2573.

17. Johnston KC, Connors AF, Jr., Wagner DP, Knaus WA, Wang X, Haley EC Jr. A predictive risk model for outcomes of ischemic stroke. Stroke 2000; 31(2):448–455.

18. Formisano R, Barbanti P, Catarci T, De Vuono G, Calisse P, Razzano C. Prolonged muscular flaccidity: frequency and association with unilateral spatial neglect after stroke. Acta Neurol Scand 1993; 88(5):313–315.

19. Pantano P, Formisano R, Ricci M, Di P, V, Sabatini U, Barbanti P, et al. Prolonged

muscular flaccidity after stroke. Morphological and functional brain alterations. Brain 1995; 118(Pt 5):1329–1338.

20. Paolucci S, Antonucci G, Pratesi L, Traballesi M, Lubich S, Grasso MG. Functional outcome in stroke inpatient rehabilitation: predicting no, low and high response patients. Cerebrovasc Dis 1998; 8(4):228–234.

21. Pedersen PM, Jorgensen HS, Nakayama H, Raaschou HO, Olsen TS. Aphasia in acute stroke: incidence, determinants, and recovery. Ann Neurol 1995; 38(4):659–666.

22. Di Carlo A, Lamassa M, Pracucci G, Basile AM, Trefoloni G, Vanni P, et al. Stroke in the very old: clinical presentation and determinants of 3-month functional outcome: A European perspective. European BIOMED Study of Stroke Care Group. Stroke 1999; 30(11):2313–2319.

23. Marini C, Totaro R, Carolei A. Long-term prognosis of cerebral ischemia in young adults. National Research Council Study Group on Stroke in the Young. Stroke 1999; 30(11):2320–2325.

24. Rothwell JC, Traub MM, Day BL, Obeso JA, Thomas PK, Marsden CD. Manual motor performance in a deafferented man. Brain 1982; 105(Pt 3):515–542.

25. Wolf SL, LeCraw DE, Barton LA, Jann BB. Forced use of hemiplegic upper extremities to reverse the effect of learned nonuse among chronic stroke and head-injured patients. Exp Neurol 1989; 104(2):125–132.

26. Taub E, Crago JE, Burgio LD, Groomes TE, Cook EW, III, DeLuca SC, et al. An operant approach to rehabilitation medicine: overcoming learned nonuse by shaping. J Exp Anal Behav 1994; 61(2):281–293.

27. Kalra L, Perez I, Gupta S, Wittink M. The influence of visual neglect on stroke rehabilitation. Stroke 1997; 28(7):1386–1391.

28. Seitz RJ, Azari NP, Knorr U, Binkofski F, Herzog H, Freund HJ. The role of diaschisis in stroke recovery. Stroke 1999; 30(9):1844–1850.

29. Jorgensen HS, Kammersgaard LP, Houth J, Nakayama H, Raaschou HO, Larsen K, et al. Who benefits from treatment and rehabilitation in a stroke unit? A community-based study. Stroke 2000; 31(2):434–439.

30. Kozlowski DA, James DC, Schallert T. Use-dependent exaggeration of neuronal injury after unilateral sensorimotor cortex lesions. J Neurosci 1996; 16(15):4776–4786.

31. Risedal A, Zeng J, Johansson BB. Early training may exacerbate brain damage after focal brain ischemia in the rat. J Cereb Blood Flow Metab 1999; 19(9):997–1003.

32. Bütefisch C, Hummelsheim H, Denzler P, Mauritz KH. Repetitive training of isolated movements improves the outcome of motor rehabilitation of the centrally paretic hand. J Neurol Sci 1995; 130(1):59–68.

33. Hesse S, Bertelt C, Jahnke MT, Schaffrin A, Baake P, Malezic M, et al. Treadmill training with partial body weight support compared with physiotherapy in nonambulatory hemiparetic patients. Stroke 1995; 26(6):976–981.

34. Hummelsheim H, Hauptmann B, Neumann S. Influence of physiotherapeutic facilitation techniques on motor evoked potentials in centrally paretic hand extensor muscles. Electroencephalogr Clin Neurophysiol 1995; 97(1):18–28.

35. Kwakkel G, Wagenaar RC, Twisk JW, Lankhorst GJ, Koetsier JC. Intensity of leg

and arm training after primary middle-cerebral-artery stroke: a randomised trial [see comments]. Lancet 1999; 354(9174):191–196.

36. Thaut MH, McIntosh GC, Rice RR. Rhythmic facilitation of gait training in hemiparetic stroke rehabilitation. J Neurol Sci 1997; 151(2):207–212.

37. Aisen ML, Krebs HI, Hogan N, McDowell F, Volpe BT. The effect of robot-assisted therapy and rehabilitative training on motor recovery following stroke. Arch Neurol 1997; 54(4):443–446.

38. Volpe BT, Krebs HI, Hogan N, Edelsteinn L, Diels CM, Aisen ML. Robot training enhanced motor outcome in patients with stroke maintained over 3 years. Neurology 1999; 53(8):1874–1876.

39. Hauptmann B, Hummelsheim H. Facilitation of motor evoked potentials in hand extensor muscles of stroke patients: correlation to the level of voluntary contraction. Electroencephalogr Clin Neurophysiol 1996; 101(5):387–394.

40. Azari NP, Binkofski F, Pettigrew KD, Freund H-J, Seitz RJ. Enhanced regional cerebral metabolic interactions in thalamic circuitry predicts motor recovery in hemiparetic stroke. Hum Brain Mapping 1996; 4:240–253.

41. Seitz RJ, Hoflich P, Binkofski F, Tellmann L, Herzog H, Freund HJ. Role of the premotor cortex in recovery from middle cerebral artery infarction. Arch Neurol 1998; 55(8):1081–1088.

42. Colebatch JG, Gandevia SC. The distribution of muscular weakness in upper motor neuron lesions affecting the arm. Brain 1989; 112(Pt 3):749–763.

43. Winstein CJ, Pohl PS. Effects of unilateral brain damage on the control of goal-directed hand movements. Exp Brain Res 1995; 105(1):163–174.

44. Benecke R, Meyer BU, Freund HJ. Reorganisation of descending motor pathways in patients after hemispherectomy and severe hemispheric lesions demonstrated by magnetic brain stimulation. Exp Brain Res 1991; 83(2):419–426.

45. Carr LJ, Harrison LM, Evans AL, Stephens JA. Patterns of central motor reorganization in hemiplegic cerebral palsy. Brain 1993; 116(Pt 5):1223–1247.

46. Binkofski F, Seitz RJ, Hackländer T, Pawelec D, Mau J, Freund H-J. The recovery of motor functions following hemiparetic stroke: a clinical and MR-morphometric study. Cerebrovasc Dis 2001; 11:273–281.

47. Sunderland A, Tinson D, Bradley L. Differences in recovery from constructional apraxia after right and left hemisphere stroke? J Clin Exp Neuropsychol 1994; 16(6):916–920.

48. Sunderland A. Recovery of ipsilateral dexterity after stroke. Stroke 2000; 31(2):430–433.

49. Binkofski F, Seitz RJ, Arnold S, Classen J, Benecke R, Freund HJ. Thalamic metabolism and corticospinal tract integrity determine motor recovery in stroke. Ann Neurol 1996; 39(4):460–470.

50. Furlan M, Marchal G, Viader F, Derlon JM, Baron JC. Spontaneous neurological recovery after stroke and the fate of the ischemic penumbra [see comments]. Ann Neurol 1996; 40(2):216–226.

51. Heinsius T, Bogousslavsky J, Van Melle G. Large infarcts in the middle cerebral artery territory. Etiology and outcome patterns [published erratum appears in Neurology 1998; 50(6):1940–1943 [see comments]. Neurology 1998; 50(2):341–350.

52. DiPiero V, Chollet FM, MacCarthy P, Lenzi GL, Frackowiak RS. Motor recovery

after acute ischaemic stroke: a metabolic study. J Neurol Neurosurg Psychiatry 1992; 55(11):990–996.

53. Pedersen PM, Jorgensen HS, Nakayama H, Raaschou HO, Olsen TS. Impaired orientation in acute stroke: frequency, determinants, and time-course of recovery. The Copenhagen Stroke Study. Cerebrovasc Dis 1998; 8(2):90–96.

54. Chen CL, Tang FT, Chen HC, Chung CY, Wong MK. Brain lesion size and location: effects on motor recovery and functional outcome in stroke patients. Arch Phys Med Rehabil 2000; 81(4):447–452.

55. Warach S, Dashe JF, Edelman RR. Clinical outcome in ischemic stroke predicted by early diffusion-weighted and perfusion magnetic resonance imaging: a preliminary analysis. J Cereb Blood Flow Metab 1996; 16(1):53–59.

56. Lovblad KO, Baird AE, Schlaug G, Benfield A, Siewert B, Voetsch B, et al. Ischemic lesion volumes in acute stroke by diffusion-weighted magnetic resonance imaging correlate with clinical outcome. Ann Neurol 1997; 42(2):164–170.

57. Barber PA, Darby DG, Desmond PM, Yang Q, Gerraty RP, Jolley D, et al. Prediction of stroke outcome with echoplanar perfusion- and diffusion-weighted MRI. Neurology 1998; 51(2):418–426.

58. Tong DC, Yenari MA, Albers GW, O'Brien M, Marks MP, Moseley ME. Correlation of perfusion- and diffusion-weighted MRI with NIHSS score in acute (<6.5 hour) ischemic stroke. Neurology 1998; 50(4):864–870.

59. Tokgozoglu SL, Batur MK, Top uoglu MA, Saribas O, Kes S, Oto A. Effects of stroke localization on cardiac autonomic balance and sudden death. Stroke 1999; 30(7):1307–1311.

60. Kennard MA. Cortical reorganization of motor function. Studies on series of monkeys of various ages from infancy to maturity. Arch Neurol Psychiatry 1942; 48: 227–240.

61. Passingham RE, Perry VH, Wilkinson F. The long-term effects of removal of sensorimotor cortex in infant and adult rhesus monkeys. Brain 1983; 106(Pt 3):675–705.

62. De Ryck M, Van Reempts J, Duytschaever H, Van Deuren B, Clincke G. Neocortical localization of tactile/proprioceptive limb placing reactions in the rat. Brain Res 1992; 573(1):44–60.

63. Schneider R, Gautier JC. Leg weakness due to stroke. Site of lesions, weakness patterns and causes. Brain 1994; 117(Pt 2):347–354.

64. Miyai I, Suzuki T, Kang J, Kubota K, Volpe BT. Middle cerebral artery stroke that includes the premotor cortex reduces mobility outcome. Stroke 1999; 30(7): 1380–1383.

65. Macdonell RA, Donnan GA, Bladin PF. A comparison of somatosensory evoked and motor evoked potentials in stroke. Ann Neurol 1989; 25(1):68–73.

66. Dominkus M, Grisold W, Jelinek V. Transcranial electrical motor evoked potentials as a prognostic indicator for motor recovery in stroke patients. J Neurol Neurosurg Psychiatry 1990; 53(9):745–748.

67. Heald A, Bates D, Cartlidge NE, French JM, Miller S. Longitudinal study of central motor conduction time following stroke. 2. Central motor conduction measured within 72 h after stroke as a predictor of functional outcome at 12 months. Brain 1993; 116(Pt 6):1371–1385.

68. Stephan KM, Netz J, Homberg V. Prognostic value of MEP and SSEP in patients
     with chronic UMN lesions after stroke. Cerebrovasc Dis 1995; 5:407–412.
69. Glees P, Cole J. Recovery of skilled motor functions after small repeated lesions
     of motor cortex in macaque. J Neurophysiol 1950; 13:137–148.
70. Lawrence DG, Kuypers HG. The functional organization of the motor system in
     the monkey. I. The effects of bilateral pyramidal lesions. Brain 1968; 91(1):1–
     14.
71. Lawrence DG, Kuypers HG. The functional organization of the motor system in
     the monkey. II. The effects of lesions of the descending brain-stem pathways. Brain
     1968; 91(1):15–36.
72. Bucy PC, Ladpli R, Ehrlich A. Destruction of the pyramidal tract in the monkey.
     The effects of bilateral section of the cerebral peduncles. J Neurosurg 1966; 25(1):
     1–23.
73. Jane JA, Yashon D, Becker DP, Beatty R, Sugar O. The effect of destruction of
     the corticospinal tract in the human cerebral peduncle upon motor function and
     involuntary movements. Report of 11 cases. J Neurosurg 1968; 29(6):581–585.
74. Dum RP, Strick PL. The origin of corticospinal projections from the premotor areas
     in the frontal lobe. J Neurosci 1991; 11(3):667–689.
75. Bortoff GA, Strick PL. Corticospinal terminations in two new-world primates: fur-
     ther evidence that corticomotoneuronal connections provide part of the neural sub-
     strate for manual dexterity. J Neurosci 1993; 13(12):5105–5118.
76. Galea MP, Darian-Smith I. Multiple corticospinal neuron populations in the ma-
     caque monkey are specified by their unique cortical origins, spinal terminations,
     and connections. Cereb Cortex 1994; 4(2):166–194.
77. Armand J, Olivier E, Edgley SA, Lemon RN. Postnatal development of corticospi-
     nal projections from motor cortex to the cervical enlargement in the macaque mon-
     key. J Neurosci 1997; 17(1):251–266.
78. Foerster O. Motorische Felder und Bahnen. In: Bumke O, Foerster O, eds. Allgem-
     eine Neurologie. Berlin: Julius Springer Verlag, 1936, pp 1–357.
79. Warabi T, Inoue K, Noda H, Murakami S. Recovery of voluntary movement in
     hemiplegic patients. Correlation with degenerative shrinkage of the cerebral pedun-
     cles in CT images. Brain 1990; 113(Pt 1):177–189.
80. Fukui K, Iguchi I, Kito A, Watanabe Y, Sugita K. Extent of pontine pyramidal
     tract Wallerian degeneration and outcome after supratentorial hemorrhagic stroke.
     Stroke 1994; 25(6):1207–1210.
81. Werring DJ, Clark CA, Barker GJ, Miller DH, Parker GJ, Brammer MJ, et al. The
     structural and functional mechanisms of motor recovery: complementary use of
     diffusion tensor and functional magnetic resonance imaging in a traumatic injury
     of the internal capsule. J Neurol Neurosurg Psychiatry 1998; 65(6):863–869.
82. Witte OW, Bidmon H-J, Schiene K, Redecker C, Hagemann G. Functional differen-
     tiation of multiple perilesional zones after focal cerebral ischemia. J Cereb Blood
     Flow Metab 2000; 20:1149–1165.
83. Classen J, Schnitzler A, Binkofski F, Werhahn KJ, Kim YS, Kessler KR, et al.
     The motor syndrome associated with exaggerated inhibition within the primary
     motor cortex of patients with hemiparetic. Brain 1997; 120(Pt 4):605–619.
84. Hauptmann B, Skrotzki A, Hummelsheim H. Facilitation of motor evoked poten-

tials after repetitive voluntary hand movements depends on the type of motor activity. Electroencephalogr Clin Neurophysiol 1997; 105(5):357–364.

85. Bolay H, Dalkara T. Mechanisms of motor dysfunction after transient MCA occlusion: persistent transmission failure in cortical synapses is a major determinant. Stroke 1998; 29(9):1988–1993.

86. von Giesen HJ, Roick H, Benecke R. Inhibitory actions of motor cortex following unilateral brain lesions as studied by magnetic brain stimulation. Exp Brain Res 1994; 99(1):84–96.

87. Schnitzler A, Benecke R. The silent period after transcranial magnetic stimulation is of exclusive cortical origin: evidence from isolated cortical ischemic lesions in man. Neurosci Lett 1994; 180(1):41–45.

88. Liepert J, Storch P, Fritsch A, Weiller C. Motor cortex disinhibition in acute stroke. Clin Neurophysiol 2000; 111(4):671–676.

89. Lee LJ, Kidwell CS, Alger J, Starkman S, Saver JL. Impact on stroke subtype diagnosis of early diffusion-weighted magnetic resonance imaging and magnetic resonance angiography. Stroke 2000; 31(5):1081–1089.

90. Hossmann KA. Viability thresholds and the penumbra of focal ischemia [see comments]. Ann Neurol 1994; 36(4):557–565.

91. Heiss WD, Huber M, Fink GR, Herholz K, Pietrzyk U, Wagner R, et al. Progressive derangement of periinfarct viable tissue in ischemic stroke. J Cereb Blood Flow Metab 1992; 12(2):193–203.

92. Mohr JP, Foulkes MA, Polis AT, Hier DB, Kase CS, Price TR, et al. Infarct topography and hemiparesis profiles with cerebral convexity infarction: the Stroke Data Bank. J Neurol Neurosurg Psychiatry 1993; 56(4):344–351.

93. Hossmann KA, Fischer M, Bockhorst K, Hoehn-Berlage M. NMR imaging of the apparent diffusion coefficient (ADC) for the evaluation of metabolic suppression and recovery after prolonged cerebral ischemia. J Cereb Blood Flow Metab 1994; 14(5):723–731.

94. Li F, Liu KF, Silva MD, Omae T, Sotak CH, Fenstermacher JD, et al. Transient and permanent resolution of ischemic lesions on diffusion-weighted imaging after brief periods of focal ischemia in rats: correlation with histopathology. Stroke 2000; 31(4):946–954.

95. Brunberg JA, Frey KA, Horton JA, Kuhl DE. Crossed cerebellar diaschisis: occurrence and resolution demonstrated with PET during carotid temporary balloon occlusion [see comments]. Am J Neuroradiol 1992; 13(1):58–61.

96. Hakim AM, Pokrupa RP, Villanueva J, Diksic M, Evans AC, Thompson CJ, et al. The effect of spontaneous reperfusion on metabolic function in early human cerebral infarcts. Ann Neurol 1987; 21(3):279–289.

97. Heiss WD, Grond M, Thiel A, von Stockhausen HM, Rudolf J. Ischaemic brain tissue salvaged from infarction with alteplase [letter]. Lancet 1997; 349(9065): 1599–1600.

98. Ringelstein EB, Biniek R, Weiller C, Ammeling B, Nolte PN, Thron A. Type and extent of hemispheric brain infarctions and clinical outcome in early and delayed middle cerebral artery recanalization. Neurology 1992; 42(2):289–298.

99. Toni D, Fiorelli M, Bastianello S, Falcou A, Sette G, Ceschin V, et al. Acute ischemic strokes improving during the first 48 hours of onset: predictability, outcome,

and possible mechanisms. A comparison with early deteriorating strokes. Stroke 1997; 28(1):10–14.

100. Toni D, Fiorelli M, Zanette EM, Sacchetti ML, Salerno A, Argentino C, et al. Early spontaneous improvement and deterioration of ischemic stroke patients. A serial study with transcranial Doppler ultrasonography. Stroke 1998; 29(6):1144–1148.

101. Heiss WD, Grond M, Thiel A, von Stockhausen HM, Rudolf J, Ghaemi M, et al. Tissue at risk of infarction rescued by early reperfusion: a positron emission tomography study in systemic recombinant tissue plasminogen activator thrombolysis of acute stroke. J Cereb Blood Flow Metab 1998; 18(12):1298–1307.

102. Kidwell CS, Saver JL, Mattiello J, Starkman S, Vinuela F, Duckwiler G, et al. Thrombolytic reversal of acute human cerebral ischemic injury shown by diffusion/perfusion magnetic resonance imaging. Ann Neurol 2000; 47(4):462–469.

103. Alexandrov AV, Demchuk AM, Felberg RA, Christou I, Barber PA, Burgin WS, et al. High rate of complete recanalization and dramatic clinical recovery during tPA infusion when continuously monitored with 2-MHz transcranial doppler monitoring. Stroke 2000; 31(3):610–614.

104. Jander S, Kraemer M, Schroeter M, Witte OW, Stoll G. Lymphocytic infiltration and expression of intercellular adhesion molecule-1 in photochemically induced ischemia of the rat cortex. J Cereb Blood Flow Metab 1995; 15(1):42–51.

105. Barone FC, Feuerstein GZ, Inflammatory mediators and stroke: new opportunities for novel therapeutics. J. Cereb Blood Flow Metab 1999; 19(8):819–834.

106. Jean WC, Spellman SR, Nussbaum ES, Low WC. Reperfusion injury after focal cerebral ischemia: the role of inflammation and the therapeutic horizon. Neurosurgery 1998; 43(6):1382–1396.

107. Jander S, Sitzer M, Schumann R, Schroeter M, Siebler M, Steinmetz H, et al. Inflammation in high-grade carotid stenosis: a possible role for macrophages and T cells in plaque destabilization. Stroke 1998; 29(8):1625–1630.

108. Sitzer M, Muller W, Siebler M, Hort W, Kniemeyer HW, Jancke L, et al. Plaque ulceration and lumen thrombus are the main sources of cerebral microemboli in high-grade internal carotid artery stenosis. Stroke 1995; 26(7):1231–1233.

109. Sette G, Baron JC, Young AR, Miyazawa H, Tillet I, Barre L, et al. In vivo mapping of brain benzodiazepine receptor changes by positron emission tomography after focal ischemia in the anesthetized baboon. Stroke 1993; 24(12):2046–2057.

110. Marchal G, Young AR, Baron JC. Early postischemic hyperperfusion: pathophysiologic insights from positron emission tomography. J Cereb Blood Flow Metab 1999; 19(5):467–482.

111. Schulz JB, Weller M, Moskowitz MA. Caspases as treatment targets in stroke and neurodegenerative diseases. Ann Neurol 1999; 45(4):421–429.

112. Weiller C, Ringelstein EB, Reiche W, Thron A, Buell U. The large striatocapsular infarct. A clinical and pathophysiological entity. Arch Neurol 1990; 47(10):1085–1091.

113. Neumann-Haefelin T, Wittsack HJ, Wenserski F, Siebler M, Seitz RJ, Modder U, et al. Diffusion- and perfusion-weighted MRI. The DWI/PWI mismatch region in acute stroke. Stroke 1999; 30(8):1591–1597.

114. Rordorf G, Koroshetz WJ, Copen WA, Cramer SC, Schaefer PW, Budzik RF Jr, et al. Regional ischemia and ischemic injury in patients with acute middle cerebral

artery stroke as defined by early diffusion-weighted and perfusion-weighted MRI. Stroke 1998; 29(5):939–943.

115. Wittsack HJ, Ritzl A, Fink GR, Wenserski F, Siebler M, Seitz RJ, Modder U, Freund HJ. MR Imaging in Acute Stroke: Diffusion-weighted and Perfusion Imaging Parameters for Predicting Infarct Size. Radiology 2002; 222(2):397–403.

116. Beaulieu C, de Crespigny A, Tong DC, Moseley ME, Albers GW, Marks MP. Longitudinal magnetic resonance imaging study of perfusion and diffusion in stroke: evolution of lesion volume and correlation with clinical outcome [see comments]. Ann Neurol 1999; 46(4):568–578.

117. Schwamm LH, Koroshetz WJ, Sorensen AG, Wang B, Copen WA, Budzik R, et al. Time course of lesion development in patients with acute stroke: serial diffusion- and hemodynamic-weighted magnetic resonance imaging. Stroke 1998; 29(11): 2268–2276.

118. Neumann-Haefelin T, Wittsack HJ, Fink GR, Wenserski F, Li TQ, Seitz RJ, et al. Diffusion- and perfusion-weighted MRI: influence of severe carotid artery stenosis on the DWI/PWI mismatch in acute stroke. Stroke 2000; 31(6):1311–1317.

119. Baird AE, Benfield A, Schlaug G, Siewert B, Lovblad KO, Edelman RR, et al. Enlargement of human cerebral ischemic lesion volumes measured by diffusion-weighted magnetic resonance imaging [see comments]. Ann Neurol 1997; 41(5): 581–589.

120. Vogel J, Hermes A, Kuschinsky W. Evolution of microcirculatory disturbances after permanent middle cerebral artery occlusion in rats. J Cereb Blood Flow Metab 1999; 19(12):1322–1328.

121. van Everdingen KJ, Visser GH, Klijn CJ, Kappelle LJ, van der GJ. Role of collateral flow on cerebral hemodynamics in patients with unilateral internal carotid artery occlusion [see comments]. Ann Neurol 1998; 44(2):167–176.

122. Powers WJ. Hemodynamics and metabolism in ischemic cerebrovascular disease. Neurol Clin 1992; 10(1):31–48.

123. Sette G, Baron JC, Mazoyer B, Levasseur M, Pappata S, Crouzel C. Local brain haemodynamics and oxygen metabolism in cerebrovascular disease. Positron emission tomography. Brain 1989; 112(Pt 4):931–951.

124. Henderson RD, Eliasziw M, Fox AJ, Rothwell PM, Barnett HJ. Angiographically defined collateral circulation and risk of stroke in patients with severe carotid artery stenosis. North American Symptomatic Carotid Endarterectomy Trial (NASCET) Group. Stroke 2000; 31(1):128–132.

125. Reichenbach JR, Rother J, Jonetz-Mentzel L, Herzau M, Fiala A, Weiller C, et al. Acute stroke evaluated by time-to-peak mapping during initial and early follow-up perfusion CT studies. Am J Neuroradiol 1999; 20(10):1842–1850.

126. Ostergaard L, Smith DF, Vestergaard-Poulsen P, Hansen SB, Gee AD, Gjedde A, et al. Absolute cerebral blood flow and blood volume measured by magnetic resonance imaging bolus tracking: comparison with positron emission tomography values. J Cereb Blood Flow Metab 1998; 18(4):425–432.

127. Rempp KA, Brix G, Wenz F, Becker CR, Guckel F, Lorenz WJ. Quantification of regional cerebral blood flow and volume with dynamic susceptibility contrast-enhanced MR imaging. Radiology 1994; 193(3):637–641.

128. Schlaug G, Benfield A, Baird AE, Siewert B, Lovblad KO, Parker RA, et al. The

ischemic penumbra: operationally defined by diffusion and perfusion MRI. Neurology 1999; 53(7):1528–1537.

129. Feeney DM, Baron JC. Diaschisis. Stroke 1986; 17(5):817–830.
130. Seitz RJ, Schlaug G, Kleinschmidt A, Knorr U, Nebeling B, Wirrwar A, et al. Remote depressions of cerebral metabolism in hemiparetic stroke: topography and relation to motor and somatosensory functions. Hum Brain Mapping 1994; 1:81–100.
131. von Giesen HJ, Schlaug G, Steinmetz H, Benecke R, Freund HJ, Seitz RJ. Cerebral network underlying unilateral motor neglect: evidence from positron emission tomography. J Neurol Sci 1994; 125(1):29–38.
132. Serrati C, Marchal G, Rioux P, Viader F, Petit-Taboue MC, Lochon P, et al. Contralateral cerebellar hypometabolism: a predictor for stroke outcome? J Neurol Neurosurg Psychiatry 1994; 57(2):174–179.
133. Juhasz C, Kamondi A, Szirmai I. Spectral EEG analysis following hemispheric stroke: evidences of transhemispheric diaschisis. Acta Neurol Scand 1997; 96(6):397–400.
134. Rossini PM, Tecchio F, Pizzella V, Lupoi D, Cassetta E, Pasqualetti P, et al. On the reorganization of sensory hand areas after mono-hemispheric lesion: a functional (MEG)/anatomical (MRI) integrative study. Brain Res 1998; 782(1–2):153–166.
135. Siebler M, Nachtmann A, Neumann-Haefelin T, Steinmetz H, Wittsack H-J, Theiss S. Interhemispheric EEG synchronization in acute stroke patients. In press.
136. Mori S, Sadoshima S, Ibayashi S, Lino K, Fujishima M. Relation of cerebral blood flow to motor and cognitive functions in chronic stroke patients. Stroke 1994; 25(2):309–317.
137. Platz T, Denzler P, Kaden B, Mauritz KH. Motor learning after recovery from hemiparesis. Neuropsychologia 1994; 32(10):1209–1223.
138. Weder B, Seitz RJ. Deficient cerebral activation pattern in stroke recovery. Neuroreport 1994; 5(4):457–460.
139. Heiss WD, Emunds HG, Herholz K. Cerebral glucose metabolism as a predictor of rehabilitation after ischemic stroke. Stroke 1993; 24(12):1784–1788.
140. Schmidt R, Fazekas F, Koch M, Kapeller P, Augustin M, Offenbacher H, et al. Magnetic resonance imaging cerebral abnormalities and neuropsychologic test performance in elderly hypertensive subjects. A case-control study. Arch Neurol 1995; 52(9):905–910.
141. Brain Mapping. The Systems. Toga AW, Mazziotta JC (eds.). San Diego: Academic Press, 2000.
142. Price CJ, Friston KJ. Scanning patients with tasks they can perform. Hum Brain Mapping 1999; 8(2–3):102–108.
143. Merzenich MM, Sameshima K. Cortical plasticity and memory. Curr Opinion Neurobiol 1993; 3:187–196.
144. Pons TP, Garraghty PE, Mishkin M. Lesion-induced plasticity in the second somatosensory cortex of adult macaques. Proc Natl Acad Sci USA 1988; 85(14):5279–5281.
145. Nudo RJ, Wise BM, SiFuentes F, Milliken GW. Neural substrates for the effects of rehabilitative training on motor recovery after ischemic infarct [see comments]. Science 1996; 272(5269):1791–1794.

146. Chollet F, DiPiero V, Wise RJ, Brooks DJ, Dolan RJ, Frackowiak RS. The functional anatomy of motor recovery after stroke in humans: a study with positron emission tomography. Ann Neurol 1991; 29(1):63–71.

147. Weiller C, Chollet F, Friston KJ, Wise RJ, Frackowiak RS. Functional reorganization of the brain in recovery from striatocapsular infarction in man. Ann Neurol 1992; 31(5):463–472.

148. Marshall RS, Perera GM, Lazar RM, Krakauer JW, Constantine RC, DeLaPaz RL. Evolution of cortical activation during recovery from corticospinal tract infarction. Stroke 2000; 31(3):656–661.

149. Weder B, Knorr U, Herzog H, Nebeling B, Kleinschmidt A, Huang Y, et al. Tactile exploration of shape after subcortical ischaemic infarction studied with PET. Brain 1994; 117(Pt 3):593–605.

150. Roland PE, Larsen B, Lassen NA, Skinhoj E. Supplementary motor area and other cortical areas in organization of voluntary movements in man. J Neurophysiol 1980; 43(1):118–136.

151. Stephan KM, Fink GR, Passingham RE, Silbersweig D, Ceballos-Baumann AO, Frith CD, et al. Functional anatomy of the mental representation of upper extremity movements of healthy subjects. J Neurophysiol 1995; 73(1):373–386.

152. Seitz RJ, Canavan AG, Yaguez L, Herzog H, Tellmann L, Knorr U, et al. Representations of graphomotor trajectories in the human parietal cortex: evidence for controlled processing and automatic performance. Eur J Neurosci 1997; 9(2):378–389.

153. Weiller C, Ramsay SC, Wise RJ, Friston KJ, Frackowiak RS. Individual patterns of functional reorganization in the human cerebral cortex after capsular infarction. Ann Neurol 1993; 33(2):181–189.

154. Honda M, Nagamine T, Fukuyama H, Yonekura Y, Kimura J, Shibasaki H. Movement-related cortical potentials and regional cerebral blood flow change in patients with stroke after motor recovery. J Neurol Sci 1997; 146(2):117–126.

155. Seitz RJ, Huang Y, Knorr U, Tellmann L, Herzog H, Freund HJ. Large-scale plasticity of the human motor cortex. Neuroreport 1995; 6(5):742–744.

156. Wunderlich G, Knorr U, Herzog H, Kiwit JC, Freund HJ, Seitz RJ. Precentral glioma location determines the displacement of cortical hand representation. Neurosurgery 1998; 42(1):18–26.

157. Seitz RJ, Azari NP. Cerebral reorganization in man after acquired lesions. Adv Neurol 1999; 81:37–47.

158. Traversa R, Cicinelli P, Bassi A, Rossini PM, Bernardi G. Mapping of motor cortical reorganization after stroke. A brain stimulation study with focal magnetic pulses. Stroke 1997; 28(1):110–117.

159. Powers WJ, Fox PT, Raichle ME. The effect of carotid artery disease on the cerebrovascular response to physiologic stimulation. Neurology 1988; 38(9):1475–1478.

160. Cholet N, Seylaz J, Lacombe P, Bonvento G. Local uncoupling of the cerebrovascular and metabolic responses to somatosensory stimulation after neuronal nitric oxide synthase inhibition. J Cereb Blood Flow Metab 1997; 17(11):1191–1201.

161. Binkofski F, Buccino G, Posse S, Seitz RJ, Rizzolatti G, Freund H. A fronto-parietal circuit for object manipulation in man: evidence from an fMRI-study. Eur J Neurosci 1999; 11(9):3276–3286.

162. Dettmers C, Fink GR, Lemon RN, Stephan KM, Passingham RE, Silbersweig D, et al. Relation between cerebral activity and force in the motor areas of the human brain. J Neurophysiol 1995; 74(2):802–815.
163. Dettmers C, Stephan KM, Lemon RN, Frackowiak RSJ. Reorganization of the executive motor system after stroke. Cerebrovasc Dis 1997; 7:187–200.
164. Jahanshahi M, Jenkins IH, Brown RG, Marsden CD, Passingham RE, Brooks DJ. Self-initiated versus externally triggered movements. I. An investigation using measurement of regional cerebral blood flow with PET and movement-related potentials in normal and Parkinson's disease subjects [see comments]. Brain 1995; 118 (Pt 4):913–933.
165. MacKinnon CD, Kapur S, Hussey D, Verrier MC, Houle S, Tatton WG. Contributions of the mesial frontal cortex to the premovement potentials associated with intermittent hand movements in humans. Hum Brain Mapping 1996; 4:1–22.
166. Freund HJ, Hummelsheim H. Lesions of premotor cortex in man. Brain 1985; 108(Pt 3):697–733.
167. Fisher CM. Concerning the mechanism of recovery in stroke hemiplegia. Can J Neurol Sci 1992; 19(1):57–63.
168. Cao Y, D'Olhaberriague L, Vikingstad EM, Levine SR, Welch KM. Pilot study of functional MRI to assess cerebral activation of motor function after poststroke hemiparesis. Stroke 1998; 29(1):112–122.
169. Durwen HF, Herzog AG. Electromyographic investigation of mirror movements in normal adults. Variation of frequency with side of movements, handedness, and dominance. Brain Dysfunct 1989; 2:84–92.
170. Durwen HF, Herzog AG. Electromyographic investigation of mirror movements in normal adults. Variation of frequency with site, effort and repetition of movements. Brain Dysfunct 1992; 5:310–318.
171. Turton A, Wroe S, Trepte N, Fraser C, Lemon RN. Contralateral and ipsilateral EMG responses to transcranial magnetic stimulation during recovery of arm and hand function after stroke. Electroencephalogr Clin Neurophysiol 1996; 101(4): 316–328.
172. Netz J, Lammers T, Homberg V. Reorganization of motor output in the non-affected hemisphere after stroke. Brain 1997; 120(Pt 9):1579–1586.
173. Zülch KJ, Müller N. Associated Movements in Man. Amsterdam: Elsevier, 1969, pp 404–426.
174. Hopf HC, Schlegel HJ, Lowitzsch K. Irradiation of voluntary activity to the contralateral side in movements of normal subjects and patients with central motor disturbances. Eur Neurol 1974; 12(3):142–147.
175. Aizawa H, Mushiake H, Inase M, Tanji J. An output zone of the monkey primary motor cortex specialized for bilateral hand movement. Exp Brain Res 1990; 82(1): 219–221.
176. Cramer SC, Finklestein SP, Schaechter JD, Bush G, Rosen BR. Activation of distinct motor cortex regions during ipsilateral and contralateral finger movements. J Neurophysiol 1999; 81(1):383–387.
177. Farmer SF, Harrison LM, Ingram DA, Stephens JA. Plasticity of central motor pathways in children with hemiplegic cerebral palsy. Neurology 1991; 41(9):1505–1510.

178. Lewine JD, Astur RS, Davis LE, Knight JE, Maclin EL, Orrison WW Jr. Cortical organization in adulthood is modified by neonatal infarct: a case study. Radiology 1994; 190(1):93–96.

179. Lemon RN, Johansson RS, Westling G. Modulation of corticospinal influence over hand muscles during gripping tasks in man and monkey. Can J Physiol Pharmacol 1996; 74(4):547–558.

180. Jones RD, Donaldson IM, Parkin PJ. Impairment and recovery of ipsilateral sensory-motor function following unilateral cerebral infarction. Brain 1989; 112(Pt 1):113–132.

181. Rossini PM, Caltagirone C, Castriota-Scanderbeg A, Cicinelli P, Del Gratta C, Demartin M, et al. Hand motor cortical area reorganization in stroke: a study with fMRI, MEG and TCS maps. Neuroreport 1998; 9(9):2141–2146.

182. Knopman DS, Rubens AB, Selnes OA, Klassen AC, Meyer MW. Mechanisms of recovery from aphasia: evidence from serial xenon 133 cerebral blood flow studies. Ann Neurol 1984; 15(6):530–535.

183. Karbe H, Kessler J, Herholz K, Fink GR, Heiss WD. Long-term prognosis of poststroke aphasia studied with positron emission tomography. Arch Neurol 1995; 52(2):186–190.

184. Weiller C, Isensee C, Rijntjes M, Huber W, Muller S, Bier D, et al. Recovery from Wernicke's aphasia: a positron emission tomographic study. Ann Neurol 1995; 37(6):723–732.

185. Schlaug G, Knorr U, Seitz R. Inter-subject variability of cerebral activations in acquiring a motor skill: a study with positron emission tomography. Exp Brain Res 1994; 98(3):523–534.

186. Jenkins IH, Brooks DJ, Nixon PD, Frackowiak RS, Passingham RE. Motor sequence learning: a study with positron emission tomography. J Neurosci 1994; 14(6):3775–3790.

187. Seitz RJ, Roland PE. Learning of sequential finger movements in man: a combined kinematic and positron emission tomography study. Eur J Neurosci 1992; 4:154–165.

188. Muller F, Kunesch E, Binkofski F, Freund HJ. Residual sensorimotor functions in a patient after right-sided hemispherectomy. Neuropsychologia 1991; 29(2):125–145.

189. Sabatini U, Toni D, Pantano P, Brughitta G, Padovani A, Bozzao L, et al. Motor recovery after early brain damage. A case of brain plasticity. Stroke 1994; 25(2):514–517.

190. Feys H, Van Hees J, Bruyninckx F, Mercelis R, De Weerdt W. Value of somatosensory and motor evoked potentials in predicting arm recovery after a stroke. J Neurol Neurosurg Psychiatry 2000; 68(3):323–331.

191. Naito E, Ehrsson HH, Geyer S, Zilles K, Roland PE. Illusory arm movements activate cortical motor areas: a positron emission tomography study. J Neurosci 1999; 19(14):6134–6144.

192. Xerri C, Merzenich MM, Peterson BE, Jenkins W. Plasticity of primary somatosensory cortex paralleling sensorimotor skill recovery from stroke in adult monkeys. J Neurophysiol 1998; 79(4):2119–2148.

193. Taub E, Uswatte G, Pidikiti R. Constraint-induced movement therapy: a new family

of techniques with broad application to physical rehabilitation—a clinical review [see comments]. J Rehabil Res Dev 1999; 36(3):237–251.

194. Liepert J, Miltner WH, Bauder H, Sommer M, Dettmers C, Taub E, et al. Motor cortex plasticity during constraint-induced movement therapy in stroke patients. Neurosci Lett 1998; 250(1):5–8.
195. Nelles G, Spiekramann G, Jueptner M, Leonhardt G, Muller S, Gerhard H, et al. Evolution of functional reorganization in hemiplegic stroke: a serial positron emission tomographic activation study. Ann Neurol 1999; 46(6):901–909.
196. Nudo RJ, Friel KM, Delia SW. Role of sensory deficits in motor impairments after injury to primary motor cortex. Neuropharmacology 2000; 39(5):733–742.
197. Clark RE, Delay ER. Reduction of lesion-induced deficits in visual reversal learning following cross-modal training. Restor Neurol Neurosci 1991; 3:247–255.
198. Neville HJ, Bavelier D. Neural organization and plasticity of language. Curr Opin Neurobiol 1998; 8(2):254–258.
199. Cohen LG, Celnik P, Pascual-Leone A, Corwell B, Falz L, Dambrosia J, et al. Functional relevance of cross-modal plasticity in blind humans. Nature 1997; 389(6647):180–183.
200. Sadato N, Pascual-Leone A, Grafman J, Deiber MP, Ibanez V, Hallett M. Neural networks for Braille reading by the blind [see comments]. Brain 1998; 121(Pt 7): 1213–1229.
201. von Monakow C. Lokalisation im Gehirn und funktionelle Störungen induziert durch kortikale Läsionen. Wiesbaden, Germany: Bergmann, J.F., 1914.
202. Heilman KM, Valenstein E, Watson RT. The Neglect Syndrome. Clinical Neuropsychology. Amsterdam: Elsevier, 1985, pp 153–183.
203. Freund H-J. The apraxias. In: Asbury AK, Mckhann GM, McDonald WI, eds. Diseases of the Nervous System. Philadelphia: Saunders, 1994, pp 751–767.
204. Barton JJ, Sharpe JA, Raymond JE. Retinotopic and directional defects in motion discrimination in humans with cerebral lesions. Ann Neurol 1995; 37(5):665–675.
205. Classen J, Kunesch E, Binkofski F, Hilperath F, Schlaug G, Seitz RJ, et al. Subcortical origin of visuomotor apraxia [published erratum appears in Brain 1996; 119 (Pt 2):697]. Brain 1995; 118(Pt 6):1365–1374.
206. Hier DB, Mondlock J, Caplan LR. Recovery of behavioral abnormalities after right hemisphere stroke. Neurology 1983; 33(3):345–350.
207. Kertesz A, Ferro JM. Lesion size and location in ideomotor apraxia. Brain 1984; 107(Pt 3):921–933.
208. Basso A, Capitani E, Della SS, Laiacona M, Spinnler H. Recovery from ideomotor apraxia. A study on acute stroke patients. Brain 1987; 110(Pt 3):747–760.
209. Pedersen PM, Jorgensen HS, Nakayama H, Raaschou HO, Olsen TS. Hemineglect in acute stroke—incidence and prognostic implications. The Copenhagen Stroke Study. Am J Phys Med Rehabil 1997; 76(2):122–127.
210. Cassidy TP, Lewis S, Gray CS. Recovery from visuospatial neglect in stroke patients. J Neurol Neurosurg Psychiatry 1998; 64(4):555–557.
211. Jehkonen M, Ahonen JP, Dastidar P, Koivisto AM, Laippala P, Vilkki J, et al. Visual neglect as a predictor of functional outcome one year after stroke. Acta Neurol Scand 2000; 101(3):195–201.
212. Poeck K, De Bleser R, von Keyserlingk DG. Neurolinguistic status and localization

of lesion in aphasic patients with exclusively consonant-vowel recurring utterances. Brain 1984; 107(Pt 1):199–217.

213. Ojemann G, Ojemann J, Lettich E, Berger M. Cortical language localization in left, dominant hemisphere. An electrical stimulation mapping investigation in 117 patients. J Neurosurg 1989; 71(3):316–326.

214. Alexander MP, Naeser MA, Palumbo C. Broca's area aphasias: aphasia after lesions including the frontal operculum. Neurology 1990; 40(2):353–362.

215. Friel KM, Nudo RJ. Recovery of motor function after focal cortical injury in primates: compensatory movement patterns used during rehabilitative training. Somatosens Mot Res 1998; 15(3):173–189.

216. Binkofski F, Seitz RJ, Kunesch E, Dohle C, Freund H-J. Tactile apraxia. Unimodal apractic disorder of tactile exploration associated with parietal lobe lessions. Brain 2001; 124:132–144.

217. Sato KC, Tanji J. Digit-muscle responses evoked from multiple intracortical foci in monkey precentral motor cortex. J Neurophysiol 1989; 62(4):959–970.

218. Schieber MH, Hibbard LS. How somatotopic is the motor cortex hand area? Science 1993; 261(5120):489–492.

219. Sanes JN, Donoghue JP, Thangaraj V, Edelman RR, Warach S. Shared neural substrates controlling hand movements in human motor cortex [see comments]. Science 1995; 268(5218):1775–1777.

220. Sutherling WW, Levesque MF, Baumgartner C. Cortical sensory representation of the human hand: size of finger regions and nonoverlapping digit somatotopy. Neurology 1992; 42(5):1020–1028.

221. Zihl J, von Cramon D. Visual field recovery from scotoma in patients with postgeniculate damage. A review of 55 cases. Brain 1985; 108(Pt 2):335–365.

222. Pommerenke K, Markowitsch HJ. Rehabilitation training of homonymous visual field defects in patients with postgeniculate damage of the visual system. Restor Neurol Neurosci 1989; 1:47–63.

223. Dubowitz V. Muscle Disorders in Childhood. London: Saunders, 1978.

224. Marsden CD. The mystery of the basal ganglia. The Robert Wartenberg Lecture. Neurology 1982; 32, 514–539.

225. Schneider JS, Diamond SG, Markham CH. Parkinson's disease: sensory and motor problems in arms and hands. Neurology 1987; 37(6):951–956.

226. Montgomery EB, Jr., Nuessen J, Gorman DS. Reaction time and movement velocity abnormalities in Parkinson's disease under different task conditions. Neurology 1991; 41(9):1476–1481.

227. Schiene K, Bruehl C, Zilles K, Qu M, Hagemann G, Kraemer M et al. Neuronal hyperexcitability and reduction of GABAA-receptor expression in the surround of cerebral photothrombosis. J Cereb Blood Flow Metab 1996; 16(5):906–914.

228. Hagemann G, Redecker C, Neumann-Haefelin T, Freund HJ, Witte OW. Increased long-term potentiation in the surround of experimentally induced focal cortical infarction [see comments]. Ann Neurol 1998; 44(2):255–258.

229. Schroeter M, Franke C, Stoll G, Hoehn M. Dynamic changes of magnetic resonance imaging abnormalities in relation to inflammation and glial responses after photothrombotic cerebral infarction in the rat brain. Acta Neuropathol (Berl) 2001; 101(2):114–122.

230. Hatazawa J, Satoh T, Shimosegawa E, Okudera T, Inugami A, Ogawa T, et al. Evaluation of cerebral infarction with iodine 123-iomazenil SPECT. J Nucl Med 1995; 36(12):2154–2161.

231. Hayashida K, Hirose Y, Tanaka Y, Miyashita K, Ishida Y, Miyake Y, et al. Reduction of ^{123}I-iomazenil uptake in haemodynamically and metabolically impaired brain areas in patients with cerebrovascular disease. Nucl Med Commun 1996; 17(8): 701–705.

232. Takahashi W, Ohnuki Y, Ohta T, Hamano H, Yamamoto M, Shinohara Y. Mechanism of reduction of cortical blood flow in striatocapsular infarction: studies using [123]Iiomazenil SPECT. Neuroimage 1997; 6(2):75–80.

233. Heiss WD, Grond M, Thiel A, Ghaemi M, Sobesky J, Rudolf J, et al. Permanent cortical damage detected by flumazenil positron emission tomography in acute stroke. Stroke 1998; 29(2):454–461.

234. Pizzamiglio L, Perani D, Cappa SF, Vallar G, Paolucci S, Grassi F, et al. Recovery of neglect after right hemispheric damage: H2(15)O positron emission tomographic activation study. Arch Neurol 1998; 55(4):561–568.

235. Cao Y, Vikingstad EM, George KP, Johnson AF, Welch KM. Cortical language activation in stroke patients recovering from aphasia with functional MRI. Stroke 1999; 30(11):2331–2340.

236. Heiss WD, Kessler J, Thiel A, Ghaemi M, Karbe H. Differential capacity of left and right hemispheric areas for compensation of poststroke aphasia [see comments]. Ann Neurol 1999; 45(4):430–438.

237. Thulborn KR, Carpenter PA, Just MA. Plasticity of language-related brain function during recovery from stroke. Stroke 1999; 30(4):749–754.

238. Warburton E, Price CJ, Swinburn K, Wise RJ. Mechanisms of recovery from aphasia: evidence from positron emission tomography studies [see comments]. J Neurol Neurosurg Psychiatry 1999; 66(2):155–161.

239. Moore RY. Catecholamine neuron systems in brain. Ann Neurol 1982; 12(4):321–327.

240. Mesulam MM, Mufson EJ, Levey AI, Wainer BH. Cholinergic innervation of cortex by the basal forebrain: cytochemistry and cortical connections of the septal area, diagonal band nuclei, nucleus basalis (substantia innominata), and hypothalamus in the rhesus monkey. J Comp Neurol 1983; 214(2):170–197.

241. McCormick DA. Neurotransmitter actions in the thalamus and cerebral cortex and their role in neuromodulation of thalamocortical activity. Prog Neurobiol 1992; 39(4):337–388.

242. Boyeson MG, Jones JL, Harmon RL. Sparing of motor function after cortical injury. A new perspective on underlying mechanisms. Arch Neurol 1994; 51(4):405–414.

243. Feeney DM, Gonzalez A, Law WA. Amphetamine, haloperidol, and experience interact to affect rate of recovery after motor cortex injury. Science 1982; 217(4562):855–857.

244. Feeney DM, Hovda DA. Amphetamine and apomorphine restore tactile placing after motor cortex injury in the cat. Psychopharmacology (Berl) 1983; 79(1):67–71.

245. Crisostomo EA, Duncan PW, Propst M, Dawson DV, Davis JN. Evidence that amphetamine with physical therapy promotes recovery of motor function in stroke patients. Ann Neurol 1988; 23(1):94–97.

246. Lipton SA, Kater SB. Neurotransmitter regulation of neuronal outgrowth, plasticity and survival. Trends Neurosci 1989; 12(7):265–270.

247. Sutton RL, Feeney DM. Alpha-adrenergic agonists and antagonists affect recovery and maintenance of beam-walking ability after sensorimotor cortex ablation in the rat. Restor Neurol Neurosci 1992; 4:1–11.

248. Goldstein LB, Davis JN. Restorative neurology. Drugs and recovery following stroke. Stroke 1990; 21(11):1636–1640.

249. Dietz V. Locomotor training in paraplegic patients [letter; comment]. Ann Neurol 1995; 38(6):965.

250. Loubinoux I, Boulanouar K, Ranjeva JP, Carel C, Berry I, Rascol O, et al. Cerebral functional magnetic resonance imaging activation modulated by a single dose of the monoamine neurotransmission enhancers fluoxetine and fenozolone during hand sensorimotor tasks. J Cereb Blood Flow Metab 1999; 19(12):1365–1375.

251. Neumann-Haefelin T, Witte OW. Periinfarct and remote excitability changes after transient middle cerebral artery occlusion. J Cereb Blood Flow Metab 2000; 20(1): 45–52.

252. Tailarach, J., Tournoux, P. Co-planar Stereotaxic Atlas of the Human Brain. 3-Dimensional Proportional System: An Approach to Cerebral Imaging. Stuttgart, New York: Thieme Verlag, 1988.

7
Recovery from Cognitive and Behavioral Deficits

José M. Ferro and Sofia Madureira
Hospital Santa Maria, Lisbon, Portugal

I. INTRODUCTION

Cognitive and behavioral deficits are present in the majority of hemispheral stroke survivors. Although they cause significant disability, they are often overlooked or paid less attention than motor deficits. Commonly used disability scales, such as the Barthel Scale, do not consider the impact of language, cognitive, or behavioral impairments on the daily life of stroke victims. Patients afflicted with communication deficits, demented, or with behavioral disturbances pose additional difficulties for their caregivers and consequently some will end up in institutions. Many of these patients will receive speech therapy or neurocognitive rehabilitation and may need pharmacological interventions. Paradoxically, they are less likely to receive appropriate secondary prevention measures.

In this chapter recovery from deficits in individual domains will be presented, focusing on data from follow-up series. Transcranial Doppler (TCD), SPECT, PET, and fMRI performed during the recovery process have been instrumental in improving our understanding of the intra- and interhemispheric mechanisms underlying recovery.

II. RECOVERY FROM APHASIA

About one-third of acute stroke patients are aphasic (1). Aphasia has an adverse influence on functional outcome (2), mood (3), quality of life (4,5), and ability to return to work. Most studies on the natural recovery of language deficits after stroke were carried out in the 1970s and 1980s (6–18). We will briefly review several aspects of recovery from aphasia, namely its time course, the influence of biographical (age, gender, education, handedness), language (aphasia type and language components), and lesion factors (etiology, location, size).

A. The Recovery Curves of Stroke Aphasia

Almost all studies agree that most of the recovery takes place during the first 1– 3 months. Within the first month the greatest improvement was observed during the first 2 weeks after onset (18). After the first 3 months there will be some improvement up to 6 and not so frequently up to 12 months post onset (19,20). After 1 year very little, if any, spontaneous recovery is to be expected and language proficiency may even decline later (21). About 40% of acute aphasics eventually recover completely or almost completely in 12 months (8). In the Copenhagen Stroke study (1) (one of the few community studies on the recovery of aphasia), the percentage of aphasic patients dropped from 38% at the time of admission to 18% at discharge. The remission curve was steep: stationary language function was reached within 2 weeks for those with initial mild aphasia, within 6 weeks for those with moderate aphasia, and within 10 weeks for those with severe aphasia.

B. Biographical Factors: Gender, Handedness, Education, Age

Some studies state that females recover better than males in oral production (22) and auditory comprehension (23), but no gender differences were noticed in the majority of other series. Left-handers, ambidextrous persons, and those with a familial story of left-handedness are more likely to have a bilateral representation of language. They might also have a better recovery than right-handers. However, the evidence for such claims is rather limited (24,25). Atypical skull asymmetries (large left frontal or right occipital torque) were associated with a better prognosis in one study (26), but this was not confirmed by subsequent investigations (27,28). It is often stated that higher education might be a favorable prognostic factor. Again the evidence for that is scarce and the opposite may even be true (15). There is no evidence for a relationship between IQ and language recovery (29).

Aphasia secondary to stroke in children recovers much better than in adults and often completely (30). The upper age limit of this superior recovery in younger patients is not known. Although some series failed to show an association between the intensity of improvement and age, at least five studies that compared language recovery in young and older stroke patients demonstrated that young and middle-aged (6,31–34) aphasic stroke patients have a better recovery than older aphasics. A different distribution of infarcts with age (35), decreased cerebral plasticity, and subclinical dementia with limited capacity for learning are plausible explanations for this difference.

C. Motivational and Emotional Factors

Motivational factors are also important in the recovery and in the rehabilitation process. Several studies (36,37) indicate that poststroke mood and anxiety disorders have a negative influence on outcome. It seems likely that depression may impact the patient's recovery from aphasia and aphasia may impact on the severity and duration of depression.

D. Language Factors: Severity, Type of Aphasia, and Language Components

Severity of aphasia at first evaluation correlates with and is a significant indicator of the intensity of the residual permanent deficit (1,10,15). Statistical prediction of outcome based on initial severity is possible using multiple regression (38) or connectionist networks (39). Type of aphasia is a major determinant of the outcome and of the pattern of evolution (8–10,15). Broadly speaking, anomic and conduction aphasia syndromes have the better outcome, transcortical and Broca's aphasia a intermediate prognosis, while Wernicke's and global aphasia have a worse prognosis.

Severe nonfluent aphasia recovers to less severe forms of nonfluent aphasia and eventually to anomic aphasia or dysarthria/dysprosody, but not to fluent aphasia. From a transient period of muteness and anarthria the patient starts producing steretyped utterances and emotional expressions. The utterances differentiate by intonation following communication intent and become more varied. If recovery continues, agrammatical speech follows. The initiation of word production may be hampered by oral apraxia. Eventually, only hesitancy in word finding and minor syntactical or phonological errors can be noticed.

Similarly, severe Wernicke's aphasia usually evolves to transcortical sensory, anomic, or, less often, conduction type. From a copious neologistic jargon with anosognosia, the patient improves to a lower-frequency semantic jargon and eventually to anomia with occasional paraphasias.

Of the four major components of the classic aphasic syndromes, comprehension usually shows the more rapid and complete recovery, at least for everyday communication and simple tasks such as word comprehension, yes-no questions, and sequential commands. Repetition also improves faster. Naming and fluency recovery curves are slower and often incomplete. The percentage of patients improving in comprehension is higher than in production. Similarly, more patients improve in oral language than in written language.

E. Lesion Factors: Type, Location, and Size

Aphasia secondary to intracerebral hemorrhage usually recovers better than that due to infarcts of similar size (19). After deep intracerebral hemorrhages (40–42), recovery goes along with the disappearance of diaschisis and the improvement of cortical hypoperfusion and hypometabolism (43,44). Following left putaminal hemorrhage patients with fluent speech are likely to have a better outcome than patients who are initially nonfluent (42). In lobar hemorrhages (45), improvement of aphasia follows reabsorption of the hematoma. The residual language deficit should be correlated with the remaining lesion after the absorption of the hematoma. After a hemorrhagic stroke, the residual lesion is much smaller than the initial hematoma; it usually spares the cortex and it is of smaller size than an infarct causing an aphasia of similar acute severity.

Following subarachnoid haemorrhage, aphasia can be due to delayed cerebral ischemia or to lesions related to the surgical or neuroradiological intervention. Language deficits are more frequent after middle cerebral artery or posterior communicating aneurysms (46). Language deficits after subarachnoid haemorrhage show wide variation in recovery rate, because improvement is influenced by the number, location, and size of infarcts on relevant anatomical structures (47). Language deficits that are not related to cerebral infarcts are in general due to cortical hypoperfusion and usually recover well.

Little information is available on recovery of aphasia following cerebral vein thrombosis (48,49), but in general its prognosis is very favorable because the language deficit is usually due to edema or hemorrhagic lesions.

Lesion size had an inverse correlation with the improvement rate (10,13,14,28), the highest negative correlation being found with the recovery of fluency (10), while comprehension recovery may even have a positive correlation with lesion size. Actually, even patients with extremely large middle cerebral artery cortical-subcortical infarcts recover their verbal comprehension to some extent and are able to understand verbal emotional expressions, single spoken or written words, and some one-step commands. A PET study indicated that metabolic activity in left hemispheric (LH) speech-relevant brain regions measured early after stroke was a predictor of the outcome of aphasia, when evaluated by the Token test and a word fluency task (50).

The relationship between lesion location and aphasia recovery is rather complex and should be considered separately for each individual aphasic syndrome. To determine the role of a particular area for aphasia recovery, the evolution of positive (with damage to that area) and negative (with that area spared) cases should be examined and longitudinally investigated. The interaction between damage to different areas, the cumulative effect of simultaneous damage to more than one area, and the fact that vascular lesions have some topographical restrictions, as they are confined to the vascular territories, must be considered (51,52). When founded only on linguistic-radiological correlations of a single case or small case series of chronic patients, statements that certain areas are critical to the recovery of particular linguistic functions should be read with caution.

Several longitudinal studies demonstrated the crucial role of the anatomical areas surrounding and connected to the classic language areas in the recovery process. An infarct limited to Broca's area generally produces a nonfluent aphasia with a good prognosis (53). However, if the infarct also involves the insulae, the rolandic operculum, the white matter underlying Broca's area, or the anterior striatum, the likelihood of complete recovery decreases. Large prerolandic infarcts involving simultaneously several of the above-mentioned anatomical structures usually produce a persisting Broca's aphasia (15). Persistent nonfluency is associated with extensive corticosubcortical rolandic damage (14).

In the acute stage, a global aphasia is the monotonous presentation of several types of infarcts (28): type 1—whole middle cerebral artery (MCA) territory (with or without lenticulostriate involvement); type 2—dual embolic simultaneous lesion of Broca's and Wernicke's area (54); type 3—frontal corticosubcortical infarct; 4—frontosubcortical-parietal infarct; types 3 and 4 are located on superior division of the middle cerebral artery territory; 5—lenticulostriate infarct. The first type has an ominous prognosis. There are few reported follow-up evaluations of patients with the dual-infarct type, and the prognosis is variable (54–57). The third and fourth types evolve to Broca's or transcortical motor aphasia, while the fifth has the better outcome and evolves either to a transcortical or an anomic aphasia and eventually to complete recovery (28).

In Wernicke's aphasia recovery is rather limited if the lesion also extends to the areas surrounding Wernicke's area, i.e., the second temporal gyrus, the posterior insula, and the supramarginal and angular gyrus (15). Persistent impairment of oral naming is associated with lesion size (>60 cm^2) and with damage to the posterior-superior temporal and the inferior parietal areas (semantic paraphasic errors) or to the insula-putamen (phonological paraphasic errors) (58). Persistent deficits in sentence repetition are associated with lesions destroying parts or all of Wernicke's area (59). In what concerns the recovery of auditory comprehension for commands, lesions in the posterior superior temporal and infrasylvian supramarginal regions (13) or damage to more than half of Wernicke's area, particularly if with additional extension into the middle temporal gyrus (16), indicates a poor prognosis for recovery. Late recovery of auditory comprehension in global aphasics is superior after subcortical temporal isthmus lesions, in contrast to Wernicke's cortical area lesions (60). However, damage to Wernicke's area did not preclude complete recovery of single-word comprehension. Only patients with very extensive left hemispheric lesions had incomplete recovery of single-word comprehension (61).

We described general anatomical rules for recovery. However, considerable interindividual variability exists, reflecting individual differences in the cortical extent of language areas (62) and the variable contribution of subcortical structures and corticosubcortical loops and of the nondominant hemisphere for language processing.

F. Intra- and Interhemispheric Reorganization and Aphasia Recovery

The role of the LH and right hemisphere (RH) in aphasia recovery may be investigated analyzing the evolution of language deficits in patients with sequential lesions and by using functional imaging methods.

1. Sequential Lesions

A few case reports have been published of aphasic patients who sustained a second lesion after a left hemispheric stroke that rendered them aphasic. The language deficits of these partly or completely recovered aphasics increased irrespective of the hemispheric side of the second stroke (63).

2. Functional Imaging Methods

The contributions of the right hemisphere and of the spared areas of the left hemisphere to the recovery of language have been investigated using functional imaging methods, such as rCBF, SPECT, TCD, or PET. In the acute phase, these methods show an area of abnormal circulation/metabolism larger than the infarct depicted by CT/MR. This can be observed in (1) ipsilesional zones with the same territorial blood supply, representing hypoperfusion, (2) functional connected ipsilesional areas, representing diaschisis (64), and (3) contralesional homotopic areas, representing transcallosal diaschisis (65).

These in vivo studies of recovery mechanisms use in general two types of experimental designs: (1) measurements at rest, comparing baseline and follow-up, (2) measurements during activation tasks, when the recovery of the performance on such task is under study. The interpretation of abnormal activation during recovery is not straightforward, because it can represent either new emerging functional proprieties responsible for the recovery or a maladaptive process that can explain the persistence of the deficits (66). Most of the functional studies found a circulatory or metabolic enhancement both on the nondamaged areas of the left hemisphere and on the homotopic frontal and temporal regions of the right hemisphere. They showed that there is a greater potential for homotopic interhemispheric reorganization for language than for motor functions (67).

Knopman et al. (68) used serial Xenon 133 CBF studies and observed that good recovery of comprehension was associated with early diffuse activation of the RH and late activation of the left posterior parietotemporal region, while incomplete recovery was associated with activation of right frontal areas. Weiller et al. (69) studied the recovery of six patients with Wernicke's aphasia with PET and observed bilateral activation (left prefrontal and areas of RH homotopic to language areas) during tasks of repetition of pseudowords and verb generation. This observation indicates: (1) parallel processing of LH language areas, a strategy different from the usual sequential processing, and (2) bilateral network (bitemporal or RH for the lexical-semantic processing, prefrontal LH for the speech production and syntactic processing) as the central mechanism in functional reorganization of language areas after stroke. No new areas were found to be involved in language processing during recovery. Silvestrini et al. (70) used TCD to investigate the effect of a word fluency task on the flow velocity of the middle cerebral artery of chronic patients. They found a significant increase of right MCA mean flow velocity in patients with previous aphasia (now recovered), indicating a participation of the RH in recovery. Cappa et al. (71) studied nine aphasic patients within 2 weeks and after 6 months of stroke onset with PET. They found an association between the regression of functional deactivation of intact anatomical areas in both hemispheres and spontaneous recovery. They concluded that language recovery in the first months is associated with regression of intra- and transhemispheric functional depression. Belin et al. (66) investigated seven chronic nonfluent cases with PET receiving melodic intonation therapy (MIT) in hearing, repetition, and repetition of MIT-loaded words. They observed reactivated Broca's area and left prefrontal and deactivated right Wernicke's counterpart and concluded that abnormal activation patterns are not necessarily related to recovery, because in some cases they coincide with the persistence rather than the recovery of aphasia. This observation also shows that these activations are modifiable by treatment. In fact they could be used as surrogates to evaluate whether a pharmacological or a speech therapy intervention has the potential to modify the pattern of activation that is usually found during recovery.

Two recent studies indicate that preserved left hemispheric speech area (or the cortex surrounding it) plays a crucial role in aphasia improvement. Heiss et al. (72) investigated word repetition with PET in 23 aphasic patients (with frontal, subcortical, and temporal lesions) 2 weeks and 8 months after onset. The subcortical and the frontal group improved substantially. They activated the right inferior frontal gyrus and the right superior temporal gyrus at baseline and regained left superior temporal gyrus activation at follow-up. The temporal group improved only in word comprehension. It activated the left Broca area and supplementary motor areas at baseline and the percentral gyrus bilaterally as well as the right superior temporal gyrus, but could not reactivate the left superior temporal gyrus. Activation of the right hemispheric regions was not efficacious for a considerable recovery from aphasia. Warburton et al. (73) used PET to study six patients who had at least some recovery from aphasia and found left inferotemporal activation, but little evidence of right hemispheric activation, on a word retrieval task.

In summary, in the early period after stroke, recovery, namely, comprehension recovery, reflects the regression of diaschisis in areas that usually participate in language processing. In the long term, the outcome of aphasia is mainly dependent on the size and location of the left hemispheric lesion. Reorganization of RH (mainly for language decoding and semantic tasks) and LH speech areas (mainly for speech output, syntax, and lexical tasks) constitutes the functional basis for late recovery. Good recovery seems to correlate with the possibility to activate left temporal areas.

III. RECOVERY FROM NEGLECT

Neglect is a failure to attend, represent, orient, or respond to stimuli on a hemispace (74). In neglect there is a defect of alerting, of nonlateralized nonspatial sustained attention, of lateralized spatial attention, and of motor activation and preparation to respond (74–76). Neglect is the most common cognitive dysfunction after RH strokes. It is detected in about 25% of acute stroke patients (77). Almost all investigations that have addressed recovery from neglect have studied RH lesions; therefore, we will concentrate on the recovery of left hemispatial inattention.

It can be rather misleading to indicate or to interpret figures on the prevalence of neglect, or the proportion of patients affected by or recovered from that sign, unless the definition of neglect, the methods used to evaluate it, and the setting of the study can be clearly identified. While the majority of neuropsychological disturbances are relatively stable at a given moment, neglect is a dynamic phenomenon. Performance on neglect tests can be affected by several variables that should be controlled in studies of neglect recovery (78). Shortening the presentation time (79), simultaneous performance of stepping (80) or of an attentional task (81), increasing the number of distractors (82) or the perceptual difficulty of the stimuli, using visuospatial stimuli instead of verbal (83), performing line bisection instead of line extension (84), all increase the severity of neglect. Increasing the number of trials, background leftward movements (85), priming (86), using a passive nonverbal auditory stimuli (87), performing passive or purposeful movements of the left limbs (88), an explicit verbal instruction (89), voluntary orientation (90) or gaze deviation to the left (91), pointing toward the left side with the right hand (92), all decrease the intensity of neglect. Even the same patient tested twice on the same day may show fluctuations in visual neglect after stroke.

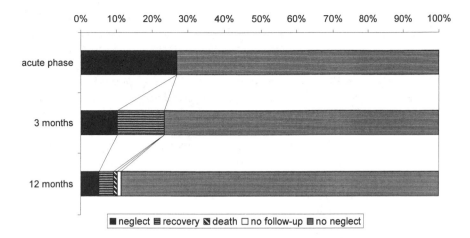

Fig. 1 Recovery from neglect on a consecutive series of 93 right hemispheric stroke patients followed during 12 months.

Follow-up studies are reported of single cases, case series, or cohorts (Fig. 1) (93–106), case reports of patients with sequential strokes, intervention studies, and functional studies of patients with neglect during the recovery period.

The setting of the different studies must be considered when reading the literature on the recovery of neglect. Of the series including acute stroke patients, only one was performed in a community setting (101); the remaining were acute hospital or rehabilitation center series. Some included only subacute or chronic stroke patients and were performed at rehabilitation centers (98,100). Generalization of the results of recovery studies from rehabilitation centers has strong limitations, because they have referral bias and miss the early course of spontaneous neglect recovery. Other methodological problems in many of these studies are patient selection (how many patients could not be assessed at entry and why not?) and patient attrition, i.e., lost during follow-up. The sample size was rather limited in other studies and very few used multivariate analysis to identify predictors of neglect recovery.

A. Neglect as an Unfavorable Prognostic Factor

Several studies indicate that neglect is an unfavorable sign for overall prognosis, improvement on rehabilitation, length of hospital stay, and discharge home (2,98,105–116). Patients with neglect have more inpatient falls and more left-sided wheelchair collisions (117). A recent study on the outcome of RH patients admitted to a stroke unit showed that patients with neglect had higher duration of hospitalization and lower Barthel scores (despite higher therapy input) but similar discharge destinations (116). However, the only community-based study yet performed failed to confirm these previous findings (77). While patients with neglect had a worse prognosis than patients without neglect, on multivariate analysis neglect was not an independent predictor of bad outcome. This means that large, severe RH strokes have poor prognosis and usually present neglect, but otherwise neglect does not have an independent influence on recovery of acute RH strokes. In a cohort of 1630 first-ever strokes in subjects under 65 years of age neglect was not identified as a predictor of independent survival (118), although patients with neglect had a worse outcome than patients without neglect. A different view is given by patients with severe strokes and neglect who are admitted to a rehabilitation center with neglect. They usually have a poor prognosis, not only because they have severe strokes but also because neglect makes rehabilitation more difficult. However, a recent study showed that patients with neglect admitted to a rehabilitation center showed significantly higher gains during rehabilitation, but had longer in-hospital stays (119). Concerning anosognosia, in the Copenhagen Stroke Study, anosognosia was found to be an independent predictor of no recovery and persistence of unawareness of the left-sided symptoms was an ominous sign (77). Anosognosia was recognized as an inhibitory factor hampering rehabilitation in another study (120).

During recovery, brief remission periods during follow-up examination in visuospatial neglect have been described (121). Conversely, subjects apparently recovered from neglect may show subtle deficits such as extinction on double simultaneous stimulation with brief presentation of stimuli or right attentional bias, e.g., when analyzing chimeric figures (122).

B. Recovery Pattern and Profile

The most evident and conspicuous manifestations of neglect usually vanish within 1 month after onset. By 12 months only a minority of patients have a clinically apparent hemispatial innattention (123). The percentage of recovered RH stroke patients in available follow-up series ranges from 0 to 100%. This variation is mainly related to patient selection and variation in the tests used to evaluate neglect. The Hier et al. study (99) is the only one to indicate the recovery time of the individual clinical manifestations of neglect. Median time to recovery was 8 weeks on drawing, 9 weeks on visual and auditory orienting, 11 weeks for anosognosia, and 43 weeks for double simultaneous tactile stimulation. Sunderland et al. detected neglect in 8–11% of patients 3 weeks after stroke, but significant neglect was rarely observed by 6 months, although further recovery was noticed between 6 months and 1 year (101). Stone et al. used quantitated neglect recovery with the visual neglect recovery index and showed that most of the recovery occurs in the first 10 days, reaching a plateau by 3 months (103). In the early phase patients with neglect also make errors or are slow in responding on the nonneglected hemispace. Improvement on cancellation tasks is observed in both the right and left half hemispaces (123). Cassidy et al. showed that recovery on a crossing-out task was maximal in the rightmost third (106).

C. Factors Influencing the Severity and Duration of Neglect

Early anatomoclinical correlations of neglect emphasized the crucial role of parietal lobe lesions in the production of neglect (124,125). After the advent of modern neuroimaging, neglect was described in association with other cortical (frontal) (126) and subcortical (thalamus, striatum) (127,128) locations (15,74,129). PET studies (130) also indicate that spatial attention is subserved by a distributed network, including the cingulum, the frontal and parietal cortices, and several subcortical structures. Mesulam's model (131,132) followed that evidence and considered that the anatomical basis of spatial attention was a distributed large-scale network, with different anatomical structures playing different roles in the network. The posterior parietal component provides a sensory representation of the extrapersonal space, the frontal component provides a map for the distribution of orienting and exploratory movements, the cingulate component gives a map to assign value to spatial coordinates, and the reticulothalamic component modifies the level of arousal or activation bias. A problem with that model is that although some cases of pure perceptual, attentional, or intentional neglect can be found, the location of their lesions does not always follow the pattern predicted by the model. Furthermore, in most patients the manifestations of neglect are mixed and monotonous regardless of the lesion location (93). As a lesion in any of the components or their reciprocate projections can produce neglect, recovery can be explained by undamaged areas taking over the function of lesioned modules. Thus persistent neglect would require large lesions damaging more than one component.

Voluntary orientation of spatial attention includes three steps: orienting (whose anatomical bases are posterior parietal-pulvinar-colliculus), selecting (cingulate gyrus), and maintaining sustained attention, also described as "disengage, move, and engage" (76). A multicomponent model of neglect (122,133) postulates three separate deficits: (1) an initial automatic orienting of attention toward the ipsilesional side, (2) impairment of disengaging attention from that side and reorienting of spatial attention toward stimuli on the contralesional side, and (3) generalized reduction of attentional/information processing capacity. The second of these disturbances seems to recover faster (122).

Parietal lesions usually produce more severe (129) and stable neglect, while after lesions with other locations, neglect is in general less severe and transient (15,79). Hier et al. (99) analyzed the effect of lobar sparing on recovery rate. They found that recovery from neglect to left-sided visual and auditory stimuli on drawing and extinction were more rapid in patients without injury to the right frontal lobe. Patients without injury to the parietal lobe also recovered more quickly from extinction. Persistent neglect is usually associated with large fronto-parietal infarcts (99). Factors with negative influence on neglect recovery include age over 65 (99), cortical lesion (vs. subcortical), ischemic lesions (vs. hemor-rhagic) lesion size (99,100), brain atrophy (100), neglect severity (94,97,100, 104), anosognosia (104), and neglect on the line cancellation test (106).

D. Intra- and Interhemispheric Reorganization and Neglect Recovery

The role of the RH and LH in the recovery of neglect can be appreciated when analyzing patients with sequential strokes and data from functional studies.

1. Sequential Strokes

There are very few reported cases of sequential strokes with neglect. Daffner et al. (134) described a case where sequential right frontal and parietal hemispheri-cal strokes worsened the neglect caused by the first stroke. Vuilleumier et al. (135) reported a patient with a right parietal stroke whose neglect showed abrupt recovery following a left hemispheric area 8 stroke. This observation seems in accordance with Kinsbourne's theory of functional interhemispheric imbal-ance (136).

2. Functional Studies

In humans, recovery from neglect caused by subcortical RH lesions is associated with disappearance of ipsilesional diaschisis on the relevant cortical areas of the RH (cingulate, frontal, parietal) (137–140). We emphasized cortical regional di-aschisis and the role of ambi- or left-hemispheric dominance on subcortical ne-glect. In fact, neglect was observed in a patient with persistent frontal diaschisis but not parietal hypometabolism, and in another patient with persisting cortical diachisis, suggesting ambi- or left-hemispheric dominance.

Few cases of neglect recovery were investigated with PET (140,141). Per-ani et al. (140) studied two cases, but only one had follow-up. Bihemispheric metabolic depression was found in the acute phase. Paralleling almost complete recovery, PET demonstrated return of LH metabolism to normal and partial RH metabolic recovery. These findings suggest a bihemispheric role in neglect recovo-ery. The LH may be important for early and RH for late recovery. Pizzamiglio et al. (141) studied neglect recovery in three patients and showed that regions notably more active after recovery were almost exclusively found in the RH cortical area, and overlapped with those observed in normal subjects performing the same task.

IV. RECOVERY FROM APRAXIA

The information available on the recovery of praxis is limited. Recovery of apraxia was studied mainly in aphasic patients (142). Kertesz et al. found that the recovery rate of praxis was similar to that of language, in particular of comprehension, except for global aphasics, who showed a somewhat better recovery of praxis than of language. Follow-up studies showed that 50% of acute apraxic patients are recovered between 3 and 6 months (15,143). In the long term the recovery from ideomotor apraxia is striking, very few patients remaining permanently affected (144), more often in buccofacial praxis. The ipsilateral nonparetic limb can show sympathetic apraxia and impaired dexterity. Ipsilateral dexterity recovers significantly during the first 6 months and about 60% of the patients will perform within the normal range (145).

Long-term recovery of apraxia is predicted by initial severity (143,144) and by LH lesion site, posterior lesions having a worse prognosis for limb apraxia (143) and extensive anterior opercular lesions for buccofacial apraxia (15). Recovery may be less complete in old patients (146). The presence of a lesion on the RH does not influence recovery (143) nor does lesion size. Even global aphasics with infarcts of the whole MCA territory can have normal praxis, showing that language and praxis are subserved by partly overlapping, but independent, neural networks (147). Apraxic patients with parietal infarcts can often recognize gestures and distinguish between correct and incorrect performances, showing that gestures have multiple and bilateral representations. There are several alternative pathways (e.g., occipitofrontal fasciculus, superior longitudinal fasciculus, external capsule) connecting the left posterior and anterior areas participating in praxis. These anatomofunctional features contribute to the superior recovery of apraxia when compared to disorders of spoken or written language. Impairment in drawing and other two- or three-dimensional constructional tasks has less functional impact than limb apraxia. LH patients show better average recovery than RH ones. The improvement in constructional tasks is superior to that of language (142) but considerable individual variability exits within the LH group (148). Some global and Wernicke's aphasics and subjects with large left parietotemporal or parieto-occipital infarcts can remain permanently impaired. After RH lesions the median duration to recovery was 16 weeks in one study (99), and the probability of recovery was between 60 and 80%. Age, lesion size, and type (infarction) had a negative effect on recovery. Recovery in the Block Design Test was more rapid in patients without injury to the right frontal lobe.

The probability of recovery from dressing apraxia following a RH stroke was 60% at the tenth week. Dressing apraxia could no longer be detected after 50 weeks. The mean duration for recovery was 32 weeks (99).

V. RECOVERY FROM ALEXIA, AGRAPHIA, AND CALCULATION DISORDERS

Very few data exist from follow-up series analyzing the recovery from alexia, agraphia, and calculation disorders following stroke. Kotila et al. (149) found that 61% and 37% of stroke survivors had either dyslexia, dysgraphia, or dyscalculia at 3 and 12 months respectively. A number of longitudinal case studies detailed the modifications of neurolinguistic processes during recovery, but they cannot provide information to establish the prognosis of individual patients. An additional difficulty are the different classification systems (150), considering either an anatomical-clinical or a neurolinguistic-neurocognitive approach. The improvement of reading and calculation is comparable to that of aphasia, while that of writing is inferior (142).

The prognosis of acalculia is better after postrolandic than after prerolandic or pre- and postrolandic lesions (151). If impairment in calculation is still present at 3 months, complete restoration of function is unlikely. Pure acute acalculia from a frontal or parietal infarct is usually short-lived.

Writing disorders in aphasic patients after left middle cerebral artery infarcts have a poor prognosis. Many patients regain the ability to write their name or copy single words even with their nondominant hand. Writing by dictation remains hard and frequently incorrect. Writing a text or letter spontaneously is usually impossible. Agraphia secondary to left prerolandic lesions had a worse prognosis than writing disorders due to post postrolandic lesions in 25 agraphic patients with left MCA infarcts followed up for 3–6 months. Of the two patients with extensive, rolandic infarcts, one remained completely agraphic and the other could not write on dictation. None of the 11 agraphic subjects with prerolandic lesions improved, while out of 12 patients with postrolandic lesions, seven recovered fully and four remained impaired, writing only on dictation (15).

Left posterior cerebral artery infarcts and occipital hemorrhages can cause hemialexia and visual-form alexia (pure or without agraphia). The prognosis for reading recovery in the latter is limited, in particular in patients with large infarcts involving the splenium of the corpus callosum. Initially patients use a letter-by-letter strategy, and if they improve they start using the whole word visual form recognition system, but this process remains slow and often inaccurate, with frequent visual errors and confabulation of the right half of the words. Very few patients improve enough to be able to read a book or a newspaper.

In temporoparietal alexia, patients usually recover the comprehension of written single words, but reading aloud and text comprehension remain impaired. In some cases of transcortical aphasia reading words aloud can become normal but without comprehension of their meaning. Of the three types of central alexia, deep dyslexia occasionally resolves into phonological dyslexia, as semantic errors decrease during recovery. This may be due to gradual recovery of the semantic reading route or a partial recovery of the phonological route, which would inhibit the production of semantic paralexias (152). Small et al. (153) studied with fMRI a patient with phonological dyslexia before and after treatment. The patient became able to read nonwords and functional words, preferring a decompositional sublexical strategy. Meanwhile the main activated area shifted from the left angular gyrus to the lingual gyrus.

VI. RECOVERY FROM AGNOSIA AND BALINT'S SYNDROME

There is almost no systematic information on the prognosis of visual agnosia and Balint's syndrome and its components, namely optic or visuomotor ataxia. The prognosis of visual agnosia is worse in the case of bilateral lesions and for the apperceptive than for the associative type of visual agnosia. Apperceptive visual agnosia often results from the improvement of cortical blindness. Associative visual agnosia can evolve favorably to include only certain classes of stimuli, such as colours or faces, or to misnaming of visual presented objects, so-called optic aphasia (154). Similarly in color agnosia, color-naming defects take longer to recover than the ability to match seen color to color name given verbally (155). A visual-speech disconnection syndrome is reported of a patient with optic aphasia, agnosia alexia, and color anomia (154).

Prosopagnosia after a unilateral RH lesion is usually transient (99). Persistent innability to recognize familiar faces is in general secondary to bilateral lesions.

Optic ataxia, even when prominent in the first day after stroke, usually recovers quickly (156) and has no long-standing functional impact. Complete Balint's syndrome when it persists for a few weeks is usually persistent and disabling, although some patients may show some improvement with rehabilitation (157).

VII. RECOVERY FROM DISORIENTATION

Disorientation regarding time, location, or identity is common in acute stroke patients. Wade et al. and Desmond et al. (158,159) found that 41% of acute stroke patients were disoriented 7–10 days after stroke and 39 patients remained disoriented 3 months later. Disorientation was associated with severe hemispheral stroke syndromes. Disorientation was an inaccurate marker of dementia or deficits in memory or attention, but intact orientation suggests that cognitive functions are likely to be preserved. In the Copenhagen Stroke Study (160) impaired orientation was found in 23% of alert nonaphasic patients on admission and in 12% of the survivors after complete rehabilitation. A stationary level of orientation was achieved by 80% of the patients within 2 weeks and by 95% within 6 weeks. Stroke severity and comorbidity were independent determinants of disorientation on admission. Lesions of the anterior or medial thalamus and of any of the cerebral lobes were associated with impaired orientation. Decreased orientation at 6 months still exerted a marked negative influence on ADL and social functions (160).

VIII. RECOVERY FROM AMNESIA

Medial temporal posterior cerebral artery infarcts, thalamic and caudate infarcts and hemorrhages, capsular genu infarcts, and intraventricular and subarachnoid hemorrhages can produce amnesia. Little systematic information exists on the follow-up of patients who suffered from memory impairment following strokes in those sites.

After temporal infarcts the recovery of memory can be almost complete or fair if the lesion is unilateral, but the prognosis is ominous when the damage is bilateral. Memory loss can then be very severe and permanent, leading to dependency in everyday life. Bilateral PCA infarcts are one of the mechanisms of "focal" or "strategic infarct" vascular dementia (161).

Although not all authors would agree (162), amnesia is considered to be more severe and stable after polar than after dorsomedial thalamic infarcts (163), owing to the simultaneous lesion of the mammillothalamic tract, the anterior thalamic nuclei, and its projections to the frontal lobe. After dorsomedial infarcts memory impairment is usually transient, unless the lesion extends rostrally to include the mammillothalamic tract, the ventral portion of the laminamedullaris interna (164), or the inferior thalamic peduncle, which includes the ventral amygdalofugal pathway (165). After unilateral infarcts memory disturbances usually show considerable recovery, but occasionally the defect persists (166). After dorsomedial infarctions abulia followed by memory impairment is the dominant residual symptom, often preventing return to work (167). Patients with bilateral lesions have a more severe and long-lasting memory defect. Bilateral paramedian thalamic infarcts are another form of strategic infarct vascular dementia. In caudate lesions abulia and "frontal lobe-like" abnormalities predominate over memory troubles (168). Confusion and memory loss due to infarct of the inferior capsular genu is also considered a strategic infarct form of vascular dementia. However, the neuropsychological defects improve with time and patients are left with minor residual cognitive and moderate memory troubles that do not in general interfere with previous lifestyle (123). Mild memory problems remain in about 30% of the survivors of primary intraventricular haemorrhage (169). They display a learning defect more important for novel words or associations (170).

A. Recovery of Cognitive Functions after Stroke

The prognosis of cognitive deficits and dementia associated with stroke was investigated longitudinally in a few studies. The prevalence of cognitive impairment 3 months after stroke ranges from 35% (171) to 70% (172). The more frequently impaired domains are memory, orientation, language, and attention (171), visuospatial and visuoconstructive tasks, arithmetic, and speed of information processing (172). Cognitive impairment was associated with major cortical syndromes and infarctions in the left anterior and posterior cerebral artery territories in one study (171) and with hemorrhagic strokes, left hemisphere lesions, female sex, and presence of aphasia in another (172).

The prevalence of dementia observed 3 months after the stroke varies between 14% (173) and 32% (174) and has been associated with: (1) stroke-related factors such as major stroke syndromes (174), stroke location and vascular territory (175), presence of aphasia (173), and confusional state in the acute phase (176); (2) vascular risk factors like diabetes (173) and prior stroke (175,177); (3) host characteristics such as higher age, lower education (174–178), nonwhite race (175,178), and preexisting dementia (179).

Table 1 shows recent studies that used comprehensive neuropsychological batteries to assess cognitive functions on at least two evaluations after stroke (176,180–183). In these studies the prevalence of cognitive impairment at baseline ranged from 32% to 35%, while dementia was observed in 6–33% of the patients. Improvement in cognitive functions occurred in 21–36% of the patients in the first year and the risk of dementia seems to be lower in subsequent years. No improvement or cognitive decline was associated with diabetes, reinfarction, acute confusional state, and presence of aphasia. Improvement in some cognitive domains was associated with major hemisphere stroke syndromes.

B. Recovery of Cognitive Deficits after Specific Types of Stroke

The pattern of cognitive deficits after the stroke is not homogeneous and varies according to the location, number, size, and pathophysiology of the brain insult.

Table 1 Follow-up Studies on Cognitive Impairment After Stroke

Author	Sample	Follow-up	Long-term cognitive impairment	Impairment criteria	Frequently impaired cognitive domains	Associated factors for cognitive impairment in the first evaluation	Predictive factors of improvement/decline on follow-up
Desmond et al., 1996	151	3, 12, 24, 36 months	Generalized cognitive impairment found in 35% at baseline. Improvement in first year: 36%	DSM III-R modified	Memory;[a] orientation,[a] visuospatial function,[a] attention,[a] language,[a] and abstract reasoning		Improvement on the first year is associated with left hemisphere infarction and major hemisphere syndrome. Diabetes mellitus associated with difficulty to improve
Andersen et al., 1996	103	1, 6, 12 months	General intellectual impairment: 32% 1st month; 26% 6th month; 26% 12th month. Recovery Improvement in the three evaluations: 16%	Cut-off score of 2SD below the mean of a population sample in the MDRS	Attention, initiation, perseveration, construction ability, memory,[a] and abstract reasoning	Age; lower prestroke social and physical activities	Decline of cognitive functions associated with reinfarction

Study	N	Time points	Outcome	Criteria	Cognitive domains	Risk factors	Notes
Treves et al., 1997	158	3, 6, 12, 24, 36 months	Dementia 0.29% 1st year; 1.3–3.4% subsequent years	DSM-III-R	Not specified	Less schooling; atrial fibrillation; diabetes mellitus	Decline associated with acute confusional state and aphasia
Hénon et al., 1999	110	6, 12, 24 months	Dementia 6 months: 33% (31% preexisting dementia) 12 months: 32% (36% preexisting dementia) 24 months: 27% (32% preexisting dementia)	DSM-IV, NINCDS-ADRDA, NINDS-AIREN	Not specified	Poststroke dementia associated with preexisting cognitive decline	
Madureira and Ferro, 1999	148	3, 12 months	Dementia 3 months: 6% 12 months: 6% Recovery Improved: 21% Stabilized: 64%	NINDS-AIREN	Verbal fluency, motor initiative, memory,[a] orientation,[a] and language	Cognitive decline associated with higher age and low education level	

DSM = Diagnostic and Statistical Manual of Mental Disorders; MDRS = Mattis Dementia Rating Scale; NINCDS-ADRDA = National Institute of Neurological and Communicative Disorders and Stroke-Alzheimer's Disease and Related Disorders Association; NINDS-AIREN = National Institute of Neurological Disorders and Stroke-Association Internationale pour la Recherche et l'Enseignement en Neurosciences.

[a] Cognitive domains that were significantly improved in the second evaluation.

Following unilateral strategic infarcts (thalamic, capsular genu, anterior cerebral artery, or posterior cerebral artery) considerable improvement occurs, but bilateral strategic lesions usually cause nonreversible dementia.

By definition, single lacunar infarcts do not produce clinically apparent cognitive deficits. In a long-term follow-up of a cohort of patients with lacunar infarction, using the Mini-Mental State Examination, Loeb et al. (184) found that 23% of the patients developed dementia. Recurrent stroke was the strongest associated factor. Guerreiro et al. (185), using a comprehensive cognitive battery to assess 66 patients with first lacunar infarction, found only one demented patient on the baseline evaluation (3 months). At the first year 4.3% of the patients were demented but by the third year, none of the evaluated patients was demented. Thus, the risk of long-term cognitive impairment appears to be low after a single lacunar infarct, but increases after recurrent strokes.

In a 2-year follow-up study of 55 patients with intracerebral haemorrhage, Guerreiro et al. (186) found dementia in 5% of the patients at the first year and other types of cognitive impairment in 51%. At the second evaluation improvement was observed in 15%. Aphasia in the acute phase, previous functional deficit, and the severity of neurological deficits were predictive factors for cognitive decline.

Subtle cognitive and behavioral impairments are common in subarachnoid haemorrhage (SAH) patients, even in the absence of other neurological deficits. Rupture of anterior communicating artery aneurysms (ACoA) can be associated with amnesia, confabulation, and personality changes referred as "ACoA syndrome" (187). The pattern of cognitive deficits in these patients may differ according to the lesion site. Irle et al. (188) showed that patients with combined lesions in the basal forebrain and striatum or basal forebrain, striatum, and ventral frontal cortex had severe memory deficits while patients with basal forebrain or striatum lesions alone had no deficits. Emotional changes were most pronounced in patients with striate lesions alone. Böttger et al. (189) also found different patterns of cognitive deficits in ACoA aneurysm patients: memory deficits, executive function deficits, and attentional deficits. Memory and attentional disorders had a better prognosis.

Cross-sectional studies are the most frequently used method for long-term evaluation of patients surviving an acute SAH. In these works there is a wide variation in the interval from the bleeding to the evaluation of individual patients. The prevalence of cognitive impairment in patients with good neurological recovery after SAH varies between 30% (190) and 83% (191), depending on the number of cognitive impaired functions considered. Frequent impairment is observed in memory, visuospatial and visuoconstructive abilities, conceptualization, attention, orientation, and cognitive speed. Cognitive impairment has been associated with a number of clinical factors such as aneurysm location (190), late surgery

(192), worse neurological condition on admission (193), and severity of the initial bleeding (194). However, age seems to be the most crucial determinant for cognitive impairment (190,191,194,195). Regarding longitudinal studies, McKenna et al. (196) compared SAH patients with and without neurological deficits at discharge, 3 and 12 months after the event. Residual confusion and generalized impairment in cognitive functions were seen in both groups at discharge. At 3 months patients with no neurological deficits were almost recovered, and at 1 year no evidence of cognitive deficits was found in this group of patients. Long-term impairment was associated with neurological deficits at discharge. Maurice-Williams et al. (197) assessed SAH patients before surgery, at discharge, and 1 year after. Four of the five patients (18.5%) who worsened considerably on the postsurgery psychometric assessment recovered at 1 year. Cognitive impairment was related to postsurgery complications such as delayed ischemia or hydrocephalus. However, residual psychological symptoms, such as irritability, forgetfulness, depression, dizziness, and headaches, were mentioned by 52% of the patients.

Ogden et al. (198), in a prospective study of 89 SAH patients, showed that notable improvement in verbal memory occurred in more than 80% of the patients 10 weeks after the SAH and continued to improve throughout a 12-month period. In contrast, nonverbal memory deficits were more frequent and persistent for 47% of the patients. Patients who showed mild or severe deficits in tests requiring sustained attention, psychomotor speed, and mental flexibility had no significant improvement at 12 months. The presence or site of the aneurysm was not associated with long-term cognitive impairment. The best predictor of impairment at follow-up was a poor grade at discharge. Germanò et al. (199) studied a group of patients enrolled according to the following criteria: age between 18 and 60 years, Hunt and Hess grade $\leq$ 2, no intracerebral or intraventricular bleeding, single aneurysm, early surgery, and no symptomatic vasospasm. In these patients they found no cognitive or emotional disturbance 1 year after the surgery.

Nonaneurysmal SAH patients are reported as having better outcome compared with aneurysmal SAH patients (200–202). Hütter et al. (203) found that patients with nonaneurysmal SAH scored worse in attention tests than aneurysmal SAH patients. Germanò et al. (204) found no significant long-term alterations after nonaneurysmal SAH. In summary, after SAH memory, orientation, attention, or subtle language disturbances have better prognosis than executive functions or visuospatial disabilities. Recovery occurs predominantly between the third and twelfth months. Subtle emotional effects may last longer.

Prospective studies to evaluate the course of cognitive impairment after different stroke types are needed to understand the mechanisms related to cognitive recovery and to identify the determinants of lack of improvement or deterioration, including prevalent subcortical white matter changes and "assymptomatic'' degenerative dementia. It is important to stress that some poststroke cognitive impairment and dementia diagnosed in early stages of recovery (i.e., 3 months) are expected to improve in a substantial proportion of patients.

REFERENCES

1. Pedersen PM, Jorgensen HS, Nakayama H, Raaschou HO, Olsen TS. Aphasia in acute stroke: incidence, determinants, and recovery. Ann Neurol 1995;38:659–666.
2. Paolucci S, Antonucci G, Pratesi L, Traballesi M, Lubich S, Grasso MG. Functional outcome in stroke inpatient rehabilitation: predicting no, low and high response patients. Cerebrovasc Dis 1998;8:228–234.
3. Starkstein SE, Robinson RG. Aphasia and depression. Aphasiology 1988;2:1–20.
4. Sarno MT. Quality of life in aphasia in the first post-stroke year. Aphasiology 1997; 11:665–679.
5. Melo TP, Ferro JM, Guerreiro S. Quality of life in 3 years survivors of intracerebral hematoma. Cerebrovasc Dis 1998;8(suppl 4):93 (abstr).
6. Vignolo LA. Evolution of aphasia and language rehabilitation: a retrospective exploratory study. Cortex 1964;1:344–367.
7. Yarnell P, Monroe P, Sobel L. Aphasia outcome in stroke: a clinical neuroradiological correlation. Stroke 1976;7:516–522.
8. Kertesz A, McCabe P. Recovery patterns and prognosis in aphasia. Brain 1977; 100:1–18.
9. Lomas J, Kertesz A. Patterns of spontaneous recovery in aphasic groups: a study of adult stroke patients. Brain Lang 1978;5:388–401.
10. Kertesz A, Harlock W, Coates R. Computer tomographic localization, lesion size, and prognosis in aphasia and nonverbal impairment. Brain Lang 1979;8:34–50.
11. Sarno MT, Levita E. Natural course of recovery in severe aphasia. Arch Phys Med Rehabil 1971;51:175–179.
12. Demeurisse G, Demol O, Derouck M, De Deuckelaer R, Coekaerts MJ, Capon A. Quantitative study of the rate of recovery from aphasia due to ischemic stroke. Stroke 1980;11:455–458.
13. Selnes OA, Knopman DS, Niccum N, Rubens AB, Larson D. Computed tomographic scan correlates of auditory comprehension deficits in aphasia: a prospective recovery study. Ann Neurol 1983;13:558–566.
14. Knopman DS, Selnes OL, Niccum N, Rubens AB, Yock D, Larson D. A longitudinal study of speech fluency in aphasia: CT correlates of recovery and persistent nonfluency. Neurology 1983;33:1170–1178.
15. Ferro JM. Neurologia do comportamento. Estudo da correlação com a tomografia axial compotorizada. Doctoral thesis. Faculdade de Medicina de Lisboa, Lisboa, 1986.
16. Naeser MA, Helm-Estabrooks N, Haas G, Auerbach S, Srinivasan M. Relationship between lesion extent in ''Wernicke's area'' on computed tomographic scan and

predicting recovery of comprehension in Wernicke's aphasia. Arch Neurol 1987; 44:73–82.

17. Pashek GV, Holland AL. Evolution of aphasia in the first year post-stroke. Cortex 1988;24:411–423.

18. Hartman J. Measurement of early spontaneous recovery from aphasia with stroke. Ann Neurol 1981;9:89–91.

19. Basso A. Prognostic factors in aphasia. Aphasiology 1992;6:337–348.

20. Kertesz A. Recovery and treatment. In: Heilman KM, Valenstein E, eds. Clinical Neuropsychology, 1993:647–674.

21. Hanson WR, Metter J, Riege EH. The course of chronic aphasia. Aphasiology 1989; 3:19–29.

22. Basso A, Capitani E, Moraschini S. Sex differences in recovery from aphasia. Cortex 1982;18:469–475.

23. Pizzamiglio L, Mammucari A, Razzano C. Evidence for sex differences in brain organization in recovery in aphasia. Brain Lang 1985;25:213–223.

24. Subirana A. Handedness and cerebral dominance. In: Vinken BJ, Bruyn GW, eds. Handbook of Clinical Neurology. Amsterdam: North-Holland, 1969:248–272.

25. Gloning K, Trappl R, Heiss WD, Quatember R. Prognosis and speech therapy in aphasia. In: Lebrun Y, Hoops R, eds. Recovery in Aphasics. Amsterdam: Swets & Zeitlinger, 1976:57–64.

26. Pieniadz JM, Naeser MA, Koff E, Levine HL. CT scan cerebral hemispheric asymmetry measurements in stroke cases with global aphasia: atypical asymmetries associated with improved recovery. Cortex 1983;19:371–391.

27. Kertesz A, Black SE, Polk M, Howell J. Cerebral asymmetries on magnetic resonance imaging. Cortex 1986;22:177–418.

28. Ferro JM. The influence of infarct location on recovery from global aphasia. Aphasiology 1992;6:415–430.

29. David RM, Skilbeck CE. Raven IQ and language recovery following stroke. J Clin Neuropsychol 1984;6:302–308.

30. Martins IP, Ferro JM. Recovery of acquired aphasia in children. Aphasiology 1992; 6:431–438.

31. Sands E, Sarno MT, Shankweiler D. Long term assessment of language function in aphasia due to stroke. Arch Phys Med Rehabil 1969;50:202–206.

32. Marshall RC, Thompkins CA, Phillips DS. Improvement in treated aphasia: examination of selected prognostic factors. Folia Phoniatr 1982;34:304–315.

33. Ferro JM, Crespo M. Young adult stroke: neuropsychological dysfunction and recovery. Stroke 1988;19:982–986.

34. Taylor MS. Preliminary findings in a study of age, linguistic evolution and quality of life in recovery from aphasia. Scand J Rehabil Med 1992;26:43–59.

35. Ferro JM, Madureira S. Aphasia type, age and cerebral infarct localisation. J Neurol 1997;244:505–509.

36. Robinson RG. Relationship of aphasia to depression. In: Robinson RG, ed. The Clinical Neuropsychiatry of Stroke. Cognitive, Behavioral and Emotional Disorders Following Vascular Brain Injury. Cambridge: Cambridge University Press, 1998: 177–185.

37. Robinson RG. The relationship of anxiety disorder to outcome. In: Robinson RG, ed. The Clinical Neuropsychiatry of Stroke. Cognitive, Behavioural and Emotional Disorders Following Vascular Brain Injury. Cambridge: Cambridge University Press, 1998:368–373.

38. Porch BE, Collins M, Wertz RT, Friden TP. Statistical prediction of change in aphasia. J Speech Hear Res 1980;23:312–321.

39. Code C, Rowley D, Kertesz A. Predicting recovery from aphasia with connectionist networks: preliminary comparisons with multiple regression. Cortex 1994;30:527–532.

40. Mohr JP, Watters WC, Duncan GW. Thalamic hemorrhage and aphasia. Brain Lang 1975;2:3–17.

41. Alexander MP, Lo Verme SR. Aphasia after left hemispheric intracerebral hemorrhage. Neurology 1980;30:1193–1202.

42. D'Esposito M, Alexander MP. Subcortical aphasia distinct profiles following left putaminal hemorrhage. Neurology 1995;45:38–41.

43. Démonet J-F, Celsis P, Puel M, Cardebat D, Marc-Vergnes JP, Rascol A. Thalamic and non-thalamic subcortical aphasia: a neurolinguistic and SPECT approach. In: Vallar G, Cappa SF, Wallesch C-W, eds. Neuropsychological Disorder Associated with Subcortical Lesions. New York: Oxford University Press, 1992:397–411.

44. Alexander MP. Speech and language deficits after subcortical lesions of the left hemisphere: a clinical, CT, and PET study. In: Vallar G, Cappa SF, Wallesch C-W eds. Neuropsychological Disorder Associated with Subcortical Lesions. New York: Oxford University Press, 1992:455–477.

45. Kase CS, Williams JP, Wyatt DA, Mohr JP. Lobar intracerebral hematomas: clinical and CT analysis of 22 cases. Neurology 1982;32:1146–1150.

46. Barbarotto R, De Santis A, Laiacona M, Basso A, Spagnoli D, Capitani E. Neuropsychological follow-up of patients operated for aneurysms of the middle cerebral artery and posterior communicating artery. Cortex 1989;25:275–288.

47. Stoltenburg-Didinger G. Neuropathology of subarachnoid hemorrhage. In: Bederson JB, ed. Subarachnoid Hemorrhage: Pathophysiology and Management. Neurological Topics. Illinois: American Association of Neurological Surgeons, 1997:41–60.

48. Bousser MG, Russel RS. Cerebral Venous Thrombosis. London: WB Saunders, 1977:136.

49. Baumgartner RW, Landis T. Venous thalamic infarction. Cerebrovasc Dis 1992; 2:353–358.

50. Karbe H, Kessler J, Herholz K, Fink GR, Heiss WD. Long-term prognosis of poststroke aphasia studied with positron emission tomography. Arch Neurol 1995; 52:186–190.

51. Ferro JM. Analysis of lesion localization and size. In: Martins IP, Castro-Caldas A, van Dongen HR, van Hout A, eds. Acquired Aphasia in Children. Acquisition and Breakdown of Language in the Developing Brain. Dordrecht: Kluwer Academic Publishers, 1991:35–44.

52. Kertesz, A. Issues in localization. In: Kertesz A, ed. Localization in Neuropsychology. New York: Academic Press, 1983:1–20.

53. Mohr JP, Pessin MS, Finkelstein S, Funkenstein HH, Duncan GW, Davis KR. Broca aphasia: pathologic and clinical. Neurology 1978;28:311–324.

54. Van Hoen G, Hawes A. Global aphasia without hemiparesis: a sign of embolic encephalopathy. Neurology 1982;32:403–406.
55. Tranel D, Biller J, Damasio H. Global aphasia without hemiparesis. Arch Neurol 1987;44:304–308.
56. Legatt AD, Rubin MJ, Kaplan LR, Healton EB, Brust JCM. Global aphasia without hemiparesis: multiple etiologies. Neurology 1987;37:201–205.
57. Bogousslavsky J. Global aphasia without other signs lateralizing signs. Arch Neurol 1988;45:143.
58. Knopman DS, Selnes OA, Niccum N, Rubens AB. Recovery of naming in aphasia: relationship to fluency, comprehension and CT findings. Neurology 1984;34:1461–1471.
59. Selnes OA, Knopman DS, Niccum N, Rubens AB. The critical role of Wernicke's area in sentence repetition. Ann Neurol 1985;17:549–557.
60. Naeser MA, Gaddie A, Palumbo CL, Stiassny-Eder D. Late recovery of auditory comprehension in global aphasia. Improved recovery observed with subcortical temporal isthmus lesion vs Wernicke's cortical area lesion. Arch Neurol 1990;47:425–432.
61. Selnes OA, Niccum N, Knopman DS, Rubens AB. Recovery of single word comprehension: CT-scan correlates. Brain Lang 1984;21:72–84.
62. Ojemann GA, Whitaker HA. Language location and variability. Brain Lang 1978;6:239–260.
63. Cappa SF, Vallar G. The role of the left and right hemispheres in recovery from aphasia. Aphasiology 1992;6:359–372.
64. Feenoy DM, Baron JC. Diaschisis. Stroke 1986;17:817–830.
65. Andrews RJ. Transhemispheric diaschisis. A review and comment. Stroke 1991;22:943–949.
66. Belin P, Van Eeckhout P, Zilbovicius M, Remy P, François C, Guillaume S, Chain F, Rancurel G, Samson Y. Recovery from nonfluent aphasia after melodic intonation therapy: a PET study. Neurology 1996,47:1504–1511.
67. Müller RA, Rothermel RD, Behen ME, Muzik O, Mangner TJ, Chugani HT. Differential patterns of language and motor reorganization following early left hemisphere lesion. Arch Neurol 1998;55:1113–1119.
68. Knopman DS, Rubens AB, Selnes OA, Klassen AC, Meyer MW. Mechanisms of recovery from aphasia: evidence from serial xenon 133 cerebral blood flow studies. Ann Neurol 1984;15:530–535.
69. Weiller C, Isensee C, Rijntjes M, Huber W, Muller S, Bier D, Dutschka K, Woods RP, Noth J, Diener HC. Recovery from Wernicke's aphasia: a positron emission tomographic study. Ann Neurol 1995;37:723–732.
70. Silvestrini M, Troisi E, Matteis M, Cupini LM, Caltagirone C. Involvement of the healthy hemisphere in recovery from aphasia and motor deficit in patients with cortical ischemic infarction: a transcranial Doppler study. Neurology 1995;45:1815–1820.
71. Cappa SF, Perani D, Grassi F, Bressi S, Alberoni M, Franceschi M, Bettinardi V, Todde S, Fazio F. A PET follow-up study of recovery after stroke in acute aphasics. Brain Lang 1997;56:55–67.
72. Heiss WD, Kessler J, Thiel A, Ghaemi M, Karbe H. Differential capacity of left

and right hemispheric areas for compensation of poststroke aphasia. Ann Neurol 1999;45:430–438.

73. Warburton E, Price CJ, Swinburn K, Wise RSJ. Mechanisms of recovery from aphasia: evidence from positron emission tomography studies. J Neurol Neurosurg Psychiatry 1999;66:155–161.

74. Heilman KM, Watson RT, Valenstein E. Neglect and related disorders. In: Heilman KM, Valenstein E, eds. Clinical Neuropsychology. New York: Oxford University Press, 1993:279–336.

75. Watson RT, Heilman KM, Miller BD, King FA. Neglect after mesencephalic reticular formation lesions. Neurology 1974;24:294–298.

76. Posner MI, Walker J, Friedrich FJ, Rafal RD. Effects of parietal lobe injury on covert orienting of visual attention. J Neurosci 1984;4:163–187.

77. Pedersen PM, Jorgensen HS, Nakayama H, Raaschou HO, Olsen TS. Hemineglect in acute stroke—incidence and prognostic implications. The Copenhagen Stroke Study. Am J Phys Med Rehabil 1997;76:122–127.

78. Pizzamiglio L, Bergego C, Halligan P, Homberg V, Robertson I, Weber E, Wilson B, Zoccolotti P, Deloche G. Factors affecting the clinical measurement of visuospatial neglect. Behav Neurol 1992;5:233–240.

79. Kaplan RF, Cohen RA, Rosengart A, Elsner AE, Hedges III TR, Caplan LR. Extinction during time controlled direct retinal stimulation after recovery from right hemispheric stroke. J Neurol Neurosurg Psychiatry 1995;59:534–536.

80. Suzuki E, Chen W, Kondo T. Measuring unilateral spatial neglect during stepping. Arch Phys Med Rehabil 1997;78:173–178.

81. Rapcsak SZ, Varfaellie M, Fleet WS, Heilman KM. Selective attention in hemispatial neglect. Arch Neurol 1989;46:178–182.

82. Kaplan RF, Verfaellie M, Meadows M, Caplan LR, Pessin MS, De Witt D. Changing attentional demands in left hemispatial neglect. Arch Neurol 1991;48:1263–1266.

83. Heilman KM, Watson RT. Changes in the symptoms of neglect induced by changing task strategy. Arch Neurol 1978;35:47–49.

84. Ishiai S, Sugishita M, Watabiki S, Nakayama T, Kotera M, Gono S. Improvement of left unilateral spatial neglect in a line extension task. Neurology 1994;44:294–298.

85. Mattingley JB, Bradshaw JL, Bradshaw JA. Horizontal visual motion modulates focal attention in left unilateral spatial neglect. J Neurol Neurosurg Psychiatry 1994;57:1228–1235.

86. Ladavas E, Paladini R, Cubelli R. Implicit associative priming in a patient with left visual neglect. Neuropsychologia 1993;31:1307–1320.

87. Hommel M, Peres B, Pollack P, Memin B, Besson G, Gaio J-M, Perret J. Effects of passive tactile and auditory stimuli on left visual neglect. Arch Neurol 1990;47:573–576.

88. Robertson IH, North N. Active and passive stimulation of left limbs: influence on visual and sensory neglect. Neuropsychologia 1993;31:293–300.

89. Ishiai S, Seki Keiko, Koyama Y, Izumi Y. Disappearance of unilateral spatial neglect following a simple instruction. J Neurol Neurosurg Psychiatry 1997;63:23–27.

90. Riddoch MJ, Humphreys GW. The effect of cueing on unilateral neglect. Neuropsychologia 1983;21:589–599.

91. Larmande P, Cambier J. Influence de l'état d'activation hémisphérique sur le phénomène d'extinction sensitive chez 10 patients atteints de lesions hémisphèriques droites. Rev Neurol 1981;137:285–290.

92. Joanette Y, Brouchon M, Gauthier L, Samson M. Pointing with left vs right hand in left visual neglect. Neuropsychologia 1986;24:391–396.

93. Ferro JM, Kertesz A, Black SE. Subcortical neglect: quantitation, anatomy, and recovery. Neurology 1987;37:1487–1492.

94. Black S, Erbert P, Leibovitch F, Szalai JP, Blair N. Recovery in hemispatial neglect. Neurology 1995;45(supple 4):A178 (abstr).

95. Campbell DC, Oxbury JM. Recovery from unilateral visuo-spatial neglect? Cortex 1976;13:303–312.

96. Kinsella G, Ford B. Acute recovery patterns in stroke patients. Neuropsychological factors. Med J Aust 1980;2:663–666.

97. Colombo A, De Renzi E, Gentilini M. The time course of visual hemi-inattention. Arch Psychiatr Nervenkr 1982;231:539–546.

98. Denes G, Semenza C, Stoppa E, Lis A. Unilateral spatial neglect and recovery from hemiplegia. A follow-up study. Brain 1982;105:543–552.

99. Hier DB, Mondlock J, Caplan LR. Recovery of behavioural abnormalities after right hemisphere stroke. Neurology 1983;33:345–350.

100. Levine DN, Warach JD, Benowitz L, Calvanio R. Left spatial neglect: effects of lesion size and premorbid brain atrophy on severity and recovery following right cerebral infarction. Neurology 1986;36:362–366.

101. Sunderland A, Wade DT, Langton HR. The natural history of visual neglect after stroke. Indications from two methods of assessment. Int Disabil Stud 1987;9:55–59.

102. Wade DT, Wood VA, Hewer RL. Recovery of cognitive function soon after stroke: a study of visual neglect, attention span and verbal recall. J Neurol Neurosurg Psychiatry 1988;51:10–13.

103. Stone SP, Patel P, Greenwood RJ, Halligan PW. Measuring visual neglect in acute stroke and predicting its recovery: the visual neglect recovery index. J Neurol Neurosurg Psychiatry 1992;55:431–436.

104. Stone SP, Patel P, Greenwood RJ. Selection of acute stroke patients for treatment of visual neglect. J Neurol Neurosurg Psychiatry 1993;56:463–466.

105. Mattingley JB, Bradshaw JL, Bradshaw JA, Nettleton NC. Recovery from directional hypokinesia and bradykinesia in unilateral neglect. J Clin Exp Neuropsychol 1994;16:861–876.

106. Cassidy TP, Lewis S, Gray CS. Recovery from visuospatial neglect in stroke patients. J Neurol Neurosurg Psychiatry 1998;64:555–557.

107. Feigenson MD, Fletcher H, McDowell MD, Meese P, MacCarthy ML. Factors influencing outcome and length of stay in a stroke rehabilitation unit. Part 1. Analysis of 248 unscreened patients—medical and functional prognostic indicators. Stroke 1977;8:651–656.

108. Wade DT, Hewer RL, Wood VA. Stroke: influence of patients sex and side of weakness on outcome. Arch Phys Med Rehabil 1984;65:513–516.

109. Kinsela G, Ford B. Hemi-inattention and the recovery patterns of stroke patients. Int Rehabil Med 1985;7:102–106.
110. Kotila M, Niemi ML, Laaksonen R. Four year prognosis of stroke patients with visuospatial inattention. Scand J Rehabil Med 1986;18:177–179.
111. Lincoln NB, Blackburn M, Ellis S, Jackson J, Edmans JA, Nouri FM, Walker MF, Haworth H. An investigation of factors affecting progress of patients on a stroke unit. J Neurol Neurosurg Psychiatry 1989;52:493–496.
112. Edmans JA, Towle D, Lincon NB. The recovery of perceptual problems after stroke and the impact on daily life. Clin Rehabil 1991;5:301–309.
113. Ween JE, Alexander MP, Desposito M, Roberts M. Factors predictive of stroke outcome in a rehabilitation setting. Neurology 1996;47:388–392.
114. Dombovy ML, Sandok BA, Basford JR. Rehabilitation for stroke: a review. Stroke 1986;17:363–369.
115. Jongbloed L. Prediction of function after stroke: a critical review. Stroke 1986;17: 765–776.
116. Kalra L, Perez I, Gupta S, Wittink M. The influence of visual neglect on stroke rehabilitation. Stroke 1997;28:1386–1391.
117. Webster JS, Roades LA, Morrill B, Rapport LJ, Abadee PS, Sowa MV, Dutra R, Godlewski MC. Rightward orienting bias, wheelchair maneuvering, and fall risk. Arch Phys Med Rehabil 1995;76:924–928.
118. Ferro JM, Correia M, Freire A, Valente P, Melo TP, Falcão JM, for the "Stroke before 65" study group. Predictors of early death and disability after acute stroke: results from the "Stroke before age 65" study. Cerebrovasc Dis. 1999; 9(suppl 1): 31. (Abstract)
119. Ring H, Feder M, Schwartz J, Samuels G. Functional measures of first-stroke rehabilitation inpatients: usefulness of the functional independence measures total score with a clinical rationale. Arch Phys Med Rehabil 1997;78:630–635.
120. Maeshima S, Dohi N, Funahashi K, Nakai K, Itakura T, Komai N. Rehabilitation of patients with anososognosia for hemiplegia due to intracerebral haemorrhage. Brain Inj 1997;11:691–697.
121. Small M, Ellis S. Brief remission periods in visuospatial neglect: evidence from long-term follow-up. Eur Neurol 1994;24:147–154.
122. Mattingley JB, Bradshaw JL, Bradshaw JA, Nettleton NC. Residual rightward attentional bias after apparent recovery from right hemisphere damage: implications for a multicomponent model of neglect. J Neurol Neurosurg Psychiatry 1994;57: 597–604.
123. Madureira S, Ferro JM. Cognitive decline associated with stroke. Cerebrovasc Dis. 1999; 9(suppl 1):91. (Abstract)
124. Hécaen H, Angelergues R. Étude anatomo-clinique de 280 cas de lésions rétrolandiques unilatérales des hémisphères cérébraux. Encéphale 1961;6:533–562.
125. Critchley M. The Parietal Lobes. New York: Hafner, 1966.
126. Heilman KM, Valenstein E. Frontal lobe neglect in man. Neurology 1971;22:660–664.
127. Watson RT, Heilman KM. Thalamic neglect. Neurology 1979;29:690–694.
128. Damasio AR, Damasio H, Chang Chui H. Neglect following damage to frontal lobe or basal ganglia. Neuropsychologia 1980;22:685–696.

129. Vallar G, Perani D. The anatomy of unilateral neglect after right-hemisphere stroke lesions. A clinical/CT-scan correlation study in man. Neuropsychologia 1986;24: 609–622.

130. Nobre AC, Sebestyen GN, Gitelman DR, Mesulam MM, Frackowiak RSJ, Frith CD. Functional localization of the system for visuospatial attention using positron emission tomography. Brain 1997;120:515–533.

131. Mesulam MM. Large-scale neurocognitive networks and distributed processing for attention, language, and memory. Ann Neurol 1990;28:597–613.

132. Mesulam MM. A cortical network for directed attention and unilateral neglect. Ann Neurol 1981;10:309–325.

133. Karnath H-O. Deficits of attention in acute and recovered visual neglect. Neuropsychologia 1988;26:27–43.

134. Daffner KR, Ahern GL, Weintraub S, Mesulam M-M. Dissociated neglect behavior following sequential strokes in the right hemisphere. Ann Neurol 1990;28:97–101.

135. Vuilleumier P, Hester D, Assal G, Regli F. Unilateral spatial neglect recovery after sequential strokes. Neurology 1996;19:184–189.

136. Kinsbourne M. A model for the mechanism of unilateral neglect of space. Trans Am Neurol Assoc 1970;95:143.

137. Perani D, Vallar G, Cappa SF, Messa C, Fazio F. Aphasia and neglect after subcortical stroke. A clinical/cerebral perfusion correlation study. Brain 1987;110:1211–1229.

138. Vallar G, Perani D, Cappa SF, Messa C, Lenzi GL, Fazio F. Recovery from aphasia and neglect after subcortical stroke: neuropsychological and cerebral perfusion study. J Neurol Neurosurg Psychiatry 1988;51:1269–1276.

139. Ferro J, Cantinho G, Levy A, Godinho F. Subcortical neglect: is cortical diaschisis relevant? In: Vallar G, Cappa SF, Wallesch C-W, eds. Neuropsychological Disorder Associated with Subcortical Lesions. New York: Oxford University Press, 1992: 427–436.

140. Perani D, Vallar G, Paulesu E, Alberoni M, Fazio F. Left and right hemisphere contribution to recovery from neglect after right hemisphere damage—an [18F]FDG PET study of two cases. Neuropsychologia 1993;31:115–125.

141. Pizzamiglio L, Perani D, Cappa SF, Vallar G, Paolucci S, Grassi F, Paulesu E, Fazio F. Recovery of neglect after right hemispheric damage. $H_2^{15}O$ Positron Emission Tomographic Activation Study. Arch Neurol 1998;55:561–568.

142. Kertesz A, Harlock W, Coates R. Computer tomographic localization, lesion size, and prognosis in aphasia and nonverbal impairment. Brain Lang 1979;8:34–50.

143. Basso A, Capitani E, Della Sala S, Laiacona M, Spinnler H. Recovery from ideomotor apraxia. A study on acute stroke patients. Brain 1987;110:747–760.

144. Mimura M, Fitzpatrick PM, Albert ML. Long-term recovery from ideomotor apraxia. Neuropsychiatry Neuropsychol Behav Neurol 1996;9:127–132.

145. Sunderland A. Recovery of ipsilateral dexterity after stroke. Stroke 2000;31:430–433.

146. Kertesz A, Ferro JM. Lesion size and location in ideomotor apraxia. Brain 1984; 107:921–933.

147. Kertesz A, Ferro JM, Shewan CM. Apraxia and aphasia. The functional-anatomocal basis for their dissociation. Neurology 1984;34:40–47.

148. Sunderland A, Tinson D, Bradley L. Differences in recovery from constructional apraxia after right and left hemisphere stroke? J Clin Exp Neuropsychol 1994;16: 916–920.
149. Kotila M, Waltimo O, Niemi M-L, Laaksonen R, Lempinen M. The profile of recovery from stroke and factors influencing outcome. Stroke 1984;15:1039–1044.
150. Lecours AR. Frank Benson's teachings on acquired disorders of written language (with addenda). Aphasiology 1999;56:107–110.
151. Ferro JM. Anatomical correlates of acalculia following left-hemispheric stroke. Behav Neurol 1990;3:7–17.
152. Friedman RB. Recovery from deep alexia to phonological alexia: points on a continuum. Brain Lang 1996;52:114–128.
153. Small SL, Flores DK, Noll DC. Different neural circuits subserve reading before and after therapy for acquired dyslexia. Brain Lang 1998;62:298–308.
154. Lhermitte F, Beauvois MF. A visual-speech disconnexion syndrome. Report of a case with optic aphasia, agnosic alexia and colour agnosia. Brain 1973;96:695–714.
155. Fukuzawa K, Sasanuma S, Tatsumi I, Suzuki T, Fukusako Y. Recovery process of colour naming defects in pure alexia—a five year longitudinal experimental study. Aphasiology 1998;12:267–282.
156. Ferro JM. Transient inaccuracy of reaching caused by a posterior parietal lesion. J Neurol Neurosurg Psychiatry 1984;47:1016–1019.
157. Perez FM, Tunkel RS, Lachmann EA, Nagler W. Balint's syndrome arising from bilateral posterior cortical atrophy or infarction: rehabilitation strategies and their limitation. Disabil Rehabil 1996;18:300–304.
158. Wade DT, Skilbeck C, Hewer RL. Selected cognitive losses after stroke. Frequency, recovery and prognostic importance. Int Disabil Stud 1989;11:34–39.
159. Desmond DW, Tatemichi TK, Figueroa M, Gropen TI, Stern Y. Disorientation following stroke: frequency, course, and clinical correlates. J Neurol 1994;241: 585–591.
160. Pedersen PM, Jorgensen HS, Nakayama H, Raaschou HO, Olsen TS. Orientation in the acute and chronic stroke patient: impact on ADL and social activities. The Copenhagen Stroke Study. Arch Phys Med Rehabil 1996;77:336–339.
161. Román GC, Tatemichi TK, Erkinjuntti T, Cummings JL, Masdeu JC, Garcia JH, Amaducci L, Orgogozo JM, Brun A, Hofman A, Moody DM, O'Brien DM, Yamaguchi T, Grafman J, Drayer PB, Bick KL, Pajeau AK, Bell MA, Decarli C, Culebras A, Korczyn AD, Bogousslavsky J, Hartmann A, Scheinberg P. Vascular dementia: diagnostic criteria for research studies. Report of the Ninds-Airen International Workshop. Neurology 1993;43:250–260.
162. Caplan LR. Posterior Circulation Disease: Clinical Findings, Diagnosis and Management. Oxford: Blackwell, 1996.
163. Clarke S, Assal G, Bogousslavsky J, Regli F, Townsend DW, Leenders KL, Blecic S. Pure amnesia after unilateral left polar thalamic infarct: topographic and sequential neuropsychological and metabolic (PET) correlations. J Neurol Neurosurg Psychiatry 1994;57:27–34.
164. von Cramon DY, Hebel N, Schri U. A contribution to the anatomical basis of thalamic amnesia. Brain 1985;108:993–1008.

165. Graff-Radford NR, Tranel D, van Hoesen GW, Brandt JP. Diencephalic amnesia. Brain 1990;113:1–25.
166. Sala SD, Spinnler H, Venneri A. Persistent global amnesia following right thalamic stroke: an 11-year longitudinal study. Neuropsychology 1997;11:90–103.
167. Kotila M, Hokkanen L, Laaksonen R, Valanne L. Long-term prognosis after left tuberothalamic infarction: a study of 7 cases. Cerebrovasc Dis 1994;4:44–50.
168. Kumral E, Evyapan D, Balkir K. Acute caudate vascular lesions. Stroke 1999;30: 100–108.
169. Martí-Fábregas J, Piles S, Guardia E, Márti-Vilalta JL. Spontaneous primary intraventricular haemorrhage: clinical data, etiology and outcome. J Neurol 1999;246: 287–291.
170. Darby DG, Donnan GA, Saling MA, Walsh KW, Bladin PF. Primary intraventricular haemorrhage: clinical and neuropsychological findings in a prospective stroke series. Neurology 1988;38:68–75.
171. Tatemichi TK, Desmond DW, Stern Y, Paik M, Sano M, Bagiella E. Cognitive impairment after stroke: frequency, patterns and relationship to functional abilities. J Neurol Neurosurg Psychiatry 1994;57:202–207.
172. Hochstenbach J, Mulder T, Van Limbeek J, Donders R, Schoonderwaldt H. Cognitive decline following stroke: a comprehensive study of cognitive decline following stroke. J Clin Exp Neuropsychol 1998;4:503–517.
173. Censori B, Manara O, Agostinis C, Camerlingo M, Casto L, Galavotti B, Partziguian T, Servalli MC, Cesana B, Belloni G, Mamoli A. Dementia after stroke. Stroke 1996;27:1205–1210.
174. Pohjasvaara T, Erkinjuntti T, Ylikoski R, Hietanen M, Vataja R, Kaste M. Clinical determinants of poststroke dementia. Stroke 1998;29:75–81.
175. Desmond DW, Moroney JT, Paik MC, Sano M, Mohr JP, Aboumatar S, Tseng C-L, Chan S, Williams JBW, Remien RH, Hauser WA, Stern Y. Frequency and clinical determinants of dementia after ischemic stroke. Neurology 2000;54:1124–1131.
176. Treves TA, Aronovich BD, Bornstein NM, Korczyn AD. Risk of dementia after a first-ever ischemic stroke: a 3-year longitudinal study. Cerebrovasc Dis 1997;7: 48–52.
177. Pohjasvaara T, Erkinjuntti T, Vataja R, Kaste M. Comparison of stroke features and disability in daily life in patients with ischemic stroke aged 55 to 70 and 71 to 85 years. Stroke 1997;28:729–735.
178. Tatemichi TK, Desmond DW, Mayeux R, Paik M, Stern Y, Sano M, Remien RH, Williams JBW, Mohr JP, Hauser WA, Figueroa M. Dementia after stroke: baseline frequency, risks and clinical features in a hospitalized cohort. Neurology 1992;42: 1185–1193.
179. Hénon H, Pasquier F, Durieu I, Godefroy O, Lucas C, Lebert F, Leys D. Preexisting dementia in stroke patients: baseline frequency, associated factors and outcome. Stroke 1997;28:2429–2436.
180. Desmond DW, Moroney JT, Sano M, Stern Y. Recovery of cognitive function after stroke. Stroke 1996;27:1798–1803.
181. Andersen G, Vestergaard K, Riis JO, Ingeman-Nielsen M. Intellectual impairment in the first year following stroke, compared to an age-matched population sample. Cerebrovasc Dis 1996;6:363–369.

182. Hénon H, Pasquier F, Durieu I, Guerouaou D, Leys D. Post-stroke dementia: influence of preexisting dementia. First International Congress on Vascular Dementia. Geneva, 1999, pp 7 (abstr).

183. Madureira S, Ferro JM: Cognitive decline and stroke: a one year follow-up study. First International Congress on Vascular Dementia. Geneva 1999, pp 7 (abstr).

184. Loeb C, Gandolfo C, Croce R, Conti M. Dementia associated with lacunar infarction. Stroke 1992;23:1225–1229.

185. Guerreiro M, Salgado AV, Reis A, Ferro JM. Neuropsychological study of a cohort of lacunar infarctions. Cerebrovasc Dis 1994;4 (abstr).

186. Guerreiro MM, Melo TP, Ferro JM. Cognitive impairment after spontaneous intracerebral hematoma. Cerebrovasc Dis 1997;7(suppl 4):5 (abstr).

187. Alexander MP, Freedman M. Amnesia after anterior communicating artery aneurysm rupture. Neurology 1984;34:752–757.

188. Irle E, Wowra B, Kunert HJ, Hampl J, Kunze S. Memory disturbances following anterior communicating artery rupture. Ann Neurol 1992;31:473–480.

189. Böttger S, Prosiegel M, Steiger HJ, Yassouridis A: Neurobehavioural disturbances, rehabilitation outcome, and lesion site in patients after rupture and repair of anterior communicating artery aneurysm. J Neurol Neurosurg Psychiatry 1998;65:93–102.

190. Bornstein RA, Weir BKA, Petruk KC, Disney LB. Neuropsychological function in patients after subarachnoid haemorrhage. Neurosurgery 1987;21:651–654.

191. Ljunggren B, Sonesson B, Säveland H, Brandt L. Cognitive impairment and adjustment in patients without neurological deficits after aneurysmal SAH and early operation. J Neurosurg 1985;62:673–679.

192. Desantis A, Laiacona M, Barbarotto R, Basso A, Villani R, Spagnoli D, Capitani E. Neuropsychological outcome of patients operated upon for an intracranial aneurysm: analysis of general prognostic factors and of the effects of the location of the aneurysm. J Neurol Neurosurg Psychiatry 1989;52:1135–1140.

193. Richardson JTE. Cognitive performance following rupture and repair of intracranial aneurysm. Acta Neurol Scand 1991;83:110–122.

194. Hütter B-O, Gilsbach J-M. Which neuropsychological deficits are hidden behind a good outcome (Glasgow=1) after aneurysmal subarachnoid haemorrhage? Neurosurgery 1993;33:999–1006.

195. Satzger W, Niedermeier N, Schönberger J, Engel RR, Beck OJ. Timing of operation for ruptured cerebral aneurysm and long-term recovery of cognitive functions. Acta Neurochir (Wien) 1995;136:168–174.

196. McKenna P, Willison JR, Lowe D, Neil-Dwyer G. Recovery after subarachnoid haemorrhage. Br Med J 1989;299:485–487.

197. Maurice-Williams RS, Willison JR, Hatfield R. The cognitive and psychological sequelae of uncomplicated aneurysm surgery. J Neurol Neurosur Psychiatry 1991;54:335–340.

198. Ogden JA, Mee EW, Henning M. A prospective study of impairment of cognition and memory and recovery after subarachnoid haemorrhage. Neurosurgery 1993;33:572–587.

199. Germanò A, Tisano A, Raffaele M, Munaò F, Cacciola F, La Rosa G, Tomasello F. Is there a group of early surgery aneurysmal SAH patients who can expect to

achieve a complete long-term neuropsychological recovery? Acta Neurochir (Wien) 1997;139:507–514.

200. Eskensen V, Sörensen EB, Rosenörn J, Schmidt K: the prognosis in subarachnoid haemorrhage of unknown etiology. J Neurosurg 1984;61:1029–1031.

201. Brismar J, Sundbärg G: Subarachnoid haemorrhage of unknown origin: prognosis and prognostic factors. J Neurosurg 1985;63:349–354.

202. Cioffi F, Pasqualin A, Cavazzani P, Da Pian R. Subarachnoid haemorrhage of unknown origin: clinical and tomographical aspects. Acta Neurochir (Wien) 1989; 97:31–39.

203. Hütter BO, Gilsbach JM, Kreitschmann I. Is there a difference in cognitive deficits after aneurysmal subarachnoid haemorrhage and subarachnoid haemorrhage of unknown origin? Acta Neurochir (Wien) 1994;127:129–135.

204. Germanò A, Caruso G, Caffo M, Cacciola F, Belvedere M, Tisano A, Raffaele M, Tomasello F. Does subarachnoid blood extravasation per se induce long-term neuropsychological and cognitive alterations? Acta Neurochir (Wien) 1998;140: 805–812.

8
Mood Changes and Disorders After Stroke

Antonio Carota and Julien Bogousslavsky
University of Lausanne and Centre Hospitalier Universitaire Vaudois,
Lausanne, Switzerland

I. INTRODUCTION

Mood disorders are frequently seen in stroke patients. Symptoms or signs of depression and anxiety occur at any time after stroke in about 20–60% of patients (1–4), and have a negative impact on the functional outcome. The phenomenon is even more important because of the high incidence and cost of disability of stroke.

From a theoretical point of view, stroke is an excellent field of research for mood disorders in terms of anatomicoclinical correlations, as poststroke depression is a very frequent disorder. High-resolution MRI techniques permit precise localization. In addition, advances in functional neuroimaging have allowed the visualization of brain activity during mental and motor tasks, making it possible to identify the involvement of cerebral regions that are distant from the lesion, but still part of the neural networks underlying a specific behavioral function. Thus, stroke is a highly innovative field of investigation of human behavior and, despite methodological diversity, will soon become a field of convergence for the disciplines of neurology, neuropsychology, psychology, and psychiatry (5).

Although the anatomicoclinical correlations of most neurobehavioral syndromes occurring in stroke are now recognized, the etiopathology and prognosis of poststroke mood disorders are still not completely understood (6). Many complicated factors are involved: these include the possibility of different subgroups with different etiologies for the same mood disorder; differences in the methods used for diagnosis; the location of the lesion; the poststroke delay; cognitive and physical impairment; the presence of aphasia, anosognosia, motor aprosody, amnesia, fatigue, apathy, catastrophic reaction, emotionalism, indifference reaction, loss of self psychic autoactivation, or dynamic psychological reactions to the disease itself; and the role of neurorehabilitation and behavioral or pharmacological treatments.

Neurocognitive approaches (i.e., the study of specific cognitive functions by means of double dissociation in a single patient with different lesions and/or the study of all the subgroups of functions constituting a normal function) are therefore of limited value in this field. The complexity of behavioral and cognitive symptoms and the marked interpatient variation in clinical expression also limit the use of protocol paradigms in functional neuroimaging. The physiological neural systems processing mood regulation and the neurotransmitters involved are only partially known, and there are no biological markers for diagnosis or experimental models. As a result, the best current approach to investigating mood disorders in stroke is to use very large populations in clinical studies with univocal diagnostic criteria, extensive neuropsychological measurements, and valid statistical analysis.

Many such studies (about 300 in the past 30 years) have been performed; however, because of methodological limitations and differences, the results have been contradictory and difficult to interpret, and at present, the data are not conclusive.

In this chapter, we critically summarize current knowledge on depression, anxiety, mania, and psychosis developing after stroke.

II. DIAGNOSIS OF MOOD AND BEHAVIOR CHANGES AFTER STROKE

The diagnosis of mood disorders associated with stroke and/or with other chronic medical conditions is largely based on structured interviews using DSM-IV diagnostic criteria (American Psychiatric Association, 1994). The difference between DSM-III and DSM-IV criteria for poststroke mood disorders is that in the DSM-IV definition, stroke is considered the causal factor of the mood disturbance (DSM-IV 310.1). The ICD-10 diagnostic criteria (World Health Organization, 1993) for an organic depressive disorder are comparable to those in DSM-IV. The DSM-IV diagnostic criteria for mood disorder due to a general medical condition are summarized in Table 1.

It is still a subject of controversy whether poststroke depression (''organic depression'') and endogenous depression are the result of dysfunction of the same cerebral areas and whether the behavioral signs and subjective symptoms of both conditions are equivalent (7) or at least partially different (8). In endogenous depression, the ''nonreactive'' or ''unmotivated'' (possibly biologically deter-

Table 1   DSM-IV Diagnostic Criteria

Mood disorder due to a general medical condition, mood-incongruent delusions or hallucinations, or disorganized speech. The essential feature is a prominent persistent mood judged to be due to the direct physiological effects of a general medical condition.

Subtypes

    I. With depressive features—the predominant mood is depressed, but not all criteria for a major depressive episode are met

   II. With major depressive-like episodes

      A. At least five of the following symptoms are present over at least a 2-week period; at least one of the symptoms is either (1) a depressed mood or (2) loss of interest or pleasure

         1. Depressed mood most of the day

         2. Markedly decreased interest or pleasure

         3. Significant weight loss or weight gain

         4. Insomnia or hypersomnia

         5. Psychomotor agitation or retardation

         6. Fatigue or loss of energy

         7. Feelings of worthlessness or excessive or inappropriate guilt

         8. Diminished ability to think or concentrate

         9. Recurrent thoughts of death

      B. Distress or impairment of social, occupational, or other functioning

      C. No bereavement

  III. With manic features—the predominant mood is elevated, euphoric, or irritable

  IV. With mixed features—symptoms of both mania and depression are present, but neither predominates

mined) aspects (e.g., feelings of worthlessness, guilt, and suicidal ideation) and morning aggravation prevail, while in poststroke depression, anxiety, diurnal mood fluctuation, and the "motivated" or "reactive" aspects (e.g., low mood, reduced appetite, and anergia) are prevalent (9). The motivated aspects are probably the expression of a psychological reaction to functional impairment consequent to the stroke itself (9). The Post-Stroke Depression Scale, developed to define a behavioral profile specific to depression in stroke and to differentiate it from endogenous depression (10), is a useful tool for recruiting more homogeneous samples of patients in clinical studies. Despite different behavioral profiles, the experimental and clinical data indicate that the two forms of depression share the same neurotransmitter and metabolic dysfunction (serotoninergic), the same response to specific antidepressant drugs (serotonin reuptake inhibitors), and, possibly, dysfunction of the same cerebral regions (see below).

    Differentiating between "major" and "minor" forms of depression is another aspect of great clinical relevance. The symptoms of "major depression" include low mood, insomnia or hypersomnia, reduced appetite, weight loss, anergia, psychomotor retardation, difficulty in concentrating, forgetfulness, anhedonia, loss of interest in sex, feelings of worthlessness, pathological guilt, and recurrent thoughts of death or suicide. The DSM-IV diagnosis of a "major depressive-like episode" is based on the existence of five or more of these depressive symptoms, two of which must be a depressed mood and a loss of interest and pleasure in almost all activities. "Minor depression" is defined as a less severe form of depression with the presence of two, but fewer than five, of the symptoms of major depression and including either a depressed mood or loss of interest. The DSM-IV distinction between major and minor depression seems reasonable and clinically adequate in both stroke patients (11) and endogenous depression. It is uncertain whether the two forms of depression correspond to different etiologies and outcomes.

The distinction between major and minor forms of poststroke depression has been debated in terms of the "continuum" versus the "categorical" hypothesis. The continuum hypothesis considers that in stroke patients, major and minor depression are two expressions of the same disease, which are differentiated by the severity of symptoms on a continuous gradient (10). This continuity may correspond to the same psychological reaction, varying only in its intensity according to the degree of the functional consequences of stroke. The continuum hypothesis has a psychodynamic foundation and is less congruent with neurochemical or anatomicoclinical models. The categorical hypothesis considers that the major and minor forms of poststroke depression are two syndromes with different etiologies, different outcomes, and different implications for therapeutical interventions (12), and has been mainly advanced to support a localizationist model.

DSM-IV diagnostic criteria for behavioral or personality changes due to general medical conditions are summarized in Table 2.

A. Scales and Questionnaires

In the absence of biological markers, clinical studies must rely on the use of scales and questionnaires for diagnosis and reporting symptoms of poststroke mood disorders, all of which have limitations.

Cutoff scores, indices of reliability, and the validity of the scales and the questionnaires for mood evaluation conforming to the DSM-III or DSM-IV criteria are summarized in Table 3.

The use of checklist behavioral questionnaires (Table 4) can also be proposed for predicting an organic pathology in psychiatric patients, even though psychiatric patients without organic mental disorder are expected to show some impairment in one or more of the scale items.

Table 2 DSM-IV Diagnostic Criteria for Personality Change due to a General Medical Condition (310.1)

A. A persistent personality disturbance that represents a change from the individual's previous characteristics personality pattern

B. There is evidence from the history, physical examination, or laboratory findings that the disturbance is the direct physiological consequence of a general medical condition

C. The disturbance is not better accounted for by another mental disorder, including other Mental Disorders due to a General Medical Condition

D. The disturbance does not occur exclusively during the course of a delirium and does not meet criteria for a dementia.

E. The disturbance causes clinically significant distress or impairment in social, occupational, or other important areas of functioning.

Specify type: Labile Type: the predominant feature is affective lability.

Dysinhibited Type: the predominant feature is poor impulse control as evidenced by sexual indiscretions, etc.

Aggressive Type: the predominant feature is aggressive behavior.

Apathetic Type: the predominant feature is marked apathy and indifference.

Paranoid Type: the predominant feature is suspiciousness or paranoid ideation.

Other Type: the predominant feature is not one of above.

Combined Type: more than one feature predominates in the clinical picture.

B. Diagnosis of Mood Disorders in Patients with Aphasia and Other Neurocognitive Syndromes

The neurobehavioral sequelae of stroke syndromes, such as aphasia, indifference or denial, and cognitive impairment, compromise the validity of patients' answers to the scales. Even when language and attentive functions are not involved, patients may still fail to respond in a reliable fashion to standardized tests, such as the Neurobehavioral Cognitive Status Examination (50) or the Visual Analogic Mood Scales (42). Tests to check the validity of replies in interviews are rarely performed. Even patients without cognitive deficits who show dramatic improvement of hemiplegia after thrombolysis seem unaware of the severity of the initial neurological impairment and, surprisingly, sound unemotional (51).

Caution in the use of rating scales is also required, since patients might be more sensitive to the stressor event of stroke than affected by depression and anxiety (52). For these reasons, the evaluation of mood disorders in stroke requires standardized neurological and neuropsychological measurements to assess response reliability of stress levels. The presence of misleading neurological and neurocognitive conditions (Table 5) should also be carefully evaluated.

Table 3 Methods for Assessment of Mood Disorders

Questionnaire (abbreviations)	Scoring	Comments
Hamilton Depression Rating Scales (HDRS): 17 or 21 Items versions [13–15]	>25: severe depression 18–24: moderate depression 7–17: mild depression 0–6 no depression	Most widely used Self-rating In stroke patients, cut-off of 8 or 10
Beck Depression Inventory: 21 Items (BDI-II) [16–18]	0–13: minimal, or no, depression 14–19: mild depression 20–28: moderate depression 29–63: severe depression	Most widely used Self-rating Symptoms of sadness, loss of pleasure, guilty feelings, vegetable signs. Good correlations with HDRS (0.7). It could be implemented by HDRS for somatic items.
Hospital Anxiety and Depression Scales: 14 Items (HAD) [19; 20;21]	Depression: 8–10 doubtful cases, 11 et >11: depression Anxiety: 8–10 doubtful cases, 11 et >11: anxiety	Self-rating. Easy for the patients. Excellent validity compared to HDRS.
General Health Questionnaire: 28 Items (GHQ-28) [19;22;23]	Score >12: presence of a psychiatric disorder. 4 subscales. 1) somatic symptoms, 2) anxiety and insomnia 3) social dysfunction 4) severe depression. No specific for diagnostic syndromes	No significant differences in stroke patients between the GHQ-30 and the HAD Scale in identifying depression or anxiety disorders but cut-off could be suboptimal.
Geriatric Depression Scale (GDS): 30 Items [20;24–26]	11–30: depression	More useful in geriatrci populations. It de-emphasizes somatic symptoms.
Zung Self-Rating Depression Scale (ZSRDS) (27)		Useful in patients with neurologic disorders, smilar to BDI and CES-D.
Post-Stroke Depression Scale (PSDS) [10]	No cut-off scores, but symptomatic profile	It detects: depressed mood, feelings of guilt, thoughts of death and suicide, vegetative disorders, apathy, anxiety, catastrophic reactions, emotionalism, anhedonia, diurnal mood variations.

Center for Epidemiologic Studies Depression Scale (CES-D): 20 Items [28–30]	Score >16: depression	Self-rating Correlation with HDRS: 0.44–0.69. No influence of sex, age, race, education. It could be difficult to discriminate major depression and generalized anxiety.
Goldberg Anxiety and Depression Scales (GADS): [31;32]	Nine questions	Useful as screening measures in medical setting for anxiety or depression but lacks specificity for each disorder.
Montgomery-Asberg Depression Rating Scale (MADRS): 10 Items [33,34]	Cut off of 35 to separate moderate from severe depression	Significant correlation with the HRDS. Its capacity to differentiate between responders and nonresponders to antidepressant treatment may be better than the HRS, showing a greater sensitivity to change.
Neurobehavioral Cognitive Status Examination (NCSE): 10 scales. [35–37]	Score between 10 and 40. 13 was optimal for discriminating between patients with organic mental disorder and those without the disorder.	Useful as screening tool.
Visual Analogic Mood Scales (VAMS) [18;38–42]	No cut off scores: continuous variables.	Vertical lines version to avoid bias due to hemineglect. Especially constructed for patients with language disturbancies. The utility of these scales in stroke patients is debated [38;39;42]
Stroke Aphasic Depression Questionnaire: 10 Items (SADQ) [43]	Specific for aphasic patients	Validity: 0.32–0.67 with HDRS
Modified Analogue Dysphoria Scale (MADS) [40]	Specific for patients with severe language disturbances.	Sleep and eating disturbances measured by using both self-report and nursing assessments.

Table 4   Methods for Assessment of Behavior Disorders

Questionnaire (abbreviations)	Scoring	Comments
Neuropsychiatric inventory (NPI) [44;45]	Domain-specific scores (delusions, hallucinations, agitation/aggression, dysphoria, anxiety, euphoria, apathy, disinhibition, irritability/lability, aberrant motor activity, nighttime behavioral disturbances, appetite and eating behaviors).	Structured caregiver interview Useful for behavioral changes in dementia syndromes.
Neurobehavioral Cognitive Status Examination (NCSE): 10 scales [35–37]	Score between 10 and 40. 13 is optimal for discriminating between patients with organic mental disorder and those without the disorder.	Useful as screening tool for cognitive impairment in psychiatric or medical setting.
Neurobehavioral Rating Scale: 27 subscales [46]	Subscales score (cognition/energy, metacognition [self-appraisal, planning, disinhibition] somatic conern/anxiety, depression, language, orientation, memory, reasoning, attention etc...)	Self-report. Used in closed head injury
Neuropsychology Behavior and Affect Profile: 106 statements [47]	Five scales: inappropriateness, indifference, depression, pragnosia (defect in communicative style), mania. It has questions to break the tendency of the patient among the scales.	Structured informant interview. Studies on patients with dementia and stroke.
Frontal behavioral inventory: 24 Items [48]	Operational definition with a minimal score of 27 for psychopathological diagnosis. Score range: 0–72. Evaluation of apathy, perseveration, inappropriateness, utilization behavior etc.	Informant interview. Used to enhance diagnosis of Frontal Lobe Dementia. Promitting for patients with focal brain lesions.
Revised Memory and Behavior Problems Checklist: 24 Items [49]	3 first-order factors: memory-related, depression, and disruptive behaviors, and 1 general factor of behavioral disturbance.	Questions to caregiver and patient: empirical assessment of behavior problems in dementia patients.

Table 5 Diagnostic Confounders of Depressive
Syndromes After Stroke

---

1) Indirect
Common to many severely ill hospitalized patients
   Controlled appetite (e.g., NPO and tube feeding)
   Frequently awakened
   Confined to bed
   Delirium (acute confusional states)
Of special concern in stroke patients
   Immobility (potential confusion with apathy)
   Dysphagia (interferes with eating habits)
   Slurred speech (and resultant miscommunication)
2) Direct
   Aphasia
   Amnesia and cognitive impairment
   Anosognosia and denial of depressive signs
   Aprosody
   Neurological apathy syndromes
      Isolated abulia/apathia
      Loss of psychic auto-activation
      Frontal lobe syndrome
      Klüver-Bucy syndrome
      Korsakoff's syndrome
      Poststroke fatigue
   Special behavioral syndromes
      Emotional lability or emotionalism
      Catastrophic reaction
   Dementia
   Pseudobulbar syndrome

    Most studies have excluded patients with *language disturbances* as their emotions, behavior, and mood changes cannot be reliably tested by verbal examination. Very few authors have considered the real effect of this methodological limitation by reporting the number of excluded patients and calculating its effect on the variances of the statistical analysis. Fedoroff et al. (53) suggested that the exclusion of aphasic patients did not significantly affect the results of their studies supporting a localizationistic model, but Gainotti et al. (54) showed that if the statistical analysis took into consideration those patients who could not be assessed or who could only be evaluated by nonverbal mood measurements, the role of lesion location might not be significant.

    Various scales and questionnaires have been constructed and tested to objectify mood changes in patients with aphasia. The Stroke Aphasic Depression

Questionnaire (43) and a modified Analogue Dysphoria Scale (40) make it possible to report, together with verbal items, vegetative and other symptoms independently of language ability (i.e., eating and sleep disturbances). These scales show a good validity compared to other standard mood disorder questionnaires, especially the HRDS. The Visual Analog Mood Scales (VAMS) assess mood (sad, happy, tense, afraid, tired, energetic, confused, and angry) on a 10-cm vertical line (to avoid neglect effects) with two pictures at the bottom (e.g., a smiling and a sad face for happiness and sadness). Some studies (38,39) have demonstrated their validity as standardized measurements, while others have criticized their utility because their administration is not completely independent of linguistic cues and the test-retest variability may be surprisingly great, even for short time intervals (42).

Anosognosia and denial are neurological conditions, generally consequent to right hemispheral lesions, that involve self-perception at a primitive and nonconscient level and have no apparent relation with mood disorders. Anosognosia is the patient's inability to recognize, with different degrees of severity, his own neurological deficit (i.e., hemianopsia, motor paresis, dysarthria, and sensory loss). Although the distinction with anosognosia is not always retained, denial is more dependent on the observer's interpretation of the patient's behavioral response to the disease and its consequences, and does not focus on single neurological deficits. The type of interview can influence both the degree of anosognosia and denial.

There are reports that patients with anosognosia and denial express behavioral correlates of depression (overt sadness, passivity, or vegetative symptoms), although they might deny mood changes, as they do with neurological deficits (55,56). Thus, anosognosia and neglect might surprisingly coexist with major depression, which supports a theory of depressive diseases as general arousal-attentional disorders (57). Specific scales and questionnaires (58) must be used to assess anosognosia and denial in patients with right-hemispheric lesions who are evaluated for mood disorders.

Emotional dysprosody, consequent to right-hemispheric or basal ganglia lesion, is the impaired ability to give expressional tone modulation to oral language. While talking, patients with dysprosodia give the impression of a lack of affection and are, therefore, considered depressed, even when they are not. Emotional dysprosody, which is often associated with impairment of facial emotion recognition and with anosognosia, must, therefore, be clearly distinguished from poststroke depression. The caregiver's replies to interview questions should be carefully evaluated to check whether the patient has features of dysprosody, rather than of depression. Detailed testing of emotional dysprosody is provided by the Recognition of Facial and Vocal Expression of Emotion Test (59). A test that can be used for bedside screening is the repetition of a sentence (e.g., I'm going to the cinema) in happy, sad, angry, or indifferent tones of voice, while judging the patient's ability to match the examiner's affective quality.

Patients with *amnesia* or *cognitive impairment* can provide unreliable responses to mood questionnaires and may also react with negative feelings because of inability to cope with tasks. A clinical assessment of stroke patients for mood disorders requires a complete neuropsychological evaluation, including memory testing (word and sign lists) and executive functions (i.e., Stroop test, inhibition of inappropriate responses, and Luria gestural sequences), and must include the examiner's clinical judgment regarding the reliability of a patient who shows memory or cognitive impairment.

In about 20–25% of cases, patients with stroke complain of *fatigue* or *apathy*, and these symptoms can contribute to functional and cognitive impairment (60,61).

Apathy is defined as a lack of motivation not attributable to a reduced level of consciousness, cognitive impairment, or emotional distress, which manifests as flat affect, short and delayed answers, hypophonia, reduced motor responses, fixed and blank face, perseverations, and lack of awareness of the situation. Apathy and depression are related dimensions of behavior, but can be distinguished. Apathy is related to disruption of frontosubcortical pathways at various anatomical sites, such as the right dorsolateral frontal and left frontotemporal regions (62), the cingulate gyrus (63), and the posterior limb of the internal capsule (60). Structured interviews, such as the Apathy scale (61) and the Apathy Evaluation Scale (64,65), can help in the diagnosis of apathy and in distinguishing it from depression.

Fatigue problems are reported by up to 70% of stroke patients, even at a considerable time after stroke (66), and can have a great impact on cognitive, physical, and social functions, and on rehabilitation. Fatigue is frequently independent of depressive feelings, neurological deficits, and lesion location. The Fatigue Impact Scale can be an useful tool in characterizing this symptom and its causes (66).

Loss of self-autopsychic activation (or athymormia) is a behavioral syndrome distinct from depression, characterized by apathetic, aspontaneous, indifferent behavior with loss of motor and affective drive, due to lack of motivation. In contrast to depression, it is reversible under repeated stimulation. Athymormia, which can be assessed by special interviews (67), is generally consequent either to ischemic focal lesions (68,69), such as subcortical lesions (70) involving, often bilaterally, the rostral part of the caudate nucleus, the pallidum, the putamen, the thalamus (71), and the gyrus cinguli, or to disseminated cortical and subcortical lesions, as in the case of antiphospholipid syndrome (personal observation).

The diagnosis of apathy, fatigue, and athymormia and their distinction from mood disorders is necessary to optimize therapy and maximize recovery.

Emotionalism and *catastrophic reactions* are other syndromes that can be independent of depression in patients with stroke.

Emotionalism or emotional lability is an increase in the frequency of crying or laughing that starts with little or no warning. Emotional expression is outside normal control, with the result that the patient cries or laughs in social situations in which he would not previously have done so. It affects 15–25% of patients in the first 6 months after stroke, with a declining prevalence at 1 year (72). It is one manifestation of a more general disorder of emotional control occurring after stroke and is often associated with depression (72–75), although most people with emotionalism are not depressed. The scale developed by Robinson et al. (76) is useful for measuring the intensity of pathological crying and laughing. Emotionalism must be distinguished from the pseudobulbar syndrome, because the former is provoked by stimuli that seem meaningful and is common after unilateral strokes. Various locations have been reported, e.g., anterior lesions (72) or frontal and temporal lesions (73), but a specific link between lesion location and the emergence of emotionalism has not yet been demonstrated. The underlying abnormalities may be serotoninergic, since some patients respond to antidepressant medications, such as citalopram (77), fluoxetine (78,79), or sertraline (80).

Catastrophic reaction (CR), a rare affective disorder following left-hemispheric strokes (81,82), manifests as a disruptive emotional outburst with anxiety, agitation, and aggressive behavior when the patient is confronted with a task he cannot solve because of the stroke-induced impairment. In the case of a patient with aphasia, the most frequent trigger is a linguistic task. The catastrophic reaction appears to be a specific consequence of the intense frustration and perceived loss associated with aphasia (generally nonfluent aphasia). This may explain the reported higher incidence of depression in left frontal or temporal or subcortical strokes (82).

C. Observational Methods

The use of observational methods to diagnose depression can avoid bias in patients' answers. They do not involve interviewing the patient, but instead depend on reporting apparent behavior (sadness, passivity, crying, isolation, and acts of self-harm) and vegetative symptoms (sleep or appetite disturbances, autonomic anxiety, anergia, and weight loss) (53,84).

These methods allow the diagnosis of depression in patients with aphasia or cognitive impairment and in patients who deny depression, but are "observed" to be depressed ("nonstandard depression").

The Emotional Behavior Index Form (EBIF), a simple observational method that is independent of language abilities, has been designed and employed in our center to define the emotional profile of patients during the acute phase of first-ever stroke (85). The EBIF, completed daily by the stroke unit nurses caring for the patient, consists of 38 rated items in the classes of overt sadness, passivity, aggressiveness, indifference, disinhibition, and adaptation (Table 6).

Our experience with this method is that despite a trend correlating overt sadness and passivity to diagnosis of depression with standard criteria, it does not define an early-risk profile of developing mood disorders. Most emotional reactions during the acute phase may be dissociated from the patient's subjective experience and could be the consequence of a psychological reaction to the illness.

In other studies, the identification of vegetative and behavioral signs of depression, together with psychological symptoms, seems not to overdiagnose major depression compared with the reporting of psychological symptoms alone (53,86). However, vegetative symptoms of depression alone may not make it possible to differentiate between minor depression and nondepression. Another limitation of the observational methods is that, for a valid report, the informant must be in very frequent contact with the patient and, even then, he cannot have a complete understanding of the patient's internal state of mood.

Finally, the anatomicoclinical origin of, and neurophysiological mechanisms involved in, vegetative symptoms are not completely understood. These are frequent symptoms in patients with stroke or chronic medical illness and may be dissociated from the verbal symptoms of depression.

However, to understand the etiopathology of poststroke depression, patients with only observed depression must be distinguished from those with standard depression.

D. Biological Markers

A reliable laboratory test for diagnosis of depression can avoid methodological bias in enrolling populations of stroke patients. The failure to reduce cortisol blood levels in the dexamethasone suppression test (DST) was proposed about 20 years ago as a diagnostic or screening test for depression (87,88). Its median specificity is 70–85% and its median sensitivity 50–67%, but the results can vary according to time of diagnosis of depression after stroke (89) and DST is therefore of very limited clinical value (90–94). Depressive patients with stroke may have a reduced growth hormone response to desipramine compared to patients with stroke without depression and controls (95).

The TRH stimulation test also fails to show any difference in T3 levels between depressed and nondepressed stroke patients (90,96).

Table 6   Emotional Behavior Index Form

	Not at all	Sometimes	Often	More than often
Sadness				
Cries				
Looks sad				
Complains				
Screams				
Groans				
Passivity				
Gives up				
Isolated				
Aggressiveness				
Tense				
Agitated				
Angry				
Rebellious				
Opposed				
Aggressive				
Revolted				
Indifference				
Indifferent				
Neglected				
Apathetic				
Disinhibition				
Jokes				
Disinhibited				
Laughs				
Impatient				
Denial				
Minimizes				
Total denial				
Partial denial				
Adaptation				
Smiles				
Sociable				
Quiet				
Patient				
Can make well-founded requests				
Decent				
Interested, curious				
Looks serious				
Interactive				
Accommodating				
Helpful				
Expressive				
Tidy				
Docile				

E. Electrophysiological Markers

Sleep complaints and electroencephalographic (EEG) sleep abnormalities are associated with risk of first-onset depression, illness severity, treatment outcome, and vulnerability to recurrence of depression (97). Polysomnographic measurements in patients with major depressive disorder indicate an association between depressive symptoms and sleep measurements related to delta EEG, suggesting impaired sleep drive or heightened arousal during sleep (98). Polysomnographic tests and analyses are currently too expensive and time-consuming to be used in clinical practice, but can be used for research purposes.

P300 latency increases in patients with primary major depression and could be the effect of an altered ''cognitive neuronal pool'' or of a neurotransmitter/neuropeptide imbalance in critical neural networks (99). These results have been reproduced in patients with poststroke depression (100,101); however, despite the age-related variations, stroke itself is known to increase P300 ERP latency for temporary periods (100). For this reason, the usefulness of P300 latency as a marker for poststroke depression requires further evaluation.

III. POSTSTROKE DEPRESSION

A. Incidence, Prevalence, and Demographic Data

The prevalence of depression in stroke patients is reported to be 20–40% in the first 2 weeks (53,102,103), 32–53% at 3–4 months (103–106), 26% at 6 months (107,108), 19–55% at 1 year (4,103–106,108), 19% at 2 years (103), and 9–41% at 3 years (2,103,109).

A similar prevalence is seen in community-based (27–62%) (1,4,110–112), outpatient (40%) (3,106,113), and rehabilitation patient (27.4–55%) studies (113–119).

Major depression accounts for a minority of cases, with a prevalence of 10–20% in stroke patients (102,120,121), but, depending on time elapsed after stroke and the place of residence, can increase up to 40% (103,114). The prevalence of minor depression varies between 5 and 40% in stroke patients (106,121). These large variations in epidemiological data are due to the use of different structured interviews, to the different size and selection criteria of study populations, and to different times of investigations. The incidence and prevalence of endogenous depression in the general population (15–33%) (110,122,123) are probably more elevated but, in the absence of more specific clinical and neuroradiological data about the different subtypes of depression, we suggest that a certain number of cases are due to unrecognized poststroke depression; this is certainly the case in the geriatric population.

The incidence of poststroke depression varies slightly with age (124) and gender (2,125,126). Poststroke depression is reported to be more frequent in women than men when the lesion is in the left hemisphere (127). In women, major depression correlates with a high level of education, cognitive impairment, and previous psychiatric antecedents, while in men, it is more dependent on physical impairment (127). However, Morris et al. (128) found that minor depression is more frequent in men and is associated with inadequate spousal social support.

In our opinion, there are no valid phsyiopathological theories that can explain the sexual difference according to cerebral localization, and psychological factors are probably more relevant.

Critical analysis of the epidemiological data merely indicates that the incidence and prevalence of mood disorders after stroke are very high and that the risk factors are still not clearly understood. Finally, the investigation of mood disorders in stroke patients is necessary even when several years have elapsed since the acute phase.

B. Attempts at Localization

In "primary" or "endogenous" depression, CT and MRI imaging studies are not diagnostic, but show a trend toward a reduction in volume of the basal ganglia (129,130), hyppocampus (131–133), amygdala (132), cortical and subcortical atrophy (129), white matter hyperintensities (134,135), and ventricular enlargement (136).

PET (137–139) and SPECT studies (140,141) show reduced metabolism with normalization after therapy in the left frontosubcortical and paralimbic circuits, left anterior cingulate, superior temporal and parietal cortex, and caudate.

The report of dysexecutive signs in depressed patients (142) supports the association of depression with dysfunction of frontostriatal and frontobasal limbic pathways.

Most clinical studies investigating mood changes after stroke have also tried to identify the cerebral regions the dysfunction of which causes poststroke depression. The underlying hypothesis is that the same cerebral regions are involved in poststroke and endogenous depression, but that, in the case of endogenous or primary depression, a neurotransmitter or neuropeptide abnormality, and not a structural lesion, is the main factor. These regions should be part of, or connected to, the limbic and temporal lobes and be involved in the processing of emotions and mood states that enhance or inhibit oriented-goal behaviors. The central role of the limbic and temporal regions is suggested by the strict association that exists, in the case of focal cerebral lesions, between emotional changes and memory disturbances. The amygdala and hippocampal area should be the critical systems regulating both functions. The temporal lobes, the connections of hippocampus and amygdala with the neocortex, the posterior and anterior insula are involved in the cognitive process establishing primary (right-hemisphere dominance) or social (left-hemisphere dominance) emotions. Temporal lobe hypoperfusion was found in a group of depressed patients with subcortical lesions, but not in a group with subcortical ischemic lesion without depression, suggesting that, in the case of subcortical lesions, because of a dyaschisis phenomenon, the temporal lobe may be critical for the occurrence of poststroke depression (143). The basal ganglia are also part of the pathways (frontosubcortical and temporolimbic) underlying behavioral responses. Their major role in emotion and mood state is in highly dynamic modulation, execution, spontaneity, and basic motor processing of emotional behaviors, all of which probably have side dominance. The basal ganglia also synchronize mood and motor behavior, and depression and anxiety show well-recognized patterns of abnormal motor expression (144).

Although other studies could not replicate these findings (145), several clinical and experimental studies have suggested the role of the limbic connected areas and basal ganglia in the development of poststroke depression (146–149). The results of these studies are summarized below.

Beblo et al. (150) reduced methodological bias by selecting 20 patients with poststroke depression without severe physical impairment, psychiatric antecedents, concomitant morbidity, and aphasia, and then performed complete neuropsychological measurements. Their findings again pointed out that poststroke depression may be related to dysfunction of (cortico-)striato-pallido-thalamic-cortical projections or frontal frontal/temporal lobe-basal ganglia-ventral brainstem circuits. Kim and Choi-Kwon (151) found a similar lesion distribution in patients with poststroke depression and patients with emotional lability, suggesting that both conditions may have the same origin. In patients with acute traumatic brain injury and major depression, the presence of left dorsolateral frontal lesions and/or left basal ganglia lesions is associated with an increased probability of developing major depression (152).

Patients with Parkinson's disease and Huntington's chorea affected by depression show reduced regional blood flow in the orbital frontal cortex and basal ganglia, basal temporal lobes, cingulate cortex, and thalamus (153).

The role of subcortical lesions is suggested by numerous retrospective MRI studies (154–160) that show a relationship between major unipolar depression and silent cerebral infarction, especially in the subcortical frontal area and basal ganglia (160). In these patients, the severity of depression can be greater and the response to pharmacological treatment less prompt. These studies suggest that approximately half of patients with presenile-onset major depression and probably the majority of patients with senile-onset major depression might have the diagnosis of poststroke or "secondary" depression. Health strategies aimed at preventing cerebrovascular disease (e.g., diet, physical activity/exercise, smoking cessation, and cardiovascular medication compliance) may lessen depressive vulnerability in the elderly.

Severe depressive mood disorders, together with euphoria, emotional lability, and loss of spontaneity, are also reported in patients with CADASIL (161,162). In HIV encephalopathy patients who have diffuse white matter or basal ganglia lesions, depressive symptoms are an important clinical manifestation (163,164). In patients with multiple sclerosis, severity of depression correlates with the amount of demyelinating lesions in the semiovale centers (165) and has been related to an increased lesion load of the projection areas of the basal limbic system (166).

A large number of clinical studies performed by Robinson and colleagues (148,167) (Johns Hopkins University) support the role of frontal, subcortical, and basal ganglia lesions in the development of poststroke mood changes. However, these authors indicated that the location of the lesion in the left hemisphere and the proximity of its anterior border to the frontal pole are other determinant factors for behavioral changes. According to Robinson et al. (168,169), the neuroanatomy of the biogenic amine-containing pathways in the cerebral cortex, which have a more anterior distribution, might explain the linear correlation between anterior lesion location and severity of depression. Furthermore, these authors support a categorical hypothesis, because they considered that, in stroke patients, major and minor depression have different etiologies and lesion locations (more caudal in the case of minor depression) (11). These studies were interpreted in the light of the "valence" hypothesis, which states that, in physiological states, the left hemisphere is specialized in the control of positive emotions, while the right hemisphere processes negative emotions. The valence hypothesis predicts that, in the case of dysfunction of the left hemisphere, there is an emergence of negative and paleological emotions normally processed by the right hemisphere (170).

The conclusions of the studies of Robinson et al. advancing a localizationist model for poststroke depression with left-hemispheric dominance have been the subject of great criticism. Diffuse lesions in the territory of the medial cerebral artery are frequently proximal to both poles. Small samples of patients were analyzed (30–45 subjects) and the same patients were probably reused in successive studies, and therefore the major hypothesis linking poststroke depression to lesion site appears statistically weak. The exclusion of patients with severe aphasia or cognitive impairment has probably resulted in an important selection bias. The confounding role of amnesia, anosognosia, apathia, fatigue, loss of psychic auto-activation, and emotional lability has not been completely evaluated, and these symptoms are neurobehavioral clinical correlates of basal ganglia lesions (171). Another criticism of the localizationist model is that, especially during the acute phase, the symptoms of poststroke depression can be the result of metabolic dysfunction of distant cerebral areas connected with the lesions, a well-known phenomenon in the case of neglect, aphasia, or apraxia determined by subcortical lesions. Several other clinical studies, using similar methods, failed to find any lateralization or any anteroposterior gradient for poststroke mood changes (15,114,117,121,172–175), while others found that right, rather than left, hemispheric lesions were significantly associated with poststroke depression (72,173,176). It is also possible that when depression and anxiety coexist, they may be associated with different patterns of asymmetrical hemispheric function, as shown by a lateralized processing test (i.e., the chimeric face test) in groups with only depression or anxiety and groups in which both conditions are present (177). It has also been suggested that, while a clinical syndrome similar to endogenous depression is seen in patients with right lesions, symptoms in patients with left lesions more closely resemble those of neurotic depression, despite the fact that both conditions can respond to antidepressants (178).

The Baltimore group was unable to replicate their findings at different times poststroke. In their later studies, they suggested that, during the acute phase (179–182), poststroke depression is associated with left anterior and basal ganglia lesions (183), is a function of the volume of the lesion, and is independent of language dominance (184); during short-term follow-up (several months), lesion volume and the proximity of the lesion to the frontal pole of both hemispheres are the major determinants (179); and after 1–2 years, poststroke depression is significantly associated with dysfunction of the right hemisphere and the volume of the lesion and its proximity to the occipital pole (179). Furthermore, these findings are valid only in patients with typical occipital asymmetry, while a reversal pattern is seen in cases of atypical occipital asymmetry (186). Gender could also play a role, since, in the case of left lesions, women might have a greater risk of depression than men (127). Finally poststroke delay, occipital asymmetry but not cerebral dominance for language, and gender are, according to Robinson et al., the principal factors explaining interstudy differences in anatomical correlates of poststroke depression.

In conclusion, endogenous and poststroke depression could have the same origin in the dysfunctioning of a mood-processing neural network, which includes the frontosubcortical circuits, basal ganglia, and limbic lobes, and both exhibit serotonin hyporegulation.

Methodological limitations mean that results regarding the role of a left-right and an anterior-posterior gradient may be biased and that lesion location may contribute only a small extent to the risk of developing poststroke depression (6).

C. Cognitive Impairment

A significant association between poststroke depression and cognitive deficits has been reported in several studies (108,187–192), even though stroke itself may be followed by a significant decline in cognitive performance when prestroke and poststroke measurements are compared (193).

The main question in this field is whether it is depression that negatively influences the outcome of cognitive impairment or whether cognitive impairment leads to depression. Data from numerous studies (105,145,187,191) fail to provide an insight into the problem, mainly because of methodological limitations. Many studies cannot be compared because of differences in the neuropsychological measurements adopted and the times of investigation. Another consideration is that, in the majority of these studies, the presence of cognitive impairment was evaluated using the MMSE, a test with obvious limitations, including its dependence on verbal skills to communicate the test instructions, the different degrees of sensitivity of its various items (which overestimate deficits in patients with left lesions), and its inability to accurately test frontal or executive functions (190,194). Although noncomparable, some of these studies provide evidence that depression is the main factor leading to, or aggravating, cognitive impairment due to stroke. This hypothesis induced the authors to use the term "dementia of depression" (190).

We will briefly summarize the data in favor of this hypothesis. Frontoamnesic deficits due to disruption of cortical projections to the caudate nucleus have been suggested to explain the progressive deterioration of patients with poststroke depression and lesions of the caudate nucleus (149). Working with a group of 53 patients with single stroke lesions, Bolla-Wilson et al. (190) found that patients with left-hemispheric lesions and major depression were more impaired in terms of orientation, language (naming), verbal learning, visuoperceptual and visuoconstructional tasks, and executive functions (attention, concentration, nonverbal problem solving, and psychomotor speed) than those with left lesions, but no depression, data confirmed by other studies (105,196,197). The presence of dysphasia has also been suggested to increase the risk of major depression (105). The same neuropsychological profile has been seen in elderly patients with endogenous depression (198). Greater severity and longer duration of cognitive impairment were seen in patients with depression and left lesions compared to nondepressed patients with similar cerebral lesions or depressed patients with right lesions, suggesting the possibility of "dementia of depression" in patients with left lesions and depression (190,199,200).

The results of other studies favor the opposite hypothesis that in patients with stroke and cognitive impairment, depressive symptoms are part of, or determined by, a dementia syndrome, the so-called "depression of dementia" (199).

In other community studies, using MMSE (15,108,172) or other measurements (188), no evidence was found to support a correlation between cognitive impairment and major depression 1 year after first-ever stroke (108).

In conclusion, in our opinion, despite inconclusive findings indicating depression to be a factor leading to dementia in cerebrovascular patients, sufficient data exist to support a correlation between cognitive impairment and depression. In this context, it is imperative to perform a complete cognitive and mood evaluation in patients with poststroke depression and to intervene as soon as possible with behavioral or pharmacological treatments, where indicated, to favorably enhance the functional and social rehabilitation.

D. Neurological Deficits and Outcome

Neurological deficits, which induce feelings of frustration related to acknowledgment of the handicap and its implications in daily life, contribute to the development of mood disorders that might therefore have a psychological, rather than an organic, etiology. Depressive symptoms may be the expression of the patient's strategy for coping with the handicap. Several studies have shown that the development and intensity of depressive symptoms correlate strongly with the grade of functional impairment (105,111,124) during the acute phase and the first 6 months (201), a result not confirmed in other studies when depressed patients with stroke were compared with patients with stroke but no depression (87,107,202). No definite conclusion can be made from the literature (Table 7), although the association of poststroke depression with stroke severity and functional outcome seems more likely.

Table 7 Factors Associated with Poststroke Depression in 12 Clinical Studies[a]

	Significance in 12 studies	
Factors	Significant	Nonsignificant
Age	6	6
Gender (F)	5	6
Prior stroke	3	2
Prior disability	0	2
Prior depression	3	1
Stroke severity	5	0
Stroke side	1	7
Lesion volume	1	2
Anterior circulation	3	2
Cognition	5	2
Functional outcome	9	1

[a] Wade et al., 1987 (1); Ebrahim et al., 1987 (117); Andersen et al., 1995 (118); Burvill et al., 1997 (111); Herrmann et al., 1998 (119); Kotila et al., 1998 (112); Pohjasvaara et al. 1998 (113); Kauhanen et al., 1999 (105); Robinson et al., 1999 (203); Sato et al., 1999 (145); Dennis et al., 2000 (204); Singh et al., 2000 (205).

We will report the results of some studies in which the association between poststroke depression and functional impairment was quantified using rigorous functional measurements (ADL, Barthel Index, NIH, and the Functional Independence Measure).

In the study of Neau et al. (124) of young adult patients with stroke, multivariate analysis showed a low NIH score on admission to be a significant predictor for return to work, absence of poststroke depression, and a good quality of life. The hypothesis that functional impairment could be one of the major causal factors for depression, especially in the elderly, is also based on studies that showed a similar incidence or prevalence of depression in patients with stroke and patients with similar functional disability due to other medical illness (i.e., hip fracture) (206–209). In the study of Singh et al. (205), functional measurements correlated temporally with the progress of poststroke depression and were better longitudinal predictors of depressive symptoms than lesion location.

The other unresolved issue is whether it is the functional impairment that leads to depression or whether the depression itself can compromise the motor and cognitive outcome of deficits due to the stroke. Many studies (104,112,210–212), but not all (213), report that depressive feelings themselves negatively influence the prognosis and functional outcome of patients with stroke at short- and long-term follow-up. A comparison of groups of stroke patients with or without mood disorders, but with the same functional disability, showed that physical functioning, bodily pain, somatic symptoms, and social functioning were worse in patients with affective disorders (214). Depressive patients with stroke may not have the energy or motivation to participate in rehabilitation therapy. They may also feel helpless or hopeless about the future and, therefore, fail to put any effort into rehabilitation treatments.

It is important to consider that, surprisingly, patients with great disability and depressive mood frequently express little enthusiasm about receiving psychiatric treatment. The reason for this is probably related to the negative correlation between physical impairment, reduced functional autonomy, and the lack of self-esteem that induces the patients to perceive themselves as useless and hopeless. Self-esteem has been shown to be significantly correlated to functional independence (215). The functional ability and state of self-esteem at 2 weeks, as well as the presence of heart disease, were significant predictors (55%) of functional ability at 3 months. Level of self-esteem is also a consistent factor in the prediction of the functional long-term outcome.

Other authors found that minor, rather than major, depression correlated with greater physical disability and therefore only minor depression corresponds to an adjustment reaction to physical impairment (12,172).

Depressive feelings at the time of initial inpatient evaluation result in a greater than threefold increase in the risk of subsequent mortality (over the following 10 years) in patients with poststroke depression compared to patients with stroke but no depression (216). This risk is independent of other cardiovascular risk factors, age, sex, social class, type of stroke, lesion location, and level of social functioning, but may also be associated with social isolation (216). Patients who are depressed may return to detrimental habits, such as smoking or consuming excessive alcohol, and may not comply with treatment recommendations, such as medications or health-promoting behavior. The effect of negative mood states in increasing mortality is probably also mediated by modifications of the cardiovascular system (217,218). Patients with endogenous depression experience a higher grade of arterial hypertension (219) (especially elevation of the systolic pressure) and myocardial infarction (220–222). Another possible explanation for the increased mortality is enhanced platelet aggregation caused by depression (223). The final effect is the progression of atheromatosis with an increased risk of severe or fatal cardiac and cerebrovascular events. The few studies that have examined depression as a risk factor of mortality over the period from 15 months to 2 years in patients with stroke found a significant association of mortality with either depression prior to stroke or depression during the first weeks after stroke (216,218).

E. Psychiatric Antecedents and Psychosocial Factors

It is important to have an understanding of the patient's baseline characteristics, particularly as regards a previous history of depression, to ensure that evidence of a current disorder represents a meaningful change from a premorbid level of function. The process of adjustment to serious physical illness can be understood in terms of personal vulnerability, including low self-esteem, conflict within close relationships (particularly marital), and negative experiences in the developmental history. Acting on this vulnerability are stressful life events (e.g., illness or stroke), which can have an even greater impact if the subject has preexisting psychological problems. An increased incidence of personal or familial history of psychiatric disorders in patients with poststroke depression also suggests a personal or genetic predisposition (172). Finally, in this perspective, it is understandable that physical illness could dramatically precipitate a preexisting psychiatric condition (224) or allow a genetic trait for mood disorders to emerge. Thus, the coexistence of preexisting premorbid factors and psychological factors caused by the patient's reaction to neurological impairment could result in highly complex and dynamic situations.

We will summarize some of the studies underlining the role of psychosocial factors as major determinants in the development of poststroke depression. These studies show that the quality of social functioning is strongly associated with physical and cognitive recovery, as well as with the existence of depression (128).

An impaired relationship with the patient's spouse or closest other relative prior to the stroke and limited social activities are both associated with depression immediately after stroke and depression at long-term follow-up (203,225,226).

Psychodynamic factors related to increased expectations and demands for support in marital relationships are critical. Other factors to consider are job loss or loss of job satisfaction and the lack of social support and contact, especially during the first weeks of stroke, while financial security, decreased social activity, and adequacy of living arrangements might also be important in the long-term follow-up. Difficulties in maintaining an adequate social life after stroke play a great part in reduced self-esteem and sense of self, which contribute to reduced activity, seeking of psychiatric care, and collaboration in outpatient physical rehabilitation.

Following stroke, individuals may settle for a restricted future because their expectations of life with a disability are low. Clinicians need to be aware of the effect of stroke on each aspect of the patient's life in order to maximize therapy and rehabilitation. The Social Functioning Examination is a useful tool for determining the causes of impairment in social functioning (225).

F. Treatment of Poststroke Depression

Several pharmacological treatments have been proposed for patients with poststroke depression (Table 8).

Tricyclic antidepressants are no longer the treatment of first choice (245), because of the severity and elevated frequency of adverse effects (orthostatic hypotension, atrioventricular block, delirium or confusion, drowsiness, agitation, life-threatening cardiac arrhythmias, heart block, urinary outlet obstruction, and narrow-angle glaucoma).

The first-choice drugs are currently the serotonin reuptake inhibitors (SRIs), which have been shown to be more effective than placebo and tricyclic drugs and to have fewer side effects. This also supports the hypothesis of a serotoninergic imbalance in poststroke depression. The side effects of SRIs are similar in frequency and expression in patients with poststroke and endogenous depression. Adverse reactions to SRIs are rare, and consist of gastrointestinal effects (particularly nausea), headache, and "stimulant" adverse effects, such as agitation, anxiety, and insomnia. Fluoxetine-induced mania has been described in patients with stroke (246). Male sexual dysfunction is very rare, but must be taken into account when proposing a treatment.

Only a few studies have compared the effects of two or more SRIs, and these have generally involved only a small sample of patients (227). Fluoxetine, nortriptiline, and sertraline are among the more efficacious. Fluoxetine may not be the first-choice SRI if a rapid onset is required, as steady-state concentrations are not reached until after 4–5 weeks, unlike sertraline and other SRIs, which

Table 8 Drugs Used in Poststroke
Depression (with References)

Selective serotonin reuptake inhibitors
Sertraline (80)
Fluoxetine (227–229)
Citalopram (230)
Paroxetine (231)
Psychostimulants
Methylphenidate (232–235)
Dextroamphetamine (234)
Tricyclics
Imipramine (236)
Amitriptyline (237)
Desipramine (236)
Amoxapine (238)
Nortriptyline (227,229,239–241)
MAO inhibitors
Moclobémide (242)
Others
Trazodone (243)
Maprotiline (tetracyclic) (244)
Mianserin (120,236)

require less than 1 week (247). One advantage of fluoxetine compared to other SRIs could be the long half-life, which may allow less frequent administration in noncompliant patients and result in less severe discontinuation effects. Sertraline seems to be more efficacious in the treatment of stroke-associated lability of mood and, compared to fluoxetine, is better tolerated, with minor probability of agitation, weight loss, dermatological adverse effects, and fewer interactions with drugs influencing P-450 enzymes. A recent study comparing combinations of drugs with either noradrenergic effects (desipramine plus mianserin) or noradrenergic and serotonergic effects (imipramine plus mianserin) indicated that drugs with the dual effect may be more effective (236).

Our opinion is that, given the similar pharmacology of the SRIs, the lack of sufficiently large studies, and the inconsistent differences seen in these studies, no valid guidelines can be established for the choice of any one SSRI for use in poststroke mood disorders.

Trazodone and lisuride maleate are probably good alternative treatments to SRIs for poststroke depression. Depressed mood, hypobulia, sleep disturbance, anxiety, etc., were significantly improved by these drugs compared to the baseline condition (248.)

The SRIs improve the cognitive functions related to depression, but not those directly consequent to cerebral damage (236,249); however the improvement in cognitive functions has no clear physiopathological correlates.

Some studies have demonstrated that improvement of mood disorders by SRIs can also enhance recovery of neurological function (250,251) and that this effect can be quite large (30% recovery) (250), but a close relationship between appropriate early treatment and recovery has not been noted in all studies (120,227). Palomaki et al. (120) also showed that prophylactic treatment for depression in all patients with first-ever stroke may not affect the outcome.

A placebo effect may also account for 35–75% of the therapeutic response in trials of antidepressants (252) and spontaneous remissions may be frequent in the immediate period following stroke in the case of minor depression and after a longer interval (1 or 2 years) in the case of major depression (253).

These data indicate that the natural course of poststroke depression and the effect of pharmacological therapy remain essentially undetermined. Based on evaluation of hospital populations consisting mainly of male low-social-group Afro-American patients, Robinson et al. (254,255) suggested that major poststroke depression has a natural course of less than 1 year, while minor depression is often more persistent. Similar data emerged in other studies (172,256). We also do not know whether the natural outcome, independent of therapy, could also be characterized by recurrence.

The limitations of the various studies in understanding the outcome of depression and the effect of therapy make us consider that the placebo effect and spontaneous remissions might cause a possible overestimation of the therapeutic properties of SRIs in the early phases, but are less likely to do so in the chronic phase.

The use of psychostimulant drugs seems an interesting alternative to SRIs, their beneficial effects probably being due to their overcoming the fatigue and apathy components of depression. Unfortunately, adverse reactions necessitating the interruption of therapy with drugs of this class are not rare, and consist of adrenergic-like symptoms (tachycardia and hypertension); indeed anorexia is seen infrequently at the doses normally employed.

In is interesting to note that patients show a rapid response to psychostimulants, usually within the first 1–2 days of treatment, and that the use of drugs of this class should probably be encouraged in the acute phase, despite the possible cardiovascular side effects (232–235,257,258), but probably not for chronic use.

In terms of nonpharmacological treatments, several reports show electroconvulsive therapy to be efficacious in isolated cases (259,260), although the advantages compared to other treatments are not evident. Cognitive behavior therapy may be an appropriate treatment (261), especially if cognitive and psychosocial factors contributing to depression are clearly defined in the isolated patient. Unfortunately, few studies have been performed on the effect of cognitive therapy on the outcome of poststroke depression. We suggest that patients reporting only verbal distress might respond better to cognitive therapy alone, while patients with only vegetative symptoms might be best treated with an antidepressant drug, and patients with combined symptoms might require psychological, social, and pharmacological interventions.

A report of an improved emotional outcome following acute stroke as a result of informational methods consisting of workbook-based intervention is, in our opinion, particularly interesting (262). The intervention groups exhibited lower levels of anxiety and depression 1 month after discharge, and this was not explained by differences in age, gender distribution, or initial neurological impairment, factors that could be associated with distress outcomes. The group of patients who received advice and information were more knowledgeable about, and compliant with, treatment and showed the best response.

G. Suicide

Poststroke depression can be accompanied by suicidal ideation, but reports of suicide among stroke patients are extremely rare. Risk factors for suicide include depression, severe insomnia, chronic illness, and organic brain syndrome. Some studies (263,264) showed an incidence of suicidal ideation of 6% in the acute phase and 6–12% in the following 2 years. Early clinical assessment of suicide risk factors is, therefore, essential in the rehabilitation setting and has to be evaluated together with the diagnosis of major depression.

In the acute phase, the degree of physical impairment, together with alcohol abuse, seem to be important factors, while in the chronic phase, suicidal ideation is an independent sign of major depression and mainly a result of poor social support, brooding, and self-blame (264,265). Other risk factors for suicide are a younger age, the presence of a sensory deficit, and impaired cognitive functions.

Patients who are suicidal in the acute phase seem to have lesions with a more anterior location than patients with delayed-onset suicidal ideation (265). The psychopathology of suicidal ideation in poststorke depression can be influenced by biological or organic mechanisms (such as lesion location), probably more often in the acute phase, but psychological and social factors are, in our opinion, more significant, especially in the chronic phase.

Clinicians should always look for indirect verbal cues and nonverbal behavior patterns indicating potential suicide in patients with stroke and signs of depression, however long the interval since the acute phase.

IV. ANXIETY

Anxiety is an emotional state involving physiological arousal (increased heart rate), verbal reports of feelings of distress (e.g., apprehension and worry), overt behavior (e.g., avoidance), and cognitive disruption (i.e., maladaptive shifts in attention due to off-target thinking, hyperawareness about possible threatening cues in the environment, and the perception that adverse events are occurring in an unpredictable and uncontrollable manner). It differs from fear in inducing minor mobilization for physical action and is associated with more cognitive symptoms and less visceral activation.

The incidence of anxiety is probably lower than that of poststroke depression, being about 25% in the acute phase (3,102,266), decreasing slightly at 1 year (267) and at 3 year follow-up (267). The incidence is greater in patients with previous psychiatric disorders (268).

In stroke patients, anxiety is frequently associated with depression, and the association is more significant if depression and the initial neurological impairment are severe (266). Nevertheless, factors associated with poststroke depression (stroke severity, prior stroke, poor functional status, anterior circulation lesion, and cognitive sequelae) do not predict anxiety levels (266).

Castillo et al. (3) found an association between anxiety and left cortical lesion in the case of anxiety with no concurrent depression, and between anxiety and right lesion in the case of anxiodepressive symptoms. They also indicated that patients with worries had more anterior lesions, while patients with generalized anxiety disorder had more posterior right-hemisphere lesions. There is no clear etiopathogenetic theory to support these data. In addition, Anstrom (267) found the opposite results in a small sample population. In another small population study, Starkstein et al. (269) showed that patients with poststroke anxiety have more cortical lesions, while patients with combined anxiety and depression have more subcortical lesions. Poststroke anxiety shares many features with the feelings of distress and worry expressed by patients with posttraumatic stress disorders. In both conditions, the extension and volume of the lesion do not correlate with the level of anxiety.

In the psychodynamic theory, stroke and posttraumatic stress disorders can be considered as a sudden and unpredictable occurrence of a life-threatening stressor (internal in the case of stroke and external in the case of trauma).

Finally, in our opinion, the physiopathology of poststroke anxiety remains essentially undetermined and there is little evidence that anxiety is associated with specific lesion locations. As in the case of poststroke depression, the causes of anxiety are the sum of complex psychodynamic factors and possible organic factors, and result in the interaction of individual traits of cortical arousal and autonomic nervous system reactivity under the influence of the limbic system.

While the roles of lesion location and metabolic or neurotransmitter imbalance are still largely undetermined, several psychological models have been elaborated in relation to neural substrates (Eisenck's introverted neurotics, Gray's behavioral inhibition system, and Cloninger's system of harm avoidance), behavior (Izard), or cognitive fuction (Mandler's interruption theory, Spielberger's state-trait model, Beck's cognitive schemata, and Hallam's theory of anxiety as a personal construct).

There is little information on the long-term outcome of poststroke anxiety (267) or the effect of drug therapy. No systematic studies of treatment have been performed. Benzodiazepines are the most commonly prescribed medications. Short-half-life drugs (i.e., lorazepam, oxazepam, and temazepam) are preferable. Undesirable side effects of long-acting benzodiazepines include drowsiness, cognitive impairment, confusion, psychomotor retardation, risk of falls, depression, intoxication, paradoxical reactions, amnestic syndromes, respiratory problems, abuse, dependence, and withdrawal reactions. The use of benzodiazepine for poststroke anxiety should have a clear indication and time-limited duration. SRIs and buspirone can be useful as mood stabilizers. Buspirone is better tolerated and, compared to benzodiazepines, has no addictive profile or withdrawal symptoms after discontinuation and few adverse interactions with other drugs. Psychotherapy, cognitive behavioral therapy, and relaxing techniques can be useful, but their use remains empirical in stroke patients with anxiety.

V. POSTSTROKE MANIA AND PSYCHOSIS

Stroke can produce a varied spectrum of neurobehavioral syndromes that may come to the attention of the mental health professional evaluating psychiatric symptoms, especially in elderly individuals. In an MRI study, patients with late-onset mania showed a higher incidence of silent cerebral infarcts than controls (270).

Manic or psychotic symptoms may occur immediately after the stroke or months or years later.

The incidence and lifetime prevalence of *mania* in patient with brain injury are low and appear to be no higher than in the general population (1–2%) (271). The presence of an underlying or preexisting brain disease may have an important etiological role and also an adverse effect on the resolution of the neuropsychiatric symptoms.

According to the DSM-IV diagnostic criteria (Table 9), mania is characterized by signs such as inflated self-esteem or grandiosity, decreased need for sleep, distractibility, flight of ideas, and excessive involvement in pleasurable activities with potentially painful consequences.

Manic-like behavior is also described as disinhibition syndrome, acquired sociopathy, pseudopsychopathic syndrome, and frontal lobe syndrome. Unfortunately, these various terms create confusion when comparing different studies.

The distinction between primary and secondary mania is more relevant on clinical grounds.

The DSM-IV offers three different entries for "secondary" mania (due to a general medical condition): (1) manic episode; (2) personality change classified as disinihibited or aggressive; (3) impulse control disorders not classified elsewhere and, more specifically, intermittent explosive disorder. As with primary

Table 9 Diagnostic Criteria for Manic Episodes (adapted from DSM-IV)

A. Distinct period of abnormally and persistently elevated, expansive or irritable mood lasting at least 1 week (or any duration if hospitalization is necessary)
B. During the period of mood disturbance, three (or more) of the following symptoms persist (four if the mood is only irritable) and are present to a significant degree:
   1. Inflated self-esteem or grandiosity
   2. Decreased need for sleep (e.g., feels rested after only 3 hr of sleep)
   3. More talkative than usual or under pressure to keep talking
   4. Flight of ideas or subjective experience that thoughts are racing
   5. Distractibility (i.e., attention too easily drawn to unimportant or irrelevant external stimuli)
   6. Increased goal-directed activity (socially, at work or school, or sexually)
   7. Excessive involvement in pleasurable activities that have a high potential for painful consequences (e.g., engaging in unrestrained buying sprees, sexual indiscretions, or foolish business investments)

mania, patients with poststroke mania show the symptoms of elation, pressured speech, flight of ideas, grandiose thoughts, insomnia, hallucinations, and paranoid delusions. Another issue requiring exploration is whether the symptoms of mania may be masked in the acute phase by stroke symptoms, such as denial or indifference reactions. The possible overdiagnosis of mania following stroke based on the nonspecific effects of illness, such as decreased sleep, also needs to be verified.

The incidence of mania in acute stroke is about 1% (271), but is higher (6–9%) in brain injury (272). This difference is explained by the higher prevalence of lesions involving basotemporal and orbitofrontal cortices in traumatic brain injury patients compared to stroke patients.

In another series of manic syndrome following cerebral injury, lesions were mainly located in the right hemisphere and involved the thalamus, right temporal lobe, or, bilaterally, the frontal cortex (273). Most cases of mania in stroke patients have been reported to have a right-hemispheric lesion (274–276) involving the basal medial and frontal area of the temporal lobe (273), caudate (277), thalamus (78,276–280), basal ganglia (281), and ventral pons (282). Very few cases of mania are reported to be a consequence of a left-hemispheric lesion (275,283,284). Regard and Landis (285) described a nondisabling form of hyperphagia, with a specific preference for fine food (''gourmand syndrome'') in which most patients have right anterior frontal lesions.

Ranging from mildly inappropriate social behavior to full-blown mania or aggressivity, dyscontrol syndrome may result from lesions of specific brain areas, such as the orbitofrontal and basotemporal cortices of the right hemisphere (108,174,286).

Hypometabolism involving the right inferior temporal lobe was seen in a

PET study of two patients with lesions of the right head of the caudate, leading to the hypothesis of a direct or indirect role (diaschisis) of the right inferior temporal lobe in secondary mania. In primary mania, reduced blood flow in the right temporal lobe has also been found (287).

Based on the phylogenetic origin of these cortical areas (basofrontal and temporobasal) and their main connections with dorsal regions related to visuospatial functions, somatosensation, and spatial memory, the orbitofrontal and basotemporal cortices may selectively inhibit or release motor, instinctive, affective, and intellectual behaviors processed in the dorsal cortex. This supports the hypothesis that dysfunction of these heteromodal ventral brain areas may result in disinhibited behavior. Although there have been no treatment-response studies of mania following stroke because of the rare incidence of the syndrome, the response of poststroke depression to antidepressants justifies attempts at pharmacological treatment of symptoms (288).

The clinical presentation of poststroke mania and the response to treatment seem similar to those of mania without brain injury. Clonidine (289) and lithium and carbamazepine are useful (290).

Most patients with secondary mania reported in the literature were treated with drugs frequently used for patients with primary mania, such as neuroleptics, anticonvulsants, and lithium, as well as electroconvulsive therapy (291). However, whether the usefulness of these treatment modalities is similar in patients with secondary mania to that in patients with primary mania remains to be empirically established.

A general consensus derived from the critical analysis of anecdotal cases shows that secondary mania may be more difficult to treat than primary mania, probably because stroke patients are more prone to epileptic seizures and secondary effects of neuroleptic therapy.

Behavioral symptoms of *psychosis* have been described in relation to cerebral infarctions. The prevalence of schizophrenia-like symptoms is unknown, but it is not an infrequent clinical phenomenon in the hospital setting, especially in the acute phase of stroke.

The proportion of psychiatric inpatients who have depression with melancholic and/or psychotic features is higher among elderly subjects, and this has been linked to white matter lesions and other brain changes that become more common in old age.

Elderly patients with stroke and psychotic symptoms have hallucinations and delusions. In presenile or senile patients presenting with behavioral or psychiatric manifestations without any previous history of mental illness, cerebrovascular disease should be a diagnostic consideration.

At least four symptom clusters have been identified, namely affective, paranoid delusional, confusional state, and changes in mood with behavioral disturbances, but the mechanisms involved are unclear (292).

In most cases, psychosis has been reported with right hemispheric stroke (293–300), especially in the temporo-parieto-occipital junction regions or the thalamus (278) and in aged patients with preexisting degenerative disease or cerebral atrophy.

Thus, a right-hemisphere lesion may act in combination with one or more additional factors, such as seizures, genetic vulnerability, or subcortical atrophy. Several types of hallucination can occur in patients with brain injury; these have been termed atypical psychosis, peduncular hallucinosis, release hallucinosis, organic psychosis, and agitated delirium. The term "peduncular hallucinosis," in the case of lesions in the midbrain and pons, was first used by Lhermitte to describe visual hallucinations that the patient knows not to be real. The term "hallucinosis" differentiates these visual hallucinations from hallucinations in which the patient believes the sensory perception to be real.

In the case of parieto-temporal-occipital infarcts, patients with psychosis have real hallucinations because they have no insight into the false nature of these perceptions. Seizures can precede the onset of psychosis (294). The hallucinatory experience of such patients probably reflects pathological activation of neural ensembles in the regions bordering an occipital lesion. These regions are presumed to contain records of visual feature fragments that are coactivated by feedback projections in the earliest visual association cortices, where they produce meaningful patterns during normal recall (301).

Generally patients respond to treatment with neuroleptic medications, although anticonvulsant medication can be useful in some treatment-resistant cases.

Hallucinations and delusions following brain injury are interesting clinical phenomena that may provide insights into the mechanism of hallucination in patients without brain injury and, despite their rarity, are certainly deserving of further investigation.

VI. CONCLUSIONS

Mood disorders and behavioral changes (depression, anxiety, psychosis, and mania) after stroke constitute a challenging field of research in neurology not only because of the possibility of correlating emotions, mood states, and behaviors with neural circuits, but also because they are very frequent and have a great impact on the outcome, neurorehabilitation, and social integration of patients. There is no complete consensus on anatomicoclinical correlations of poststroke mood disorders. A vast amount of scientific literature has failed to define precise anatomicoclinical correlations but, in our opinion, some notions are worthy of attention.

The key issues in this chapter will be now summarized.

In the case of poststroke depression, the role of frontosubcortical, temporolimbic, basal ganglia, and prefrontal circuits and other limbic-related areas can be retained, and appears to be mediated by a serotonin imbalance.

The physiopathology of poststroke anxiety seems even more complex and difficult to investigate. There is little evidence that anxiety is associated with specific lesion locations, at least when anxiety is not associated with depressive symptoms.

Mania and psychosis, which are more frequent in "aged brains" with underlying atrophy, could be release symptoms resulting from lesions of heteromodal cerebral regions.

Lesions accompanying mania and psychosis have been more frequently reported in the right hemisphere and involve the basal medial temporal and frontotemporal areas, caudate nucleus, and thalamus. Very few cases with left-hemispheric lesions have been described. Mania and psychosis are probably the result of critical cerebral lesions that disorganize the physiological cognitive process of matching emotions and multimodal sensorial stimuli.

Planning clinical investigations to define the etiopathology, treatment, and prognosis of behavioral or mood syndromes related to stroke is a very difficult task. The first problem is the definition of diagnostic criteria. Univocal diagnostic criteria are actually adopted (DSM-IV), but the possibility of subgroups of syndromes (major and minor, predominantly with vegetative signs or with verbal referral, or reacting to psychological or social factors) makes it problematic not only to carry out clinical investigations on large population samples, but also to maximize treatment of individual patients. A major reworking of criteria for case definition is necessary in this population, placing great emphasis on cognitive, behavioral, physiological (or vegetative) changes.

The other concern in investigating mood changes is to obtain a complete evaluation of the impact of other cognitive (i.e., aphasia, anosognosia, and amnesia), behavioral (i.e., motor aprosody, fatigue, apathy, emotionalism, catastrophic reactions, indifference reaction, and loss of psychic autoactivation), physiological (appetite, physical immobility, dysphagia, slurred speech, and noncommunication), and psychological changes due to the stroke itself.

In this context, it is important to determine the functional deficit that accounts, at least in part, for the subsequent mood disorder. It is understandable that patients with visual field deficits are prone to anxiety when away from home because of the tendency for moving people and vehicles to suddenly appear in their central vision and we must empathize with the very sad and frustrating condition of a patient with aphasia who cannot communicate with his spouse or relatives.

In the very innovative and challenging investigation field of mood changes after stroke, we suggest encouraging clinical studies involving homogeneous large sample populations and statistical analyses with a high power of predictability. We would also like to see the creation of neurobehavioral databases using homogeneous criteria to group numerous stroke centers and to avoid statistical bias due to small populations.

To reduce the possibility of behavioral or physical conditions that can be mistaken for mood changes (see Table 4), studies should be based on populations of first-ever stroke patients who are young, have no psychiatric antecedents, and have relatively mild, or no, cognitive or physical impairment.

For lesion localization, MRI (together with more valid definitions of lesion location) and functional neuroimaging (SPECT, PET, and functional MRI) are now standard approaches for evaluating mood disorders and behavioral changes. In our opinion, it would be very interesting to apply the new functional neuro-imaging studies using voxel-based statistical whole brain analysis to the study of mood disorders after stroke (302).

Using these techniques, the aim is to look for a dysfunction occurring in a cortical-subcortical system that includes different subsystems, each with specific subfunctions. A regional analysis is then necessary to identify the specific components contributing to mood state regulation, since it is likely that lesions anywhere along the pathway will produce similar symptoms. Special neurocognitive paradigm tasks need to be constructed to define the role of single cerebral structures in complex neural networks.

MRI studies, especially on populations with senile or presenile onset major depression or other mood changes, may make it possible to identify silent strokes (probably in the subcortical and basal ganglia regions) and to determine what health strategies for preventing cerebrovascular disease may reduce depressive vulnerability in the elderly.

The high prevalence of depression accompanying cerebrovascular diseases and the prolongation of disability in depressed people with stroke means that closer liaison is needed between psychiatrists, neurologists, and physicians caring for the elderly.

Another important consideration is that all psychosocial factors possibly interfering with mood changes should be evaluated. The stroke patient is coping with a serious physical illness that reduces his self-integrity in terms of personal vulnerability and low self-esteem and generates possible conflicts with close relationships (especially the spouse) or other caregivers. Strategies to increase social activity, support and contacts, financial security, job satisfaction, adequacy of living arrangements, and psychiatric care are required to obtain the collaboration of patients in physical rehabilitation.

Specific psychiatric or neurological evaluation of the depressive symptoms, including subjective distress and vegetative symptoms, can permit the choice of more specific therapies, such as cognitive or pharmacological approaches or a combination of the two.

Pharmacological therapy for poststroke mood changes, when the diagnosis is clear and pharmacological therapy is indicated, can provide great benefit to the stroke patient and improve the quality of life.

ACKNOWLEDGMENT

The authors thank Kathy Taylor, Tom Barkas, and Fabienne Staub for their suggestions.

REFERENCES

1. Wade DT, Legh-Smith J, Hewer RA. Depressed mood after stroke. A community study of its frequency. Br J Psychiatry 1987; 151:200–205.
2. Andersen G, Vestergaard K, Riis J, Lauritzen L. Incidence of post-stroke depression during the first year in a large unselected stroke population determined using a valid standardized rating scale. Acta Psychiatr Scand 1994; 90:190–195.
3. Castillo CS, Starkstein SE, Fedoroff JP, Price TR, Robinson RG. Generalized anxiety disorder after stroke. J Nerv Ment Dis 1993; 181:100–106.
4. Beekman AT, Penninx BW, Deeg DJ, Ormel J, Smit JH, Braam AW, Van Tilburg W. Depression in survivor of stroke: a community-based study of prevalence, risk factors and consequences. Soc Psychiatry Psychiatr Epidemiol 1998; 33:463–470.
5. Bogousslavsky J, Cummings JL, eds. Behavior and Mood Disorders in Focal Brain Lesions. New York: Cambridge University Press, 2000.
6. Carson AJ, Machale S, Allen K, Lawrie SM, Dennis M, House A, Sharpe M. Depression after stroke and lesion location: a systematic review [In Process Citation]. Lancet 2000; 356:122–126.
7. Robertson JT. Phenomenology and Specificity of Depressive Symptoms. The Clinical Neuropsychiatry of Stroke. New York: Cambridge University Press, 1998.
8. Lipsey JR, Spencer WC, Rabins PV, Robinson RG. Phenomenological comparison of poststroke depression and functional depression. Am J Psychiatry 1986; 143: 527–529.
9. Gainotti G, Azzoni A, Marra C. Frequency, phenomenology and anatomical-clinical correlates of major post-stroke depression [see comments]. Br J Psychiatry 1999; 175:163–167.
10. Gainotti G, Azzoni A, Razzano C, Lanzillotta M, Marra C, Gasparini F. The Post-Stroke Depression Rating Scale: a test specifically devised to investigate affective disorders of stroke patients. J Clin Exp Neuropsychol 1997; 19:340–356.
11. Paradiso S, Robinson RG. Minor depression after stroke: an initial validation of the DSM-IV construct. Am J Geriatr Psychiatry 1999; 7:244–251.
12. Morris PL, Shields RB, Hopwood MJ, Robinson RG, Raphael B. Are there two depressive syndromes after stroke? J Nerv Ment Dis 1994; 182:230–234.

13. Hamilton M. A rating scale for depression. J Neurol Neurosurg Psychiatry 1960.
14. Williams JB. A structured interview guide for the Hamilton Depression Rating Scale [see comments]. Arch Gen Psychiatry 1988; 45:742–747.
15. Malec JF, Richardson JW, Sinaki M, O'Brien MW. Types of affective response to stroke. Arch Phys Med Rehabil 1990; 71:279–284.
16. Beck AT, Steer RA, Brown GK. Manual for the Beck Depression Inventory, 2d ed. San Antonio, TX: The Psychological Corporation, 1996.
17. Gallagher D, Nies G, Thompson LW. Reliability of the Beck Depression Inventory with older adults. J Consult Clin Psychol 1982; 50:152–153.
18. House A, Dennis M, Hawton K, Warlow C. Methods of identifying mood disorders in stroke patients: experience in the Oxfordshire Community Stroke Project. Age Ageing 1989; 18:371–379.
19. O'Rourke S, Machale S, Signorini D, Dennis M. Detecting psychiatric morbidity after stroke: comparison of the GHQ and the HAD Scale. Stroke 1998; 29:980–985.
20. Johnson G, Burvill PW, Anderson CS, Jamrozik K, Stewart-Wynne EG, Chakera TM. Screening instruments for depression and anxiety following stroke: experience in the Perth community stroke study. Acta Psychiatr Scand 1995; 91:252–257.
21. Herrmann C. International experiences with the Hospital Anxiety and Depression Scale—a review of validation data and clinical results. J Psychosom Res 1997; 42: 17–41.
22. Goldberg DP, Hillier VF. A scaled version of the General Health Questionnaire. Psychol Med 1979; 9:139–145.
23. Bridges KW, Goldberg DP. The validation of the GHQ-28 and the use of the MMSE in neurological in-patients. Br J Psychiatry 1986; 148:548–553.
24. Yesavage JA, Brink TL, Rose TL, Lum O, Huang V, Adey M, Leirer VO. Development and validation of a geriatric depression screening scale: a preliminary report. J Psychiatr Res 1982; 17:37–49.
25. Yesavage JA. Geriatric Depression Scale. Psychopharmacol Bull 1988; 24:709–711.
26. Koenig HG, Meador KG, Cohen HJ, Blazer DG. Self-rated depression scales and screening for major depression in the older hospitalized patient with medical illness. J Am Geriatr Soc 1988; 36:699–706.
27. Zung WW, Richards CB, Short MJ. Self-rating depression scale in an outpatient clinic. Further validation of the SDS. Arch Gen Psychiatry 1965; 13:508–515.
28. CES-D Scale: A self-report depression scale for research in the general population. Appl Psychol Measurement 1977; 385–401.
29. Ramasubbu R, Robinson RG, Flint AJ, Kosier T, Price TR. Functional impairment associated with acute poststroke depression: the Stroke Data Bank Study. J Neuropsychiatry Clin Neurosci 1998; 10:26–33.
30. Parikh RM, Eden DT, Price TR, Robinson RG. The sensitivity and specificity of the Center for Epidemiologic Studies Depression Scale in screening for post-stroke depression. Int J Psychiatry Med 1988; 18:169–181.
31. Goldberg D, Bridges K, Duncan-Jones P, Grayson D. Detecting anxiety and depression in general medical settings. Br Med J 1988; 297:897–899.
32. Huber P, Mulligan R, Mackinnon A, Nebuloni-French T, Michel JP. Detecting

anxiety and depression in hospitalised elderly patients using a brief inventory. Eur Psychiatry 1999; 14:11–16.

33. Montgomery SA, Asberg M. A new depression scale designed to be sensitive to change. Br J Psychiatry 1979; 134:382–389.

34. Muller MJ, Szegedi A, Wetzel H, Benkert O. Moderate and severe depression. Gradations for the Montgomery-Asberg Depression Rating Scale. J Affect Disord 2000; 60:137–140.

35. Mitrushina M, Abara J, Blumenfeld A. The neurobehavioral cognitive status examination as a screening tool for organicity in psychiatric patients. Hosp Community Psychiatry 1994; 45:252–256.

36. Mitrushina M, Abara J, Blumenfeld A. Aspects of validity and reliability of the Neurobehavioral Cognitive Status Examination (NCSE) in assessment of psychiatric patients. J Psychiatr Res 1994; 28:85–95.

37. Logue PE, Tupler LA, D'Amico C, Schmitt FA. The Neurobehavioral Cognitive Status Examination: psychometric properties in use with psychiatric inpatients. J Clin Psychol 1993; 49:80–89.

38. Stern RA. Assessment of mood states in neurodegenerative disease: methodological issues and diagnostic recommendations. Semin Clin Neuropsychiatry 1996; 1:315–324.

39. Stern RA. Assessment of mood states in aphasia. Semin Speech Lang 1999; 20:33–49.

40. Stern RA, Bachman DL. Depressive symptoms following stroke. Am J Psychiatry 1991; 148:351–356.

41. Robinson RG, Szetela B. Mood change following left hemispheric brain injury. Ann Neurol 1981; 9:447–453.

42. Price CI, Curless RH, Rodgers H. Can stroke patients use visual analogue scales? Stroke 1999; 30:1357–1361.

43. Sutcliffe LM, Lincoln NB. The assessment of depression in aphasic stroke patients: the development of the Stroke Aphasic Depression Questionnaire. Clin Rehabil 1998; 12:506–513.

44. Cummings JL. The Neuropsychiatric Inventory: assessing psychopathology in dementia patients. Neurology 1997; 48:S10–S16.

45. Cummings JL, Mega M, Gray K, Rosenberg-Thompson S, Carusi DA, Gornbein J. The Neuropsychiatric Inventory: comprehensive assessment of psychopathology in dementia. Neurology 1994; 44:2308–2314.

46. Levin HS, High WM, Goethe KE, Sisson RA, Overall JE, Rhoades HM, Eisenberg HM, Kalisky Z, Gary HE. The neurobehavioural rating scale: assessment of the behavioural sequelae of head injury by the clinician. J Neurol Neurosurg Psychiatry 1987; 50:183–193.

47. Nelson LD, Satz P, Mitrushina M. Development and validation of the Neuropsychology Behavior and Affect Profile. Psychol Assess 1989; 1:266–272.

48. Kertesz A, Davidson W, Fox H. Frontal behavioral inventory: diagnostic criteria for frontal lobe dementia. Can J Neurol Sci 1997; 24:29–36.

49. Teri L, Truax P, Logsdon R, Uomoto J, Zarit S, Vitaliano PP. Assessment of behavioral problems in dementia: the revised memory and behavior problems checklist. Psychol Aging 1992; 7:622–631.

50. Toedter LJ, Schall RR, Reese CA, Hyland DT, Berk SN, Dunn DS. Psychological measures: reliability in the assessment of stroke patients. Arch Phys Med Rehabil 1995; 76:719–725.

51. Grotta J, Bratina P. Subjective experiences of 24 patients dramatically recovering from stroke. Stroke 1995; 26:1285–1288.

52. Schramke CJ, Stowe RM, Ratcliff G, Goldstein G, Condray R. Poststroke depression and anxiety: different assessment methods result in variations in incidence and severity estimates. J Clin Exp Neuropsychol 1998; 20:723–737.

53. Fedoroff JP, Starkstein SE, Parikh RM, Price TR, Robinson RG. Are depressive symptoms nonspecific in patients with acute stroke? Am J Psychiatry 1991; 148: 1172–1176.

54. Gainotti G, Azzoni A, Gasparini F, Marra C, Razzano C. Relation of lesion location to verbal and nonverbal mood measures in stroke patients. Stroke 1997; 28:2145–2149.

55. Starkstein SE, Berthier ML, Fedoroff P, Price TR, Robinson RG. Anosognosia and major depression in 2 patients with cerebrovascular lesions [see comments]. Neurology 1990; 40:1380–1382.

56. Starkstein SE, Fedoroff JP, Price TR, Leiguarda R, Robinson RG. Anosognosia in patients with cerebrovascular lesions. A study of causative factors. Stroke 1992; 23:1446–1453.

57. Ramasubbu R. Denial of illness and depression in stroke [letter; comment]. Stroke 1994; 25:226–227.

58. Dennis M, O'Rourke S, Lewis S, Sharpe M, Warlow C. A quantitative study of the emotional outcome of people caring for stroke survivors. Stroke 1998; 29:1867–1872.

59. Ekman P, Friesen WV. Constants across cultures in the face and emotion. J Pers Soc Psychol 1971; 17:124–129.

60. Starkstein SE, Fedoroff JP, Price TR, Leiguarda R, Robinson RG. Apathy following cerebrovascular lesions. Stroke 1993; 24:1625–1630.

61. Starkstein SE, Fedoroff JP, Price TR, Leiguarda R, Robinson RG. Apathy following cerebrovascular lesions. Stroke 1993; 24:1625–1630.

62. Okada K, Kobayashi S, Yamagata S, Takahashi K, Yamaguchi S. Poststroke apathy and regional cerebral blood flow. Stroke 1997; 28:2437–2441.

63. Cummings JL. Anatomic and behavioral aspects of frontal-subcortical circuits. Ann NY Acad Sci 1995; 769:1–13.

64. Marin RS, Biedrzycki RC, Firinciogullari S. Reliability and validity of the Apathy Evaluation Scale. Psychiatry Res 1991; 38:143–162.

65. Marin RS, Firinciogullari S, Biedrzycki RC. The sources of convergence between measures of apathy and depression. J Affect Disord 1993; 28:117–124.

66. Ingles JL, Eskes GA, Phillips SJ. Fatigue after stroke. Arch Phys Med Rehabil 1999; 80:173–178.

67. Habib M. Activity and motivational disorders in neurology: proposal for an evaluation scale. Encephale 1995; 21:563–570.

68. Trillet M, Croisile B, Tourniaire D, Schott B. Disorders of voluntary motor activity and lesions of caudate nuclei. Rev Neurol (Paris) 1990; 146:338–344.

69. Caplan LR, Schmahmann JD, Kase CS, Feldmann E, Baquis G, Greenberg JP,

Gorelick PB, Helgason C, Hier DB. Caudate infarcts. Arch Neurol 1990; 47:133–143.

70. Danel T, Goudemand M, Ghawche F, Godefroy O, Pruvo JP, Vaiva G, Samaille E, Pandit F. Delusional melancholia and multiple lacunar infarcts of the basal ganglia. Rev Neurol (Paris) 1991; 147:60–62.

71. Bogousslavsky J, Regli F, Delaloye B, Delaloye-Bischof A, Assal G, Uske A. Loss of psychic self-activation with bithalamic infarction. Neurobehavioural, CT, MRI and SPECT correlates. Acta Neurol Scand 1991; 83:309–316.

72. Machale SM, O'Rourke SJ, Wardlaw JM, Dennis MS. Depression and its relation to lesion location after stroke. J Neurol Neurosurg Psychiatry 1998; 64:371–374.

73. House A, Dennis M, Molyneux A, Warlow C, Hawton K. Emotionalism after stroke. Br Med J 1989; 298:991–994.

74. Calvert T, Knapp P, House A. Psychological associations with emotionalism after stroke. J Neurol Neurosurg Psychiatry 1998; 65:928–929.

75. Morris PL, Robinson RG, Raphael B. Emotional lability after stroke. Aust NZ J Psychiatry 1993; 27:601–605.

76. Robinson RG, Parikh RM, Lipsey JR, Starkstein SE, Price TR. Pathological laughing and crying following stroke: validation of a measurement scale and a double-blind treatment study [see comments]. Am J Psychiatry 1993; 150:286–293.

77. Andersen G, Vestergaard K, Lauritzen L. Effective treatment of poststroke depression with the selective serotonin reuptake inhibitor citalopram. Stroke 1994; 25:1099–1104.

78. Brown KW, Sloan RL, Pentland B. Fluoxetine as a treatment for post-stroke emotionalism. Acta Psychiatr Scand 1998; 98:455–458.

79. Panzer MJ, Mellow AM. Antidepressant treatment of pathologic laughing or crying in elderly stroke patients. J Geriatr Psychiatry Neurol 1992; 5:195–199.

80. Burns A, Russell E, Stratton-Powell H, Tyrell P, O'Neill P, Baldwin R. Sertraline in stroke-associated lability of mood. Int J Geriatr Psychiatry 1999; 14:681–685.

81. Teasell R. Catastrophic reaction after stroke. A case study. Am J Phys Med Rehabil 1993; 72:151–153.

82. Starkstein SE, Fedoroff JP, Price TR, Leiguarda R, Robinson RG. Catastrophic reaction after cerebrovascular lesions: frequency, correlates, and validation of a scale. J Neuropsychiatry Clin Neurosci 1993; 5:189–194.

83. Reference deleted.

84. Paradiso S, Ohkubo T, Robinson RG. Vegetative and psychological symptoms associated with depressed mood over the first two years after stroke. Int J Psychiatry Med 1997; 27:137–157.

85. Ghika-Schmid F, Van Melle G, Guex P, Bogousslavsky J. Subjective experience and behavior in acute stroke: the Lausanne Emotion in Acute Stroke Study. Neurology 1999; 52:22–28.

86. Fedoroff JP, Lipsey JR, Starkstein SE, Forrester A, Price TR, Robinson RG. Phenomenological comparisons of major depression following stroke, myocardial infarction or spinal cord lesions. J Affect Disord 1991; 22:83–89.

87. Finklestein S, Benowitz LI, Baldessarini RJ, Arana GW, Levine D, Woo E, Bear D, Moya K, Stoll AL. Mood, vegetative disturbance, and dexamethasone suppression test after stroke. Ann Neurol 1982; 12:463–468.

88. Harney JH, Fulton C, Ross ED, Rush AJ. Dexamethasone suppression test and onset of poststroke depression in patients with ischemic infarction. J Clin Psychiatry 1993; 54:343–348.

89. Harvey SA, Black KJ. The dexamethasone suppression test for diagnosing depression in stroke patients. Ann Clin Psychiatry 1996; 8:35–39.

90. Dam H, Pedersen HE, Dige-Petersen H, Ahlgren P. Neuroendocrine tests in depressive stroke patients. Prog Neuropsychopharmacol Biol Psychiatry 1994; 18: 1005–1013.

91. McLeer SV, Dixon JF, Henry D, Ruggiero K, Escovitz K, Niedda T, Scholle R. Psychopathology in non-clinically referred sexually abused children. J Am Acad Child Adolesc Psychiatry 1998; 37:1326–1333.

92. Grober SE, Gordon WA, Sliwinski MJ, Hibbard MR, Aletta EG, Paddison PL. Utility of the dexamethasone suppression test in the diagnosis of poststroke depression. Arch Phys Med Rehabil 1991; 72:1076–1079.

93. Dam H, Pedersen HE, Damkjaer M, Ahlgren P. Dexamethasone suppression test in depressive stroke patients. Acta Neurol Scand 1991; 84:14–17.

94. Lipsey JR, Robinson RG, Pearlson GD, Rao K, Price TR. The dexamethasone suppression test and mood following stroke. Am J Psychiatry 1985; 142:318–323.

95. Barry S, Dinan TG. Alpha-2 adrenergic receptor function in post-stroke depression. Psychol Med 1990; 20:305–309.

96. Marchesi C, Silvestrini C, Ponari O, Volpi R, Chiodera P, Coiro V. Unreliability of TRH test but not dexamethasone suppression test as a marker of depression in chronic vasculopathic patients. Biol Psychiatry 1996; 40:637–641.

97. Fulton MK, Armitage R, Rush AJ. Sleep electroencephalographic coherence abnormalities in individuals at high risk for depression: a pilot study. Biol Psychiatry 2000; 47:618–625.

98. Perlis ML, Giles DE, Buysse DJ, Thase ME, Tu X, Kupfer DJ. Which depressive symptoms are related to which sleep electroencephalographic variables? Biol Psychiatry 1997; 42:904–913.

99. Himani A, Tandon OP, Bhatia MS. A study of P300-event related evoked potential in the patients of major depression. Indian J Physiol Pharmacol 1999; 43:367–372.

100. Korpelainen JT, Kauhanen ML, Tolonen U, Brusin E, Mononen H, Hiltunen P, Sotaniemi KA, Suominen K, Myllyla VV. Auditory P300 event related potential in minor ischemic stroke. Acta Neurol Scand 2000; 101:202–208.

101. Yanai I, Fujikawa T, Osada M, Yamawaki S, Touhouda Y. Changes in auditory P300 in patients with major depression and silent cerebral infarction. J Affect Disord 1997; 46:263–271.

102. Castillo CS, Schultz SK, Robinson RG. Clinical correlates of early-onset and late-onset poststroke generalized anxiety. Am J Psychiatry 1995; 152:1174–1179.

103. Astrom M, Adolfsson R, Asplund K. Major depression in stroke patients. A 3-year longitudinal study. Stroke 1993; 24:976–982.

104. Kotila M, Numminen H, Waltimo O, Kaste M. Post-stroke depression and functional recovery in a population-based stroke register. The Finnstroke study. Eur J Neurol 1999; 6:309–312.

105. Kauhanen M, Korpelainen JT, Hiltunen P, Brusin E, Mononen H, Maatta R, Nieminen P, Sotaniemi KA, Myllyla VV. Poststroke depression correlates with cognitive impairment and neurological deficits. Stroke 1999; 30:1875–1880.

106. Burvill PW, Johnson GA, Jamrozik KD, Anderson CS, Stewart-Wynne EG, Chakera TM. Prevalence of depression after stroke: the Perth Community Stroke Study. Br J Psychiatry 1995; 166:320–327.

107. Feibel JH, Springer CJ. Depression and failure to resume social activities after stroke. Arch Phys Med Rehabil 1982; 63:276–277.

108. House A, Dennis M, Warlow C, Hawton K, Molyneux A. The relationship between intellectual impairment and mood disorder in the first year after stroke. Psychol Med 1990; 20:805–814.

109. Angeleri F, Angeleri VA, Foschi N, Giaquinto S, Nolfe G, Saginario A, Signorino M. Depression after stroke: an investigation through catamnesis. J Clin Psychiatry 1997; 58:261–265.

110. Fuh JL, Liu HC, Wang SJ, Liu CY, Wang PN. Poststroke depression among the Chinese elderly in a rural community. Stroke 1997; 28:1126–1129.

111. Burvill P, Johnson G, Jamrozik K, Anderson C, Stewart-Wynne E. Risk factors for post-stroke depression. Int J Geriatr Psychiatry 1997; 12:219–226.

112. Kotila M, Numminen H, Waltimo O, Kaste M. Depression after stroke: results of the FINNSTROKE Study. Stroke 1998; 29:368–372.

113. Pohjasvaara T, Leppavuori A, Siira I, Vataja R, Kaste M, Erkinjuntti T. Frequency and clinical determinants of poststroke depression. Stroke 1998; 29:2311–2317.

114. Schwartz JA, Speed NM, Brunberg JA, Brewer TL, Brown M, Greden JF. Depression in stroke rehabilitation. Biol Psychiatry 1993; 33:694–699.

115. Paolucci S, Antonucci G, Pratesi L, Traballesi M, Grasso MG, Lubich S. Poststroke depression and its role in rehabilitation of inpatients. Arch Phys Med Rehabil 1999; 80:985–990.

116. Ng KC, Chan KL, Straughan PT. A study of post-stroke depression in a rehabilitative center. Acta Psychiatr Scand 1995; 92:75–79.

117. Ebrahim S, Barer D, Nouri F. Affective illness after stroke. Br J Psychiatry 1987; 151:52–56.

118. Andersen G, Vestergaard K, Ingemann-Nielsen M, Lauritzen L. Risk factors for post-stroke depression. Acta Psychiatr Scand 1995; 92:193–198.

119. Herrmann N, Black SE, Lawrence J, Szekely C, Szalai JP. The Sunnybrook Stroke Study: a prospective study of depressive symptoms and functional outcome. Stroke 1998; 29:618–624.

120. Palomaki H, Kaste M, Berg A, Lonnqvist R, Lonnqvist J, Lehtihalmes M, Hares J. Prevention of poststroke depression: 1 year randomised placebo controlled double blind trial of mianserin with 6 month follow up after therapy. J Neurol Neurosurg Psychiatry 1999; 66:490–494.

121. Eastwood MR, Rifat SL, Nobbs H, Ruderman J. Mood disorder following cerebrovascular accident. Br J Psychiatry 1989; 154:195–200.

122. Mulsant BH, Ganguli M. Epidemiology and diagnosis of depression in late life. J Clin Psychiatry 1999; 60(suppl 20):9–15.

123. Butler RN, Cohen G, Lewis MI, Simmons-Clemmons W, Sunderland T. Late-life depression: how to make a difficult diagnosis. Geriatrics 1997; 52:37–41, 50.

124. Neau JP, Ingrand P, Mouille-Brachet C, Rosier MP, Couderq C, Alvarez A, Gil R. Functional recovery and social outcome after cerebral infarction in young adults. Cerebrovasc Dis 1998; 8:296–302.

125. Angeleri F, Angeleri VA, Foschi N, Giaquinto S, Nolfe G. The influence of depression, social activity, and family stress on functional outcome after stroke. Stroke 1993; 24:1478–1483.

126. Sharpe M, Hawton K, Seagroatt V, Bamford J, House A, Molyneux A, Sandercock P, Warlow C. Depressive disorders in long-term survivors of stroke. Associations with demographic and social factors, functional status, and brain lesion volume. Br J Psychiatry 1994; 164:380–386.

127. Paradiso S, Robinson RG. Gender differences in poststroke depression. J Neuropsychiatry Clin Neurosci 1998; 10:41–47.

128. Morris PL, Robinson RG, Raphael B, Samuels J, Molloy P. The relationship between risk factors for affective disorder and poststroke depression in hospitalised stroke patients. Aust N Z J Psychiatry 1992; 26:208–217.

129. Rabins PV, Pearlson GD, Aylward E, Kumar AJ, Dowell K. Cortical magnetic resonance imaging changes in elderly inpatients with major depression [see comments]. Am J Psychiatry 1991; 148:617–620.

130. Parashos IA, Tupler LA, Blitchington T, Krishnan KR. Magnetic-resonance morphometry in patients with major depression. Psychiatry Res 1998; 84:7–15.

131. Vakili K, Pillay SS, Lafer B, Fava M, Renshaw PF, Bonello-Cintron CM, Yurgelun-Todd DA. Hippocampal volume in primary unipolar major depression: a magnetic resonance imaging study. Biol Psychiatry 2000; 47:1087–1090.

132. Mervaala E, Fohr J, Kononen M, Valkonen-Korhonen M, Vainio P, Partanen K, Partanen J, Tiihonen J, Viinamaki H, Karjalainen AK, Lehtonen J. Quantitative MRI of the hippocampus and amygdala in severe depression. Psychol Med 2000; 30:117–125.

133. Bremner JD, Narayan M, Anderson ER, Staib LH, Miller HL, Charney DS. Hippocampal volume reduction in major depression. Am J Psychiatry 2000; 157:115–118.

134. Coffey CE, Wilkinson WE, Weiner RD, Parashos IA, Djang WT, Webb MC, Figiel GS, Spritzer CE. Quantitative cerebral anatomy in depression. A controlled magnetic resonance imaging study. Arch Gen Psychiatry 1993; 50:7–16.

135. Kramer T, Garralda ME. Psychiatric disorders in adolescents in primary care. Br J Psychiatry 1998; 173:508–513.

136. Pantel J, Schroder J, Essig M, Schad LR, Popp D, Eysenbach K, Jauss M, Knopp MV. Volumetric brain findings in late depression. A study with quantified magnetic resonance tomography. Nervenarzt 1998; 69:968–974.

137. Meltzer CC, Price JC, Mathis CA, Greer PJ, Cantwell MN, Houck PR, Mulsant BH, Ben-Eliezer D, Lopresti B, Dekosky ST, Reynolds CF. PET imaging of serotonin type 2A receptors in late-life neuropsychiatric disorders. Am J Psychiatry 1999; 156:1871–1878.

138. Drevets WC, Frank E, Price JC, Kupfer DJ, Holt D, Greer PJ, Huang Y, Gautier C, Mathis C. PET imaging of serotonin 1A receptor binding in depression. Biol Psychiatry 1999; 46:1375–1387.

139. Staley JK, Malison RT, Innis RB. Imaging of the serotonergic system: interactions

of neuroanatomical and functional abnormalities of depression. Biol Psychiatry 1998; 44:534–549.

140. Willeit M, Praschak-Rieder N, Neumeister A, Pirker W, Asenbaum S, Vitouch O, Tauscher J, Hilger E, Stastny J, Brucke T, Kasper S. [123I]-beta-CIT SPECT imaging shows reduced brain serotonin transporter availability in drug-free depressed patients with seasonal affective disorder. Biol Psychiatry 2000; 47:482–489.

141. Hickie I, Ward P, Scott E, Haindl W, Walker B, Dixon J, Turner K. Neo-striatal rCBF correlates of psychomotor slowing in patients with major depression. Psychiatry Res 1999; 92:75–81.

142. Degl'innocenti A, Agren H, Backman L. Executive deficits in major depression. Acta Psychiatr Scand 1998; 97:182–188.

143. Grasso MG, Pantano P, Ricci M, Intiso DF, Pace A, Padovani A, Orzi F, Pozzilli C, Lenzi GL. Mesial temporal cortex hypoperfusion is associated with depression in subcortical stroke. Stroke 1994; 25:980–985.

144. Ghika J. Mood and behavior in disorders of the basal ganglia. In: Bogousslavsky J, Cummings JL, eds. Behavior and Mood Disorders in Focal Brain Lesions. New York: Cambridge University Press, 2000, pp 22–201.

145. Sato R, Bryan RN, Fried LP. Neuroanatomic and functional correlates of depressed mood: the Cardiovascular Health Study. Am J Epidemiol 1999; 150:919–929.

146. Lauterbach EC, Jackson JG, Wilson AN, Dever GE, Kirsh AD. Major depression after left posterior globus pallidus lesions. Neuropsychiatry Neuropsychol Behav Neurol 1997; 10:9–16.

147. Herrmann M, Bartels C, Schumacher M, Wallesch CW. Poststroke depression. Is there a pathoanatomic correlate for depression in the postacute stage of stroke? Stroke 1995; 26:850–856.

148. Morris PL, Robinson RG, Raphael B, Hopwood MJ. Lesion location and poststroke depression. J Neuropsychiatry Clin Neurosci 1996; 8:399–403.

149. Bokura H, Robinson RG. Long-term cognitive impairment associated with caudate stroke. Stroke 1997; 28:970–975.

150. Beblo T, Wallesch CW, Herrmann M. The crucial role of frontostriatal circuits for depressive disorders in the postacute stage after stroke. Neuropsychiatry Neuropsychol Behav Neurol 1999; 12:236–246.

151. Kim JS, Choi-Kwon S. Poststroke depression and emotional incontinence: correlation with lesion location. Neurology 2000; 54:1805–1810.

152. Fedoroff JP, Starkstein SE, Forrester AW, Geisler FH, Jorge RE, Arndt SV, Robinson RG. Depression in patients with acute traumatic brain injury. Am J Psychiatry 1992; 149:918–923.

153. Robinson RG, Chemerinski E, Jorge R. Pathophysiology of secondary depressions in the elderly. J Geriatr Psychiatry Neurol 1999; 12:128–136.

154. Yanai I, Fujikawa T, Horiguchi J, Yamawaki S, Touhouda Y. The 3-year course and outcome of patients with major depression and silent cerebral infarction. J Affect Disord 1998; 47:25–30.

155. Fujikawa T, Yanai I, Yamawaki S. Psychosocial stressors in patients with major depression and silent cerebral infarction. Stroke 1997; 28:1123–1125.

156. Fujikawa T, Yamawaki S, Touhouda Y. Incidence of silent cerebral infarction in patients with major depression. Stroke 1993; 24:1631–1634.

157. Fujikawa T, Yokota N, Muraoka M, Yamawaki S. Response of patients with major depression and silent cerebral infarction to antidepressant drug therapy, with emphasis on central nervous system adverse reactions. Stroke 1996; 27:2040–2042.

158. O'Brien J, Desmond P, Ames D, Schweitzer I, Harrigan S, Tress B. A magnetic resonance imaging study of white matter lesions in depression and Alzheimer's disease [see comments] [published erratum appears in Br J Psychiatry 1996; 168(6): 792]. Br J Psychiatry 1996; 168:477–485.

159. Ballard C, McKeith I, O'Brien J, Kalaria R, Jaros E, Ince P, Perry R. Neuropathological substrates of dementia and depression in vascular dementia, with a particular focus on cases with small infarct volumes. Dement Geriatr Cogn Disord 2000; 11: 59–65.

160. Greenwald BS, Kramer-Ginsberg E, Krishnan KR, Ashtari M, Auerbach C, Patel M. Neuroanatomic localization of magnetic resonance imaging signal hyperintensities in geriatric depression. Stroke 1998; 29:613–617.

161. Fukutake T. Young-adult-onset hereditary subcortical vascular dementia: cerebral autosomal recessive arteriosclerosis with subcortical infarcts and leukoencephalopathy (CARASIL). Rinsho Shinkeigaku 1999; 39:50–52.

162. Chabriat H, Joutel A, Vahedi K, Iba-Zizen MT, Tournier-Lasserve E, Bousser MG. CADASIS. Cerebral Autosomal Dominant Arteriopathy with Subcortical Infarcts and Leukoencephalophathy. Rev Neurol (Paris) 1997; 153:376–385.

163. Glass JD, Wesselingh SL, Selnes OA, McArthur JC. Clinical-neuropathologic correlation in HIV-associated dementia [see comments]. Neurology 1993; 43:2230–2237.

164. Berger JR, Nath A, Greenberg RN, Andersen AH, Greene RA, Bognar A, Avison MJ. Cerebrovascular changes in the basal ganglia with HIV dementia. Neurology 2000; 54:921–926.

165. Bakshi R, Czarnecki D, Shaikh ZA, Priore RL, Janardhan V, Kaliszky Z, Kinkel PR. Brain MRI lesions and atrophy are related to depression in multiple sclerosis. Neuroreport 2000; 11:1153–1158.

166. Berg D, Supprian T, Thomae J, Warmuth-Metz M, Horowski A, Zeiler B, Magnus T, Rieckmann P, Becker G. Lesion pattern in patients with multiple sclerosis and depression. Mult Scler 2000; 6:156–162.

167. Robinson RG, Kubos KL, Starr LB, Rao K, Price TR. Mood disorders in stroke patients. Importance of location of lesion. Brain 1984; 107 (Pt 1):81–93.

168. Pearlson GD, Robinson RG. Suction lesions of the frontal cerebral cortex in the rat induce asymmetrical behavioral and catecholaminergic responses. Brain Res 1981; 218:233–242.

169. Robinson RG, Stitt TG. Intracortical 6-hydroxydopamine induced an asymmetrical behavioral response in the rat. Brain Res 1981; 213:387–395.

170. Davidson RJ. Anterior cerebral asymmetry and the nature of emotion. Brain Cogn 1992; 20:125–151.

171. Bhatia KP, Marsden CD. The behavioural and motor consequences of focal lesions of the basal ganglia in man. Brain 1994; 117 (Pt 4):859–876.

172. Morris PL, Robinson RG, Raphael B. Prevalence and course of depressive disorders in hospitalized stroke patients. Int J Psychiatry Med 1990; 20:349–364.

173. Dam H, Pedersen HE, Ahlgren P. Depression among patients with stroke. Acta Psychiatr Scand 1989; 80:118–124.
174. Sharpe M, Hawton K, House A, Molyneux A, Sandercock P, Bamford J, Warlow C. Mood disorders in long-term survivors of stroke: associations with brain lesion location and volume. Psychol Med 1990; 20:815–828.
175. House A, Dennis M, Warlow C, Hawton K, Molyneux A. Mood disorders after stroke and their relation to lesion location. A CT scan study. Brain 1990; 113 (Pt 4):1113–1129.
176. Finset A, Goffeng L, Landro NI, Haakonsen M. Depressed mood and intra-hemispheric location of lesion in right hemisphere stroke patients. Scand J Rehabil Med 1989; 21:1–6.
177. Heller W, Etienne MA, Miller GA. Patterns of perceptual asymmetry in depression and anxiety: implications for neuropsychological models of emotion and psychopathology. J Abnorm Psychol 1995; 104:327–333.
178. Kikumoto O. Clinical study on depressive state following stroke. Seishin Shinkeigaku Zasshi 1990; 92:441–434.
179. Shimoda K, Robinson RG. The relationship between poststroke depression and lesion location in long-term follow-up. Biol Psychiatry 1999; 45:187–192.
180. Robinson RG. Mood Disorders Secondary to Stroke. Semin Clin Neuropsychiatry 1997; 2:244–251.
181. Starkstein SE, Robinson RG, Berthier ML, Parikh RM, Price TR. Differential mood changes following basal ganglia vs thalamic lesions. Arch Neurol 1988; 45:725–730.
182. Starkstein SE, Robinson RG, Price TR. Comparison of patients with and without poststroke major depression matched for size and location of lesion. Arch Gen Psychiatry 1988; 45:247–252.
183. Starkstein SE, Robinson RG, Price TR. Comparison of cortical and subcortical lesions in the production of poststroke mood disorders. Brain 1987; 110 (Pt 4): 1045–1059.
184. Robinson RG, Lipsey JR, Bolla-Wilson K, Bolduc PL, Pearlson GD, Rao K, Price TR. Mood disorders in left-handed stroke patients. Am J Psychiatry 1985; 142: 1424–1429.
185. Reference deleted.
186. Starkstein SE, Bryer JB, Berthier ML, Cohen B, Price TR, Robinson RG. Depression after stroke: the importance of cerebral hemisphere asymmetries. J Neuropsychiatry Clin Neurosci 1991; 3:276–285.
187. Robinson RG, Bolla-Wilson K, Kaplan E, Lipsey JR, Price TR. Depression influences intellectual impairment in stroke patients. Br J Psychiatry 1986; 148:541–547.
188. Kase CS, Wolf PA, Kelly-Hayes M, Kannel WB, Beiser A, D'Agostino RB. Intellectual decline after stroke: the Framingham Study. Stroke 1998; 29:805–812.
189. Zerfass R, Kretzschmar K, Forstl H. Depressive disorders after cerebral infarct. Relations to infarct site, brain atrophy and cognitive deficits. Nervenarzt 1992; 63: 163–168.
190. Bolla-Wilson K, Robinson RG, Starkstein SE, Boston J, Price TR. Lateralization of dementia of depression in stroke patients. Am J Psychiatry 1989; 146:627–634.

191. Downhill JEJ, Robinson RG. Longitudinal assessment of depression and cognitive impairment following stroke. J Nerv Ment Dis 1994; 182:425–431.
192. Andersen G, Vestergaard K, Ingeman-Nielsen MW, Lauritzen LU. Risk factors for depression after apoplexy. Ugeskr Laeger 1996; 158:6107–6110.
193. Pohjasvaara T, Mantyla R, Aronen HJ, Leskela M, Salonen O, Kaste M, Erkinjuntti T. Clinical and radiological determinants of prestroke cognitive decline in a stroke cohort. J Neurol Neurosurg Psychiatry 1999; 67:742–748.
194. Feher EP, Mahurin RK, Doody RS, Cooke N, Sims J, Pirozzolo FJ. Establishing the limits of the Mini-Mental State. Examination of 'subtests.' Arch Neurol 1992; 49:87–92.
195. Reference deleted.
196. Tatemichi TK, Desmond DW, Stern Y, Paik M, Sano M, Bagiella E. Cognitive impairment after stroke: frequency, patterns, and relationship to functional abilities. J Neurol Neurosurg Psychiatry 1994; 57:202–207.
197. Veiel HO. A preliminary profile of neuropsychological deficits associated with major depression. J Clin Exp Neuropsychol 1997; 19:587–603.
198. Speedie L, Rabins P, Pearlson G, Moberg P. Confrontation naming deficit in dementia of depression. J Neuropsychiatry Clin Neurosci 1990; 2:59–63.
199. Andersen G, Vestergaard K, Riis JO, Ingeman-Nielsen M. Dementia of depression or depression of dementia in stroke? Acta Psychiatr Scand 1996; 94:272–278.
200. Starkstein SE, Robinson RG. Dementia of depression in Parkinson's disease and stroke. J Nerv Ment Dis 1991; 179:593–601.
201. Robinson RG, Starr LB, Kubos KL, Price TR. A two-year longitudinal study of post-stroke mood disorders: findings during the initial evaluation. Stroke 1983; 14: 736–741.
202. Folstein MF, Maiberger R, McHugh PR. Mood disorder as a specific complication of stroke. J Neurol Neurosurg Psychiatry 1977; 40:1018–1020.
203. Robinson RG, Murata Y, Shimoda K. Dimensions of social impairment and their effect on depression and recovery following stroke. Int Psychogeriatr 1999; 11: 375–384.
204. Dennis M, O'Rourke S, Lewis S, Sharpe M, Warlow C. Emotional outcomes after stroke: factors associated with poor outcome. J Neurol Neurosurg Psychiatry 2000; 68:47–52.
205. Singh A, Black SE, Herrmann N, Leibovitch FS, Ebert PL, Lawrence J, Szalai JP. Functional and neuroanatomic correlations in poststroke depression: the Sunnybrook Stroke Study. Stroke 2000; 31:637–644.
206. Lieberman D, Friger M, Fried V, Grinshpun Y, Mytlis N, Tylis R, Galinsky D. Characterization of elderly patients in rehabilitation: stroke versus hip fracture. Disabil Rehabil 1999; 21:542–547.
207. Wetterling T. Vascular depression—a new concise concept?. Fortschr Neurol Psychiatr 1999; 67:327–335.
208. Lieberman D, Galinsky D, Fried V, Grinshpun Y, Mytlis N, Tylis R. Geriatric Depression Screening Scale (GDS) in patients hospitalized for physical rehabilitation. Int J Geriatr Psychiatry 1999; 14:549–555.
209. Bond J, Gregson B, Smith M, Rousseau N, Lecouturier J, Rodgers H. Outcomes following acute hospital care for stroke or hip fracture: how useful is an assessment

of anxiety or depression for older people? Int J Geriatr Psychiatry 1998; 13:601–610.

210. Paolucci S, Antonucci G, Pratesi L, Traballesi M, Grasso MG, Lubich S. Poststroke depression and its role in rehabilitation of inpatients. Arch Phys Med Rehabil 1999; 80:985–990.

211. Lam CL, Lauder IJ. The impact of chronic diseases on the health-related quality of life (HRQOL) of Chinese patients in primary care. Fam Pract 2000; 17:159–166.

212. Parikh RM, Robinson RG, Lipsey JR, Starkstein SE, Fedoroff JP, Price TR. The impact of poststroke depression on recovery in activities of daily living over a 2-year follow-up. Arch Neurol 1990; 47:785–789.

213. Loong CK, Kenneth NK, Paulin ST. Post-stroke depression: outcome following rehabilitation. Aust N Z J Psychiatry 1995; 29:609–614.

214. Carson AJ, Ringbauer B, Mackenzie L, Warlow C, Sharpe M. Neurological disease, emotional disorder, and disability: they are related: a study of 300 consecutive new referrals to a neurology outpatient department. J Neurol Neurosurg Psychiatry 2000; 68:202–206.

215. Chang AM, Mackenzie AE. State self-esteem following stroke. Stroke 1998; 29:2325–2328.

216. Morris PL, Robinson RG, Andrzejewski P, Samuels J, Price TR. Association of depression with 10-year poststroke mortality. Am J Psychiatry 1993; 150:124–129.

217. Wassertheil-Smoller S, Applegate WB, Berge K, Chang CJ, Davis BR, Grimm RJ, Kostis J, Pressel S, Schron E. Change in depression as a precursor of cardiovascular events. SHEP Cooperative Research Group (Systoloc Hypertension in the elderly). Arch Intern Med 1996; 156:553–561.

218. Everson SA, Roberts RE, Goldberg DE, Kaplan GA. Depressive symptoms and increased risk of stroke mortality over a 29-year period. Arch Intern Med 1998; 158:1133–1138.

219. Jonas BS, Franks P, Ingram DD. Are symptoms of anxiety and depression risk factors for hypertension? Longitudinal evidence from the National Health and Nutrition Examination Survey I Epidemiologic Follow-up Study. Arch Fam Med 1997; 6:43–49.

220. Hippisley-Cox J, Fielding K, Pringle M. Depression as a risk factor for ischaemic heart disease in men: population based case-control study [published erratum appears in Br Med J 1998; 18; 317(7152):185]. Br Med J 1998; 316:1714–1719.

221. Ford DE, Mead LA, Chang PP, Cooper-Patrick L, Wang NY, Klag MJ. Depression is a risk factor for coronary artery disease in men: the precursors study. Arch Intern Med 1998; 158:1422–1426.

222. Pratt LA, Ford DE, Crum RM, Armenian HK, Gallo JJ, Eaton WW. Depression, psychotropic medication, and risk of myocardial infarction. Prospective data from the Baltimore ECA follow-up. Circulation 1996; 94:3123–3129.

223. Kusumi I, Koyama T, Yamashita I. Serotonin-stimulated Ca2+ response is increased in the blood platelets of depressed patients. Biol Psychiatry 1991; 30:310–312.

224. Morris PL, Raphael B. Depressive disorder associated with physical illness. The impact of stroke. Gen Hosp Psychiatry 1987; 9:324–330.

225. Robinson RG, Starr LB, Lipsey JR, Rao K, Price TR. A two-year longitudinal study of poststroke mood disorders. In-hospital prognostic factors associated with six-month outcome. J Nerv Ment Dis 1985; 173:221–226.

226. Baker AC. The spouse's positive effect on the stroke patient's recovery. Rehabil Nurs 1993; 18:30–33.

227. Robinson RG, Schultz SK, Castillo C, Kopel T, Kosier JT, Newman RM, Curdue K, Petracca G, Starkstein SE. Nortriptyline versus fluoxetine in the treatment of depression and in short-term recovery after stroke: a placebo-controlled, double-blind study. Am J Psychiatry 2000; 157:351–359.

228. Stamenkovic M, Schindler S, Kasper S. Poststroke depression and fluoxetine [letter]. Am J Psychiatry 1996; 153:446–447.

229. Gonzalez-Torrecillas JL, Mendlewicz J, Lobo A. Effects of early treatment of poststroke depression on neuropsychological rehabilitation. Int Psychogeriatr 1995; 7:547–560.

230. Andersen G, Vestergaard K, Lauritzen LU. Effective treatment of depression following apoplexy with citalopram. Ugeskr Laeger 1995; 157:2000–2003.

231. Derex L, Ostrowsky K, Nighoghossian N, Trouillas P. Severe pathological crying after left anterior choroidal artery infarct. Reversibility with paroxetine treatment [see comments]. Stroke 1997; 28:1464–1466.

232. Lazarus LW, Winemiller DR, Lingam VR, Neyman I, Hartman C, Abassian M, Kartan U, Groves L, Fawcett J. Efficacy and side effects of methylphenidate for poststroke depression [see comments]. J Clin Psychiatry 1992; 53:447–449.

233. Johnson ML, Roberts MD, Ross AR, Witten CM. Methylphenidate in stroke patients with depression. Am J Phys Med Rehabil 1992; 71:239–241.

234. Masand P, Murray GB, Pickett P. Psychostimulants in post-stroke depression. J Neuropsychiatry Clin Neurosci 1991; 3:23–27.

235. Masand P, Chaudhary P. Methylphenidate treatment of poststroke depression in a patient with global aphasia. Ann Clin Psychiatry 1994; 6:271–274.

236. Lauritzen L, Bendsen BB, Vilmar T, Bendsen EB, Lunde M, Bech P. Post-stroke depression: combined treatment with imipramine or desipramine and mianserin. A controlled clinical study. Psychopharmacology (Berl) 1994; 114:119–122.

237. Balunov OA, Sadov OG, Alemasova AY. Therapy of depressions in post-stroke patients. Alaska Med 1990; 32:20–29.

238. Shima S. The efficacy of antidepressants in post-stroke depression. Keio J Med 1997; 46:25–26.

239. Starr LB, Robinson RG, Price TR. Reliability, validity, and clinical utility of the social functioning exam in the assessment of stroke patients. Exp Aging Res 1983; 9:101–106.

240. Glassman AH, Johnson LL, Giardina EG, Walsh BT, Roose SP, Cooper TB, Bigger JTJ. The use of imipramine in depressed patients with congestive heart failure. JAMA 1983; 250:1997–2001.

241. Lipsey JR, Robinson RG, Pearlson GD, Rao K, Price TR. Nortriptyline treatment of post-stroke depression: a double-blind study. Lancet 1984; 1:297–300.

242. Tiller JW. Post-stroke depression. Psychopharmacology (Berl) 1992; 106 Suppl: S130–S133.

243. Reding MJ, Orto LA, Winter SW, Fortuna IM, DI Ponte P, McDowell FH. Antide-

pressant therapy after stroke. A double-blind trial. Arch Neurol 1986; 43:763–765.

244. Dam M, Tonin P, De Boni A, Pizzolato G, Casson S, Ermani M, Freo U, Piron L, Battistin L. Effects of fluoxetine and maprotiline on functional recovery in poststroke hemiplegic patients undergoing rehabilitation therapy [see comments]. Stroke 1996; 27:1211–1214.

245. Gustafson Y, Nilsson I, Mattsson M, Astrom M, Bucht G. Epidemiology and treatment of post-stroke depression. Drugs Aging 1995; 7:298–309.

246. Berthier ML, Kulisevsky J. Fluoxetine—induced mania in a patient with post-stroke depression [letter]. Br J Psychiatry 1993; 163:698–699.

247. Edwards JG, Anderson I. Systematic review and guide to selection of selective serotonin reuptake inhibitors [published erratum appears in Drugs 1999 Dec; 58(6): 1207–9] [see comments]. Drugs 1999; 57:507–533.

248. Hougaku H, Matsumoto M, Hata R, Handa N, Imaizumi M, Sugitani Y, Yoneda S, Etani H, Sueyoshi K, Kusunoki M. Therapeutic effect of lisuride maleate on post-stroke depression. Nippon Ronen Igakkai Zasshi 1994; 31:52–59.

249. Kimura M, Robinson RG, Kosier JT. Treatment of cognitive impairment after poststroke depression: a double-blind treatment trial. Stroke 2000; 31:1482–1486.

250. Van de Weg FB, Kuik DJ, Lankhorst GJ. Post-stroke depression and functional outcome: a cohort study investigating the influence of depression on functional recovery from stroke. Clin Rehabil 1999; 13:268–272.

251. Morris PL, Raphael B, Robinson RG. Clinical depression is associated with impaired recovery from stroke. Med J Aust 1992; 157:239–242.

252. Enserink M. Can the placebo be the cure? Science 1999; 284:238–240.

253. Parikh RM, Lipsey JR, Robinson RG, Price TR. Two-year longitudinal study of post-stroke mood disorders: dynamic changes in correlates of depression at one and two years. Stroke 1987; 18:579–584.

254. Robinson RG, Starr LB, Lipsey JR, Rao K, Price TR. A two-year longitudinal study of poststroke mood disorders. In-hospital prognostic factors associated with six-month outcome. J Nerv Ment Dis 1985; 173:221–226.

255. Robinson RG, Price TR. Post-stroke depressive disorders: a follow-up study of 103 patients. Stroke 1982; 13:635–641.

256. Astrom M, Olsson T, Asplund K. Different linkage of depression to hypercortisolism early versus late after stroke. A 3-year longitudinal study. Stroke 1993; 24: 52–57.

257. Grade C, Redford B, Chrostowski J, Toussaint L, Blackwell B. Methylphenidate in early poststroke recovery: a double-blind, placebo-controlled study. Arch Phys Med Rehabil 1998; 79:1047–1050.

258. Lingam VR, Lazarus LW, Groves L, Oh SH. Methylphenidate in treating poststroke depression. J Clin Psychiatry 1988; 49:151–153.

259. Murray GB, Shea V, Conn DK. Electroconvulsive therapy for poststroke depression. J Clin Psychiatry 1986; 47:258–260.

260. Currier MB, Murray GB, Welch CC. Electroconvulsive therapy for post-stroke depressed geriatric patients. J Neuropsychiatry Clin Neurosci 1992; 4:140–144.

261. Lincoln NB, Flannaghan T, Sutcliffe L, Rother L. Evaluation of cognitive behav-

ioural treatment for depression after stroke: a pilot study. Clin Rehabil 1997; 11: 114–122.

262. Morrison VL, Johnston M, MacWalter RS, Pollard BS. Improving emotional outcomes following acute stroke: a preliminary evaluation of work-book based intervention. Scott Med J 1998; 43:52–53.

263. Silent strokes linked to depression in the elderly [news]. Health News 1999; 5:6.

264. Kishi Y, Kosier JT, Robinson RG. Suicidal plans in patients with acute stroke. J Nerv Ment Dis 1996; 184:274–280.

265. Kishi Y, Robinson RG, Kosier JT. Suicidal plans in patients with stroke: comparison between acute-onset and delayed-onset suicidal plans. Int Psychogeriatr 1996; 8:623–634.

266. Schultz SK, Castillo CS, Kosier JT, Robinson RG. Generalized anxiety and depression. Assessment over 2 years after stroke. Am J Geriatr Psychiatry 1997; 5:229–237.

267. Astrom M. Generalized anxiety disorder in stroke patients. A 3-year longitudinal study. Stroke 1996; 27:270–275.

268. Astrom M. Depression after stroke. Antidepressive therapy enhances recovery. Lakartidiningen 1994; 91:963–966.

269. Starkstein SE, Cohen BS, Fedoroff P, Parikh RM, Price TR, Robinson RG. Relationship between anxiety disorders and depressive disorders in patients with cerebrovascular injury. Arch Gen Psychiatry 1990; 47:246–251.

270. Fujikawa T, Yamawaki S, Touhouda Y. Silent cerebral infarctions in patients with late-onset mania. Stroke 1995; 26:946–949.

271. Robinson RG. Postroke mania: prevalence and clinical symptoms. In: Robinson RG, ed. The Clinical Neuropsychiatry of Stroke. New York: Cambridge University Press, 1988, pp 297–302.

272. Jorge RE, Robinson RG, Starkstein SE, Arndt SV, Forrester AW, Geisler FH. Secondary mania following traumatic brain injury. Am J Psychiatry 1993; 150:916–921.

273. Robinson RG, Boston JD, Starkstein SE, Price TR. Comparison of mania and depression after brain injury: causal factors. Am J Psychiatry 1988; 145:172–178.

274. Bornke C, Postert T, Przuntek H, Buttner T. Acute mania due to a right hemisphere infarction. Eur J Neurol 1998; 5:407–409.

275. Liu CY, Wang SJ, Fuh JL, Yang YY, Liu HC. Bipolar disorder following a stroke involving the left hemisphere. Aust NZ J Psychiatry 1996; 30:688–691.

276. Cummings JL, Mendez MF. Secondary mania with focal cerebrovascular lesions. Am J Psychiatry 1984; 141:1084–1087.

277. Starkstein SE, Fedoroff P, Berthier ML, Robinson RG. Manic-depressive and pure manic states after brain lesions. Biol Psychiatry 1991; 29:149–158.

278. McGilchrist I, Goldstein LH, Jadresic D, Fenwick P. Thalamo-frontal psychosis [see comments]. Br J Psychiatry 1993; 163:113–115.

279. Kulisevsky J, Berthier ML, Pujol J. Hemiballismus and secondary mania following a right thalamic infarction. Neurology 1993; 43:1422–1424.

280. Bogousslavsky J, Ferrazzini M, Regli F, Assal G, Tanabe H, Delaloye-Bischof A. Manic delirium and frontal-like syndrome with paramedian infarction of the right thalamus. J Neurol Neurosurg Psychiatry 1988; 51:116–119.

281. Turecki G, Mari Jd, Del Porto JA. Bipolar disorder following a left basal-ganglia stroke [letter]. Br J Psychiatry 1993; 163:690.
282. Drake MEJ, Pakalnis A, Phillips B. Secondary mania after ventral pontine infarction. J Neuropsychiatry Clin Neurosci 1990; 2:322–325.
283. Fenn D, George K. Post-stroke mania late in life involving the left hemisphere. Aust NZ J Psychiatry 1999; 33:598–600.
284. Danel T, Comayras S, Goudemand M, Leys D, Destee A, Lauth B, Dupard T. Mood disorders and right hemisphere infarction. Encephale 1989; 15:549–553.
285. Regard M, Landis T. "Gourmand syndrome": eating passion associated with right anterior lesions [see comments]. Neurology 1997; 48:1185–1190.
286. Paradiso S, Robinson RG, Arndt S. Self-reported aggressive behavior in patients with stroke. J Nerv Ment Dis 1996; 184:746–753.
287. Migliorelli R, Starkstein SE, Teson A, De Quiros G, Vazquez S, Leiguarda R, Robinson RG. SPECT findings in patients with primary mania. J Neuropsychiatry Clin Neurosci 1993; 5:379–383.
288. Dupont RM, Cullum CM, Jeste DV. Poststroke depression and psychosis. Psychiatr Clin North Am 1988; 11:133–149.
289. Bakchine S, Lacomblez L, Benoit N, Parisot D, Chain F, Lhermitte F. Manic-like state after bilateral orbitofrontal and right temporoparietal injury: efficacy of clonidine. Neurology 1989; 39:777–781.
290. Evans DL, Byerly MJ, Greer RA. Secondary mania: diagnosis and treatment. J Clin Psychiatry 1995; 56(suppl 3).31–37.
291. Robinson RG. Treatment of mania following stroke. In: Robinson RG, ed. The Clinical Neuropsychiatry of Stroke. New York: Cambridge Press, 1998, pp 336–337.
292. Nagaratnam N, Pathma-Nathan N. Behavioural and psychiatric aspects of silent cerebral infarction. Br J Clin Pract 1997; 51:160–163.
293. Dunne JW, Leedman PJ, Edis RH. Inobvious stroke: a cause of delirium and dementia. Aust NZ J Med 1986; 16:771–778.
294. Levine DN, Finklestein S. Delayed psychosis after right temporoparietal stroke or trauma: relation to epilepsy. Neurology 1982; 32:267–273.
295. Price BH, Mesulam M. Psychiatric manifestations of right hemisphere infarctions. J Nerv Ment Dis 1985; 173:610–614.
296. Pakalnis A, Drake MEJ, Kellum JB. Right parieto-occipital lacunar infarction with agitation, hallucinations, and delusions. Psychosomatics 1987; 28:95–96.
297. Richardson JK. Psychotic behavior after right hemispheric cerebrovascular accident: a case report. Arch Phys Med Rehabil 1992; 73:381–384.
298. Berthier M, Starkstein S. Acute atypical psychosis following a right hemisphere stroke. Acta Neurol Belg 1987; 87:125–131.
299. Peroutka SJ, Sohmer BH, Kumar AJ, Folstein M, Robinson RG. Hallucinations and delusions following a right temporoparietooccipital infarction. Johns Hopkins Med J 1982; 151:181–185.
300. La Mancusa JC, Cole AR. Visual manifestations of occipital lobe infarction in three patients on a geriatric psychiatry unit. J Geriatr Psychiatry Neurol 1988; 1:231–234.

301.   Anderson SW, Rizzo M. Hallucinations following occipital lobe damage: the patho-
       logical activation of visual representations. J Clin Exp Neuropsychol 1994; 16:
       651–663.
302.   Wright IC, McGuire PK, Poline JB, Travere JM, Murray RM, Frith CD, Fracko-
       wiak RS, Friston KJ. A voxel-based method for the statistical analysis of gray and
       white matter density applied to schizophrenia. Neuroimage 1995; 2:244–252.

9

Vascular Dementia After Stroke

J. Ghika and Julien Bogousslavsky
University of Lausanne and Centre Hospitalier Universitaire Vaudois, Lausanne, Switzerland

I. DEFINITION AND DIAGNOSTIC CRITERIA

Vascular dementia (VD) is defined as a dementia syndrome occurring after stroke (1) and accounts for 10–15% of all dementias, after Alzheimer's disease (60%) and diffuse Lewy body disease (20%). Ideally, criteria for the definition of this entity should include (1) dementia, (2) vascular disease, and (3) a clear causal relationship between them, classically with sudden onset of focal neurological signs, but there is considerable variability in the clinical presentation. Various criteria have been used: NINDS-AIREN (2), ICD-10 (3,4), DSM-IV (5), or the State of California Alzheimer's Disease Diagnostic and Treatment Centers (SCADDTC) (6). All require a decline in multiple higher cortical functions, including memory, sufficient to interfere with daily living activities, and the evidence for at least one stroke, with a clearly documented temporal relationship (NINDS-AIREN: 3 months) to the onset of dementia. The ICD-10 definition represents a classification of subtypes of vascular dementia rather than diagnostic criteria. DSM-IV criteria are based on a general definition of dementias, but no criteria to establish a causal relationship between dementia and vascular disease is clearly defined. The SCADDTC was the first definition of probable, possible, or definite VD; memory deficit is not emphasized, but it does not allow much fine tuning in all subtypes. NINDS-AIREN criteria provide a better approach, including an arbitrary time relationship with vascular event(s), also adding a neuropathological classification, but it is still not satisfactory, relying heavily on memory and not allowing the exclusion of underlying Alzheimer's or other degenerative dementia. Neuroimaging is necessary (7), showing infarcts, lacunae, or white-matter lesions, but it is not certain so far that white-matter lesions really matter (7). Hemorrhages, anoxia, subdural hematomas, arteriovenous malformations (AVMs), or venous thormobosis may also be found. None of the above-mentioned definitions allow separation of mixed dementia, i.e., a pauci- or non-symptomatic Alzheimer's disease (AD) that is revealed or aggravated by a stroke or VD associated with AD.

II. EPIDEMIOLOGY

The frequency of VD highly depends on diagnostic criteria and on the sample. Hospital-based series, including memory clinics, differ from community-based or authopsy studies. The methodology is also very different from one study to the other, especially in terms of definition and neuroimaging. Lack of common diagnostic criteria limits the comparability among studies. On the whole, VD is six times less frequent than Alhzeimer's disease (AD) (8). An estimated incidence of 1.2–1.5/100 person-years at risk has been reported (8) (compared with 2.5/100 for AD), a proportion only reversed in Japan. It may concern 5–10% of patients within a year of stroke according to their age (9) with a prevalence from 1.2 to 4.2% of people over 65 years old (10,11), up to a third of the 85-year-old patients (12). VD may represent up to 10–15% of all dementias (13), even in the very old (14), and has a lifetime risk of 34.5% for men and 19.4% for women.

The frequency of poststroke cognitive dysfunction is higher (62%, increasing from 46% up to 74% from 55 to 85 years), but dementia is less frequent (26–32%) (15). The incidence of dementia after stroke in a 52-month follow-up was 8.4/100 person-years in the stroke group compared with 1.3/100 person-years in the control group. Age is a major factor in the estimation of poststroke dementia, and a stroke in an elderly person increases the freuqency of dementia by about fivefold (16). However, these figures may show a a high variation according to definition criteria: from 25% with DSM-III (the most sensitive), 20% with DSM-III-R, 18% with DSM-IV, 21% with NINDS-AIREN, 6% with the most specific ICD-10 (15,17,18). The mean age of the sample is also a major bias: from 19% to 25% respectively from 55 to 85 years. (15,19). Dementia after first-ever stroke was reported in 10–38% (9,18,20,21). It is therefore clear that stroke considerably increases the risk of dementia, and reversely, dementia in old age may be an early manifestation of cerebrovascular disease that eventually becomes clinically evident as an acute infarct. Therefore, the elevated risk of subsequent strokes in older persons with cognitive impairment suggest that cerebrovascular disease may have a role in causing cognitive impairment (22).

III. MULTIPLE ENTITIES OF VD

Six subtypes of VD have been described: (1) multi-infarct dementia, (2) strategic simple infarct dementia or focal form of VD (angular gyrus, thalamus, basal forebrain, thalamus, cingulate gyrus, anterior capsule), (3) small-vessel disease with dementia, (4) hypoperfusion dementia, (5) hemorrhagic dementia, and (6) other vascular dementias (vasculitis, dural sinus thrombosis or AVM, DIC, Spatz-Lindenberg's disease, lymphoid granulomatosis, malignant angioendotheliosis, hypoperfusion, or anoxic dementia). Genetic vascular dementias (CADASIL, British dementia, Fabry's disease, homocystinuria, sickle cell disease, Rendu-Osler disease, moya-moya disease, hemoglobin SC disease, MELAS, Sneddon's disease, Dutch and Icelandic hereditary cerebral amyloid angiopathy, coagulopathies) (23,24) should be considered separately, as well as other rare entities (25). Binswanger's disease (26) may be the end of the spectrum of hypertensive VD associating severe diffuse white-matter lesions sparing subcortical U fibers, multiple lacunar strokes, territorial strokes, and even hemorrhages as a cause of both hypertension and high variations in blood pressure.

Multi-infarct dementia is therefore not the only or the most important form of VD (26), but the the variable mixture of small- and large-vessel disease, hemodynamic, cardiac, hemorrhagic, venous, specific arteriopathies, and hematological or hereditary parameters including risk factors may be more relevant. There is a difficult border zone and a wide spectrum between so-called poststroke cognitive dysfunction and frank ICD-10, DSM-IV, or NINDS-AIREN defined dementia, both clinically and on neuroimaging. No obvious correspondence seems to exist between structural pathological changes and symptoms or signs (27). The Hatchinski Ischemic Score (cutoff 6/7) is helpful but not specific or accurate enough. It may not be able to distinguish between primary degenerative, VD, or mixed dementia, with a sensitivity of only 17–50% and a specificity of 70–82% (28–30). The features of positive history of stroke and a fluctuating course were reported as the most sensitive indices for some, but not for others who observed that the evolution of VD was faster than AD, but stepwise progression was unfrequent (31–33). Autopsy-based studies show that pure VD without AD features is exceptional (34,35). However, with pathological criteria, neither clinical nor pathological evidence of stroke means that cerebrovascular disease has anything to do with a patient's dementia (36). The role of the frequently associated Alzheimer's disease, as assessed by pathology in brain banks, adds further fuzziness to this concept and even its asserted existence. Differentiation from AD or so-called mixed dementia is far from easy on both clinical and neuroimaging criteria in the absence of biological markers. Memory impairment is emphasized as a primary criterion reflecting AD (37–39), but is also a major criterion in the present definition of VD (2 6). Ischemic scores, as already mentioned, do not help (40), but others found radioimaging (including CT, MRI, and SPECT) studies to be as useful as clinical features (41–43) and even EEG (44). However, it is well known that in patients with an underlying degenerative dementia, any lesion in the brain may precipitate dementia, with a temporal relationship. Moreover, the exact role of white-matter lesions in cognitive dysfunction, one of the most frequent features in vascular dementia, remains controversial, in both the effect of location and volume of these lesions (27). It is also possible that the cerebrovascular changes may contribute to AD evolution (45,46). Therefore, the causality between cognitive impairment and vascular brain changes is of paramount importance, and it remains so far still not settled, even in pathology-based studies. It remains unclear, so far, whether vascular lesions are the main cause, unmask or underlie preexisting degenerative changes, modify or aggravate them, and how the location, extent, type, and tempo of vascular lesions relate to cognitive and behavioral changes.

There has been growing activity in redefining vascular dementia in recent years (6,47–54). Vascular lesions seen in AD patients may have different pathophysiological processes in AD and VD and do not necessarily have cognitive consequences in AD patients (55–57). The notion of infarct and noninfarct vascular dementia has recently been proposed (58) and the difference between multiple infarcts without dementia and multi-infarct dementia lies in the presence of hypertension (HT), thalamic infarction, and perventricular hypodensities, but age, atrophy of the brain, and diabetes all seem to have a minor contribution to the dementia (59). It has also become clear that the volume of infarction does not provide an explanation for dementia and sometimes patients with small lesions can be demented whereas patients with massive lesions are not. The strategic location of stroke (bilateral, thalamic, thalamic and cortical, bilateral anterior cerebral arteries, bilateral cingulate or fornix, caudate, bilateral pallidal, anterior capsule, posterior cerebral artery, parietotemporal, dominant hemisphere, temporal) is of major importance, but the state of the remaining brain tissue "reserve capacity" may be more critical than any other factor (preexisting initial stage of a degenerative dementia, cerbral atrophy, aging, etc.) perhaps because it may explain the absence of plastic compensatory capacity or the idiosyncratic impact on the individual characteristic of intact neuronal networks (9). The source of patients included may well be more important than the actual diagnostic criteria. The presence of white-matter lesions, the total volume, pattern (patchy, confluent), or location of these nonspecific changes, which can be seen in about a third of the patients with AD, and their exact role in cognitive changes, is still not yet settled, even after many years of consideration and the improvement of radoimaging techniques. Another unresolved issue is the role of so-called "silent" or bettercalled "unrecognized" infarcts (9).

In summary, the concept of causality of vascular lesions is at the center of the debate. Authopsy series show than pure vascular dementia is a rarity (60–63), if its really exists per se. Some authors suggested calling it vascular cognitive impairment (VCI) (64) rather than dementia, with a cutoff at the fifth percentile of a normal population of each tested item, but this concept is still not yet defined by any consensus. Furthermore, distinguishing between focal, multifocal, or global cognitivobehavioral syndrome(s) and dementia is just a matter of definitions, which all rely heavily on memory and social and daily living activities' impact and suffer from the absence of biological makers.

IV. RISK FACTORS FOR VD

Risk factors for VD are supposed to be the same as those for stroke. The leading risk factor is systolic hypertension (60%) (9,65–75), but others found a significant role for diastolic blood pressure (76,77). Age is a main risk factor, as well as prior stroke episodes, TIA, smoking and alcohol consumption (68,69,78), diabetes mellitus (20%) (65,68,69,71,73,79–83), high hematocrit, hyperlipidemia, anticardiolipid antibodies, hematological disorders (sickle cell disease, hyperviscosity, thrombocytosis, polyglobuly, coagulopathies), angiitis, moya-moya disease, AVMs as well as rare genetic disease (CADASIL, Sneddon's disease, familial amyloid angiopathy, Bristih dementia, MELAS), amyloid angiopathy, history of heart condition ("cardiogenic dementia") (69,84,85), cardiac arrythmias, especially AF (76,86–89), myxoma (90), dilated cardiomyopathy (91), coronary heart disease (76,92), large-vessel disease, carotid stenosis, or dissection (93,94). Others found that hypotension (86,95) or even orthostatic hypotension or large variations in blood pressure may be responsible for watershed-zone subcortical infarcts (96,97). Conflicting results are found for apolpiprotein E4, increased in the majority of studies in VD, as well as other apolipoproteins (71,98–121). Other less-well-defined risk factors for dementia after stroke are still poorly understood, but include low level of education, social background (14), history of prior cerebrovascular disease, left hemispheric stroke, major dominant stroke syndrome, dysphasia, gait impairment and urinary incontinence (15), occupational exposure to pesticides and herbicides, plastic or rubber (69), and use of aspirin (69). No relation was found with head trauma, family history of dementia, or cigarette smoking by others (123). A protective factor was high level of education (69).

In a recent review of risk factors, Skoog et al. (71) differentiated between risk factors for stroke (as mentioned above) and risk factors for dementia. Among the latter, multiple small or large brain infarcts, extension of white-matter lesions, high alcohol consumption, psychological stress in life, lower formal education, blue-collar occupation, and occupational exposure were the main nonvascular determinants for VD. Risk factors for dementia in stroke were divided into stroke-related (cerebrovsacular risk factors) and non-stroke-related (same as AD).

V. PHYSIOPATHOLOGY OF VD

Why are stroke patients more prone to develop dementia than age- and sex-matched controls? First, poststroke dementia can be the result of the vascular lesion, can be due to an associated asymptomatic AD revealed by the stroke, or may result from white-matter changes, or all of them (124). As a whole, cerebrovascular dementia is due to osbtructive and/or hypoperfusive etiology (125). The role of autoimmunity has been considered but not settled (37,126–128). Autoantibodies and antibodies against the vascular basement membrane proteoglycan antigen and circulating immune complexes have been reported in one study (129). If white-matter disease and lacunae are the main determinant for VD to occur in the presence of a single stroke not affecting eloquent cortical areas, the location of lesions, volume of destroyed tissue, multiplicity, and bilateral occurrence might be the most important parameters (130), but there is no consensus on this issue.

Cognitive decline correlates with recurrent ''silent infarcts'' and with frontal white-matter, thalamic, internal capsular perfusional changes (131). Arteriolosclerosis in the deep white matter and the subcortical white matter showed that adventitial proliferation is more pronounced in the subcortical white matter in VD, whereas in aging it starts in deep white matter (132). Atherosclerosis and amyloid angiopathy may have larger roles than previously suspected in AD (133). In a recent study, 50% of VD cases were attributed to small-vessel infarcts, and 16% to both large and small-vessel infarcts (134). Similar figures are given in another study, with 40% of multiple lacunar strokes (78). Isolated hypertension itself in elderly patients is correlated with cognitive dysfunction, but is a weak contributor compared to age (135). Half of the patients with VD developed dementia insidiously without a single ischemic event (135). A stroke can also be the first symptom of a genetic disease leading to vascular dementia such as CADASIL (136). Lin et al. (137), in a prospective study on VD, found that the severity of overall white-matter lesions, left parietal infarct, and the number of thalamic lacunae were important factors in development of dementia after stroke. Others (138) separate various pathomechanisms (large or small-vessel disease) and brain territories involved (strategic infarctions, corticosubcortical and subcortical lacunae, watershed infarcts, white-matter lesions).

VI. CLINICAL PRESENTATION

The natural history of VD may be quite variable. The abrupt or gradual temporal relationship with stroke(s) must be recognized, not exceeding 3 months, but the question of progression, smooth, stepwise, fluctuating, static, remitting, or even reversible, is dealt with variably in the various criteria for definition.

The clinical picture of VD is not uniform. A patchy pattern of noncognitive, cognitive, and sensorimotor dysfunction, due to multiple infarcts, or the classic picture of strategic infarcts, or even more diffuse subcortical or frontosubcortical presentation with disproportionate dysexecutive dysfunction and multifocal signs as seen in multiple lacunae or diffuse white-matter abnormalities is generally representative of the clinical spectrum of the disease (139,140). Dementia is especially common after left posterior cerebral, angular gyrus, basal forebrain, bilateral subcortical, or anterior cerebral artery infarcts. More aspecific patterns, such as those seen with subdural hematomas, deep sinous thrombosis, or posthypoxic dementia, can be less frequently observed. Two decades of improving imaging techniques only further complicated the interpretation of the clinical picture, without allowing definition of clinical entities or improving the clinical diagnosis.

When studied as a whole, a specific pattern of neuropsychological dysfunction is hard to find in the many studies that have been conducted, but is generally characterized by slowing of information processing, impaired memory (forgetfulness, difficulty retrieving learned material), poor sustained attention, impairment of motivation, affective changes (especially depression and emotional lability), decreased motor and mental speed, dyscalculia, executive dysfunction, abnormal visuoconstruction, and multifocal signs including gait disorders, pseudobulbar affect, parkinsonism, and pyramidal tract deficits, gait disturbance, and urinary incontinence (141–145).

Comparisons with other entities such as AD or frontotemporal dementia (FTD) are often given, but the results are confusing, if not contradictory. In most of the papers VD has been considered as a whole rather than correlated with either of the six subtypes of VD described earlier. Furthermore, the clinical definition based on early radioimaging techniques may wildly differ from recent neuroimaging workup, even in the same reports. Sudden onset of cognitive deficits is more frequent in VD than in FTD, as well as confusion (146). VD patients are slower in information processing subtests like stimulus categorization time, omission errors, mental speed, and stimulus response intitiation (147), but patients with AD outperformed those with VD in motor speed and cognitive speed (141), which are probably the expression of frontosubcortical deficits. VD patients show more impairment in frontal executive functioning than AD patients, especially for planning, sequencing, verbal fluency, poor word list generation, impersistence, difficulty in set shifting, sensibility to intrusions, attention, motor performance (38,141,148), and motor speed (writing subtest of Wester Aphasia Battery, Picture Arrangement of the WAIS-R, and motor performance of the Mattis Dementia Rating Scale)(149).

Noncognitive psychiatric and behavior abnormalities are frequent in VD (40%) (150). Depressive symptoms (60%) seem to be more severe in VD than in AD (67,123,139,140,145,150,152–155), but this was not found by others (156,157). The most frequent psychiatric symptoms of VD were irritability (57%), apathy (44%), insomnia (43%), psychomotor agitation (41%), impatience (37%), irritability (37%), emotional lability (28%), delusions (40%), hallucinations (30%), peduncular hallucinosis and psychosis (123,140,145–149). Blunted affect, depressed mood, emotional withdrawal, motor retardation, low motivation, anxiety, unsusual thoughts, and somatic concerns occured in more than one-third (150). Emotionalism may occur (151), but elation is rare (5%) (152). Obsessive-compulsive disorders may occur in bilateral basal ganglia lesions (153). Hamilton scores are higher than in AD (150). Lack of insight and personality changes were not different from AD (157). Capgras' syndrome has been reported (158). VD patients generally have greater awareness of their cognitive deficits than AD patients (159), but this is not always the case (148); however this differentiates them from frontotemporal dementia (FTD) (146). Emotional lability is more frequent than in AD (148) as well as delirium (149). Psychiatric wandering has also been reported (150).

Executive function deficits and mood and personality changes are similar to those seen in frontosubcortical pathways lesions and are considered relatively specific in VD (139). Unilateral or bilateral primitive reflexes are often found. Patients are impaired in the Stroop interference subtest, planning ability (Tower of London test), word fluency, and shift of mental test (trail making) (146,151). Aspontaneity, apathetic behavior, and abulia are often reported (134,151). Specific clinical patterns of strategic infarcts may mimic frontosubcortical deficits (thalamopolar syndromes, paramedian thalamosubthalamic artery syndrome, right, left, and bilateral thalamic or pallidal syndromes, uni- or bilateral cingulate syndromes, uni- or bilateral caudate syndromes, frontopolar or temporopolar lesions).

Memory loss is generally less severe at onset of VD than in AD (64), but worse than in FTD (146), but after years, memory impairment of VD accelerates and catches up with AD (160). Memory loss in VD is generally characterized by poor retrieval and intact recognition (145). Free recall is better than in AD, recognition memory is better, and there are fewer recall intrusions than in AD patients (161), suggesting dysfunction of frontosubcortical circuits. Impairment of semantic memory does not differentiate between VD and AD (162). Verbal long-term memory is better than in AD (38). Declarative memory (as tested by the California Verbal Learing Test) and procedural memory (as tested by the Pursuit Rotor Learning Test) show that VD patients have higher scores than AD patients for declarative memory than for procedural memory. Episodic memory (face recognition, word recall, object recall) in VD patients does not differ on these tasks from AD patients except for word recall, which is better preserved in VD (163,164). Primary and semantic memory were not different than in AD (141), but others found category-specific semantic disorders (dissociation between living things and food versus inanimate objects) to be diagnostic for AD and absent in VD (165). Attention is deficient in VD (166).

Language deficits are also different from those of AD. Picture-naming deficits (anomia) with a semantic component are found in both AD and VD (141,167), but VD patients are better and commit fewer intrusion errors. Syntax and verbal comprehension were not different than in AD (141). Globally, language is more involved in AD than VD and starts with nominal aphasia, then transcortical sensitive and global aphasia. In VD language is relatively preserved and is rather a pure motor aphasia (168). Verbal fluency is poorer than in AD, but better than in FTD (169). Letter (FAS) or category (animal naming) does not differentiate between AD and VD (161). Verbal comprehension shows no difference with AD. Semantic fluency, as assessed by a word-list generation, is more impaired than phonemic fluency in VD, with no difference from AD (170). More naming errors are found (especially semantic errors) in AD than VD (171). More perseverations are also reported in VD, correlating with motor signs (172). Disturbances of prosody are also more frequent than in AD (173) as well as impairment of motor aspects of speech such as pitch, melody, articulation, and rate (174); VD patients also produce shorter and less grammatically complex sentences.

Visuospatial skills are deficient in VD (175), but this is not unanimously reported (141), possibly related to memory deficits (176). Deficit in Rey-Oster-reith complex figure scoring shows no difference between VD and AD (169).

VD patients are worse than FTD in digit span and constructions, but had similar performance in calculations (169). Callosal syndromes are exceptionally found, despite extensive white-matter lesions.

VD patients are more likely to have unilateral primitive reflexes (177). Gait disorders are frequent (30%) (141,178), but this was not found in another study (179). Gait disorders may be indicators of VD (138), together with parkinsonism, pyramidal tract signs, ataxia, pseudobulbar affect, and urinary incontinence (50%) (144,145,180). Sudden onset of focal neurological dysfunction, which may be transient or permanent, such as visual field deficits, brainstem, sensorimotor, or ataxic hemisyndromes, and cognitive (aphasic, agnosic, apraxic) focal deficits, are helpful indicators.

A method for clinical evaluation, combining psychiatric and neurological status examination with complex variables describing the patient's regional predominant brain syndrome (subcortical, frontosubcortical, frontal, frontoparietal, parietal, or global), may help in the differential diagnosis, VD patients having predominantly frontal and subcortical symptomatology. Neuroimaging is very helpful (181,182). Abnormal patchy areas on PET or SPECT scans, often asymmetrical, without any specific locations are reported by most series, which may separate VD from AD (bitemporoparietal) or FTD (frontotemporal) functional imaging patterns. However, multiple patterns are possible, from normal to wildely diffuse hypoperfusion or hypometabolic images. Cerebrovascular responsiveness to hypercapnia has been found useful in differentiatig AD from VD (183), as well as cerebral perfusion patterns [parietotemporal in AD, basal ganglia, thalamus, and frontal area or patchy pattern in VD (184)].

VII. BIOLOGICAL MARKERS

Biological markers for VD have been largely looked for, without much success, mainly in blood and cerebrospinal (fluid). In blood and serum, no difference with

AD has been found for plasma free radicals, superoxide dismutase (185), decrease in plasma chain-breaking antioxidants (186), or increase in neurofilament proteins levels (187). CSF tau protein and beta A4 amyloid may be helpful in differentiting VD from AD (188,189), as well as CSF and serum alpha-1 antichymotrypsin, all increased in AD but not in VD (190–192). Presenilin-1 polymorphism, which is significantly increased in AD (193), may be helpful. Ubiquitin is not increased in the CSF of VD patient (193,194). CSF chromagranin A is not helpful in differentiating VD from AD (195). Coagulation deficits (196) or dyslipidemia has been looked for, showing increased thromboxane biosynthesis (197), LDL cholesterol levels (198), and thrombin generation (199), but no change in fatty acids of plasma lipids, red cells, and platelets (200). Serum anti-GFAP and anti-S100 autoantibodies, antihistone, and anti-ds DNA are not markers for VD (201,202), but autoantibodies against GFAP have been reported (203), as well as HTLV I-positive serology (204). CSF interleukin-6 was normal in VD, while decreased in AD (205). VD has lower brain IL-1 than in AD (206). Heat shock protein HPS 70 mRNA levels in mononuclear blood cells were significantly lower in AD than VD patients in one study (207). Glial fibrillary acidic protein in the CSF is not helpful (208). Specific abnormalities in neurotransmitter systems have also been investigated. The serotonin metabolism is severely reduced in VD, as well as the activity of choline acetyltransferase and CFS acetylcholinesterase levels (209), while monoamine oxidase B is increased (210,211). CSF levels of monoamines are decreased in VD (212,213). Alterations of the noradrenergic and dopaminergic system prevail in AD and dopaminergic and serotonergic in VD (214). CSF acetylcholine and choline are generally higher in AD (215), but muscarinic acetylcholine receptors m1 and m2 are normal (216) and CSF acetylcholinesterase levels are not useful in differentiating VD from AD (217,218). Plasma serum G4 acetylcholinesterase level was increased in VD but not in AD (219). Hypothalamic neuropeptides are decreased (210). CSF neuropetides (220), GH, or response to GHRH is not helpful (221). Urinary ratio of alpha-1 microglobulin and ulinastatin may differentiate between VD and AD (222). CSF or serum neuron-specific enolase was not helpful (223) or decreased (224). CSF urate and xanthine concentrations (225), CSF amnio acid concentration, CSF fluid-serum albumin ratio (226) or alpha tocopherol (227), or CSF sulfatides are not helpful. Abnormal blood-brain barrier has been reported in VD (228–230).

Among radioimaging techniques, PET scan is useful in the differential diagnosis of VD from AD and other dementias, but this examination still does not have the value of a biological marker (231,232). Regional cerebral blood flow (rCBF), single-photon emission tomography (SPECT) with 99mTc-HMPAO, and the acetazolamide test in the evaluation of vascular and AD dementia showed in a recent study (233) that VD patients with hypoperfusion in bilateral temporal and/or parietal areas had decreased vascular reserve capacity (57% vs. 27%) as determined with acetazolamide test. SPECT scan is generally useful in the diagnosis of AD, VD, and FTD (235,236). Neuroimaging criteria have been suggested recently (237). Other studies (238,239) show the correlation of neuropsychological impairment in cerebral microangiopathy with hypoperfusion rather than with white-matter lesions on MRI, possibly leading to exhausted metabolic reserve in the whole brain as one of the main mechanisms in VD. In this respect, CSF nitric oxyde metabolites (NO_{2-} and NO_{3-}) show a steady increase in VD, whereas this increase is only seen in the early stages of AD (240); excitatory amino acids are decreased in AD but not in VD (241). Specific brain alterations in high-energy phosphate compounds, as measured by nuclear magnetic resonance spectroscopy, may contribute to separation between dementias with neurodegenerative diseases and those with ischemic or hemodynamic disorders (242). Quantitative topographical EEG has complementary value with PET (243). EEG spectral analysis (244) is generally not helpful.

VIII. PATHOLOGY

The pathology of VD is highly heterogeneous. Large- or small-vessel arterial territorial infarct(s), lacunar infarcts, watershed infarcts, granular cortical atrophy, laminar necrosis, hemorrhages, and venous thrombosis may all be found, together with white-matter demyelination, axonal loss, gliosis, and "incomplete infarcts" that underlie the so-called leukoaraiosis caused by lipohylinosis or arteriolosclerosis (for reviews see refs. 55,125,245,246).

IX. TREATMENT

Is prevention of VD possible (247)? Only through the prevention of stroke by controlling risk factors, especially hypertension, which reduces the recurrence of stroke; but on the other hand, hypotensive episodes that may result from drastic reduction in systolic blood pressure may aggravate white-matter watershed lesions. There is no effective prevention of variations in blood pressure in the elderly. Moreover, the variations of blood pressure during the night may also be important in prevention. The prevention of other risk factors such as diabetes, cigarette smoking, hyperlipidemia, and heart diseases as well as antiaggregant therapy is efficacious in the primary prevention of VD. After a first stroke, the risk of a second stroke is about 8% per year over the first 5 years. Secondary prevention with antiaggregant medication, anticoagulants, or endarterectomy is important when needed. Several drugs have been tried in VD with nonsignificant results: vinca alkaloids (vincamine, vinburnine) (248), calcium antagonists (nicardipine, cinnarizine, flunarizine) (249,250), nicergoline (251), propentofylline (252–256), pentoxyfylline (257), cerebrolysin (258), hydergine (259), buflomedil

(260,261), memantine (262), alpha-glycerylphosphorylcholine versus cytosine diphosphocholine (263), naftydofuryl (264), vinpocetine (oxygen release of hemoglobin) (265), bromocriptine (266), idebenone (267). Memantine seems to have a mild effect.

X. CONCLUSION

In conclusion VD is a heterogeneous clinical entity, still relying on clinical definitions despite good neuroimaging technique, which is infrequent and requires expertise in both neurodegenerative and cerebrovascular fields of neurology to delineate clinical entities properly. Autopsy series tend to contest even the reality of VD, except in very exceptional cases, and treatment relies essentially on secondary prevention of risk factors for stroke.

REFERENCES

1. Hachinski V. Vascular dementia: a radical definition. Dementia 1994; 5:130–132.
2. Roman GC, Tatemichi TK, Erkinjuntti T, Cummings JL, Masdeu JC, Garcia JH, Amaducci L, Orgogozo JM, Brun A, Hofman A, Moody DM, O'Brien MD, Yamaguchi T, Grafman J, Drayer BP, Bennett DA, Fisher M, Ogata J, Kokmen E, Bermejo F, Wolf PA, Gorelick PB, Bick KL, Pajeau AK, Bell MA, De Carli C, Culebras A, Korczyn AD, Bogousslavsky J, Hartmann A, Scheinberg P. Vascular dementia: diagnostic criteria for research studies. Report of the NINDS-AIREN International Workshop. Neurology 1993; 43:250–260.
3. World Health Organization. The ICD-10 Classification of Mental and Behavioural Disorders. Diagnostic Criteria for Research. Geneva: World Health Organization, 1993.
4. Wetterling T, Kanitz RD, Borgis KJ. Comparison of different diagnostic criteria for vascular dementia (ADDTC; DSM-IV, ICD-10, NINDS-AIREN). Stroke 1996; 27:30–36.
5. American Psychiatric Organization Diagnostic and Statistical Manual of Mental Disorders, 4th ed. Washington DC: American Psychiatric Association, 1994.
6. Chui HC, Victoroff JI, Margolin D, Jagust W, Shankle R, Katzman R. Criteria for the diagnosis of ischemic vascular dementia proposed by the State of California Alzheimer's Disease Diagnostic and Treatment Centers. Neurology 1992; 42:473–480.
7. Wahlund LO. Brain imaging and vascular dementia. Dementia 1994; 5:193–196.
8. Brayne C, Gill C, Huppert FA, Barkley C, Gelhauer E, Girling DM, O'Connor DW, Paykel ES. Incidence of clinically diagnosed subtypes of dementia in an elderly popuation. Project for Later life. Br J Psychiatry 1995; 167:255–262.
9. Tatemichi TK, Foulkes MA, Mohr JP et al. Dementia in stroke survivors in the

Stroke Dtat Bank cohort. Prevalence, incidence, risk factors and computed tomographic findings. Stroke 1990; 21:858–866.

10. Bickel H, Cooper B. Incidence and relative risk of dementia in an urban elderly population: findings of a prospective field study. Psychol Med 1994; 24:179–192.

11. Herbert R, Brayne C. Epidemiology of vascular dementia. Neuroepidemiology 1995; 14:240–257.

12. Skoog I, Nilsson L, Palmertz B, Andreasson LA, Svandorg A. A population-based study of dementia in 85-year-olds. N Engl J Med 1993; 328:153–158.

13. Holstein J, Chatellier G, Piette F, Moulias R. Prevalence of associated diseases in different types of dementia among elderly institutionalized patients: analysis of 3447 records. J Am Geriatr Soc 1994; 42:929–977.

14. Ebly EM, Parhad IM, Hogan DB, Fung TS. Prevalence of types of dementia in the very old: results from the Canadian Study of Health and Aging. Neurology 1994; 44:1593–1600.

15. Pohjasvaara T, Erkinjuntti T, Ylikoski R, Hietanen M, Vataja R, Kaste M. Clinical determinants of postroke dementia. Stroke 1998; 29:75–81.

16. Tatemichi TK, Paik M, Bagiella E, et al. Risk of dementia after stroke is a predictor of long-term survival. Stroke 1994; 25:1915–1919.

17. Bowler JV, Hadar U, Wade JP. Cognition in stroke. Acta Neurol Scand 1994; 90: 424–429.

18. Phojasvaara T, Erkinjuntti T, Vataja R, Kaste M. Dementia three months after stroke. Baseline frequency and effect of different definitions of dementia in the Helsinki Stroke Aging Memeory Study (SAM) cohort. Stroke 1997; 28:785 792.

19. Erkinjubtti T, Autio L, Wikstrom J. Dementia in medical wards. J Clin Epidemiol 1988; 41:123–166.

20. Tatemichi TK, Desmond DW, Stern Y, et al. Prevalence of dementia after stroke depends on the diagnostic criteria. Neurology 1992; 42(suppl 3):413.

21. Tatemichi TK, Desmond DW, Mayeux R, et al. Dementia after stroke: baseline frequency, risks and clinical features in a hospitalized cohort. Neurology 1992; 42: 1185–1193.

22. Ferrucci L, Guralnik JM, Salive ME, Pahor M, Corti MC, Baroni A, Havlik RJ. Cognitive impairment and risk of stroke in the older population. J Am Geriatr Soc 1996; 44:328–333.

23. Mendez MF, Stanley TM, Medel NM, Li Z, Tedesco DT. The vascular dementia of Fabry's disease. Dementia Geriatr Cogn Disord 1997; 8:252–257.

24. Mead S, Galton M, Revesz T, Bala Doshi R, Harwood G, Pan EL, Ghiso J, Frangione B, Plant G. Familia bristsh dementia with amyloid angiopathy. Early clinical, neuropschological and imaging findings. Brain 2000; 123:975–991.

25. Larner AJ, Kidd D, Elkington P, Rudge P, Scaravilli F. Spatz-Lindenberg disease: a rare cause of vascular dementia. Stroke 1999; 30:687–689.

26. Binswanger O. Die Abgrenzung der allgemeinen progressiven Paralysie. Berl Klin Wochenschr 1894; 31:1103–1105, 1137–1139, 1180–1186.

27. Wahlund LO, Basun H, Almqvist O, Andersson-Lundman G, Julin P, Saaf J. White matter hyperintensities in dementia: does it matter? Magnet Reson Imag 1994; 12: 387–394.

28. Sulkava R, Haltia M, Paeteau A, et al. Accuracy of clinical diagnosis of primary degenerative dementia: correlation with neuropathological findings. J Neurol Neurosurg Psychiatry 1983; 46:9–13.

29. Molsa PK, Paljarvi L, Rinne JO, et al. Validity of clinical diagnosis in dementia: a prospective pathological study. J Neurol Neurosurg Psychiatry 1985; 48:1085–1090.

30. Wade JPH, Mirsen TR, Hachisnki VC, et al. The clinical diagnosis of Alzheimer's disease. Arch Neurol 1987; 44:24–29.

31. Rosen WG, Terry RD, Fuld PA, Katzman R, Peck A. Pathological verification of ischemic score in differentiation of dementias. Ann Neurol 1980; 7:486–488.

32. Wagner O, Oesterreich K, Hoyer S. Validity of the ischemic score in degenerative and vascular dementia and depression in old age. Arch Gerontol Geriatr 1985; 4: 333–345.

33. Pantoni L, Inzitari D. Hachinski's ischemic score and the diagnosis of vascular dementia. Ital J Neurol Sci 1993; 14:539–546.

34. Hershey LA, Modic MT, Jaffe DF, Greenbough PG. Can J Neurol Sci 1986; 13(suppl):559–565.

35. Hulette C, Nochlin D, Mc Keel D, Morris JC, Mirra SS, Sumi SM, Heyman A. Clinical-neuropathological findings in multi-infarct dementia: a report of six authopsied cases. Neurology 1997; 48:668–672.

36. Fischer P, Jellinger K, Gatterer G, Danielczyk W. Prospective neuropathological validation of Hachinski's Ischemic Score in dementias. J Neurol Neurosurg Psychaitry 1991; 54:580–583.

37. Wallin A, Blennow K. The clinical diagnosis of vascular dementia. Dementia 1994; 5:181–184.

38. Looi JC, Sachdev PS. Differentiation of vascular dementia from AD on neuropsychological tests. Neurology 1999; 53:670–678.

39. Ransmayr G. Difficulties in the clinical diagnosis of vascular dementia and dementia of the Alzheimer type—comparison of clinical classifications. J Neural Transm 1998; 53:79–90.

40. Swanwick GR, Coen RF, Lawlor BA, O'Mahonny D, Walsh JB, Coakley D. Utility of ischemic scores in the differential diagnosis of Alzheimer's disease and ischemic vascular dementia. Int Psychogeraitr 1996; 8:413–424.

41. Erkinjuntti T, Sipponen JT, Iivainen M, Ketonen L, Sulkava R, Sepponen RE. Cerebral NMR and CT imaging in dementia. J Comput Assist Tomogr 1984; 8:614–618.

42. Hagiwara M. A clinical study on the usefulness of CT and MRI imaging in evaluating differential diagnosis and the degree of dementia in vascular dementia. Nippon Ika Daigaku Zasshi 1990; 57:265–275.

43. Schmidt R. Comparison of magnetic resonance imaging in Alzheimer's disease and vascular dementia and normal aging. Eur Neurol 1992; 32:164–169.

44. Erkinjuntti T, Larsen T, Sulkava R, Ketonen L, Laaksonen R, Palo J. EEG in the differential diagnosis between Alzheimer's disease and vascular dementia. Acta Neurol Scand 1988; 77:36–43.

45. Bowen BC, Barker WW, Loewenstein DA, Sheldon J, Duara R. MR signal abnormalities in memory disorder and dementia. AJR 1990; 154:1285–1292.

46. Amar K, Wilcock GK, Scott M. The diagnosis of vascular dementia in the light of new criteria. Age Aging 1996; 25:51–55.
47. Erkinjuntti T. Clinical criteria for vascular dementia: the NINDS-AIREN criteria. Dementia 1994; 5:189–192.
48. Erkinjuntti T, Ketonen L, Sulkava R, Sipponen J, Vuorialho M, Iivainen M. Do white matter changes on MRI and CT differentiate vascular dementia from Alzheimer's disease? J Neurol Neurosurg Psychiatry 1987; 50:37–42.
49. Desmond DW. Vascular dementia: a construct in evolution. Cerebrovasc Brain Metab 1996; 8:296–325.
50. Wetterling T, Kanitz RD, Borgis KJ. The ICD-10 criteria for vascular dementia. Dementia 1994; 5:185–188.
51. Erkinjuntti T. Vascular dementia: challenge of clinical diagnosis. Int Psychogeriatr 1997; 9(suppl 1):51–8, 77–83.
52. Gold G, Giannakopoulos P, Bouras C. Re-evaluating the role of vascular changes in the differential diagnosis of Alzheimer's disease and vascular dementia. Eur Neurol 1998; 40:121–129.
53. Sachdev PS, Brodaty H, Looi JC. Vascular dementia: diagnosis, management and possible prevention. Med J Aust 1999; 170:81–85.
54. Holmes C, Cairns N, Lantos P, Mann A. Validity of current criteria for Alzheimer's disease, vascular dementia and dementia with Lewy bodies. Br J Psychiatry 1999; 174:45–50.
55. Englund E. Neuropathology of white matter changes in Alzheimer's disease and vascular dementia. Dementia Geriatr Cogn Disord 1998; 9 (suppl 1):6–12.
56. Doddy RS, Massman PJ, Mawad M, Nance M. Cognitive consequences of subcortical magnetic resonance imaging changes in Alzheimer's disease: comparison to small vessel ischemic vascular dementia. Neuropsychiatry Neuropsychol Behav Neurol 1998; 11:191–199.
57. Wallin A, Edman A, Blennow K, Gottfires CG, Karlsson I, Regland B, Sjogren M. Stepwise comparative status (STEP): a tool for identification of regional brain syndromes in dementia. J Geriatr Psychiatr Neurol 1996; 9:185–189.
58. Emery VO, Gillie EX, Smith JA. Reclassification of the vascular dementias: comparison of infarct and non-infact dementias. Int Psychogeriatr 1996; 8:33–61.
59. Yanagisawa M, Kaieda M, Nagatsumi A, Terashi A. Difference in MRI findings and risk factors between multiple infarction without dementia and multi-infarct dementia. Nippon Ika Daigaku Zasshi 1995; 62:428–438.
60. Joachim CL, Morris JH, Sleoe D. Clinically diagnosed Alzheimer's disease: authopsy results in 150 cases. Ann Neurol 1988; 24:50–56.
61. Jellinger K, Danielczyk W, Fisher P, Gabriel E. Clinicopathological analysis of dementia disorders in the elderly. J Neurol Sci 1990; 95:239–258.
62. Kondo N. A study of the difference between clinical and neuropathological diagnoses of age-related dementing illnesses: correlations with Hachinski's ischemic score. Seishin Shinkeigaku Zasshi, 1995; 97:825–846.
63. Nolan KA, Lino MM, Seligmann AW, Blass JP. Absence of vascular dementia in an autopsy series from a dementia clinic. J Am Geriatr Soc 1998; 46:597–604.
64. Bowler JV, Hachinski V. Vascular cognitive impairment: a new approach to vascular dementia. Bailleres Clin Neurol 1995; 4:357–376.

65. Parnetti L, Mecocci P, Santucci C et al. Is multi-infarct dementia representative of vascular dementias? A retrospective study. Acta Neurol Scand 1990; 81:484–487.
66. Petty LA, Parker JC Jr. Hypertension and vascular dementia. Ann Clin Lab Sci 1992; 22:34–39.
67. Johansson A, Gustafson L. Psychiatric symptoms in patients with dementia treated in a psychiatric day hospital. Int Psychogeraitr 1996; 8:645–658.
68. Skoog I. Status of risk factors for vascular dementia. Neuroepidemiology 1998; 17:2–9.
69. Lindsey J, Herbert R, Rockwood K. The Canadian Study of Health and Aging: risk factors for vascular dementia. Stroke 1997; 28:526–530.
70. Ott A, Stolk RP, van Harkamp F, Grobbee DE, Breteler MM. Association of diabetes mellitus and dementia: the Rotterdam study. Diabetologia 1996; 39:1392–1397.
71. Skoog I, Hesse C, Aevarsson O, Landahl S, Wahlstrom J, Fredman P, Blennow K. A population study of apoE genotype at the age of 85: relation to dementia, cerebrovascular disease and mortality. J Neurol Neurosurg Psychiatry 1998; 64: 37–43.
72. Lis CG, Gaviria M. Vascular dementia, hyppertension, and the brain. Neurol Res 1997; 19:471–480.
73. Hogan DB, Ebly EM, Rockwood K. Weight, blood pressure, osmolarity, and glucose levels across various stages of Alzheimer's disease and vascular dementia. Dementia Geriatr Cogn Disord 1997; 8:147–151.
74. Guo Z, Viitanen M, Fratiglioni L, Winblad B. Blood pressure and dementia in the elderly: epidemiologic perspectives. Biomed Pharmacother 1997; 51:68–73.
75. Skoog I, Lernfelt B, Landahl S, Palmertz B, Andreasson LA, Nilsson L, Persson G, Oden A, Svanborg A. 15-year longitudinal study of blood pressure and dementia. Lancet 1996; 347:1141–1145.
76. Skoog I, Andreasson LA, Landahl S, Lernfelt B. A population-based study on blood pressure and brain atrophy in 85-year olds. Hypertension 1998; 32:404–409.
77. Boston PF, dennis MS, Jagger C. Factors associated with vascular dementia in an elderly population. Int J Geriatr Psychiatry 1999; 14:761–766.
78. Kiyohara Y. Prevalence, incidence, and risk factors of vascular dementia: the Hisayama study. Rinsho Shinkeigaku 1999; 39:47–49.
79. Chen CF, Chen TH, Jia HY. A study of the risk factors of Binswanger's encephalopathy. Chung-Hua Liu Hsing Hsueh Tsa Chih 1997; 18:220–223.
80. Stewart R, Liolista D. Type 2 diabetes mellitus, cognitive impairment and dementia. Diabetic Med 1999; 16:93–112.
81. Szatamari S, Fekete I, Csiba L, Kollar J, Sikula J, Bereczki D. Screening of vascular cognitive impairment on a Hungarian cohort. Psychiatry Clin Neurosci 1999; 53: 39–43.
82. Curb JD, Rodriguez BL, Abbott RD, Petrovic H, Ross GW, Masaki KH, Foley D, Blanchette PL, Harris T, Chen R, White LR. Longitudinal association of vascular and Alzheimer's dementias, diabetes, and glucose tolerance. Neurology 1999; 52: 971–975.
83. Tariot PN, Ogden MA, Cox C, Williams TF. Diabetes and dementia in long-term care. J Am Geriatr Soc 1999; 47:423–429.
84. Cardiogenic dementia. Lancet 1977; 1:27–28.

85. Thal LJ, Grundman M, Klauber MR. Dementia: characteristics of a referral population and factors associated with progression. Neurology 1988; 38:1083–1090.

86. Sulkava R, Erkinjuntti T. Vascular dementia due to cardiac arrythmias and systemic hypotension. Acta Neurol Scand 1987; 76:123–128.

87. Ohsawa N, Takahashi S, Yonezawa H. Cerebral blood flow patterns in patients with leukoaraisosis and lacunar infarction. Risho Shinkeigaku 1994; 34:443–448.

88. Ott A, Breteler MM, de Bruyne MC, van Harskamp F, Grobbee DE, Hofman A. Atrial fibrillation and dementia in a population-based study. The Rotterdam Study. Stroke 1997; 28:316–321.

89. Ramirez-Lassepas M. Stroke and the aging of the brain and the arteries. Geraitrics 1998; (suppl 1):S44–48.

90. Hutton JT. Atrial myxoma as a cause of progressive dementia. Arch Neurol 1981; 38:533.

91. Schmidt R, Fazekas F, Offenbacher H, Duselag J, Lechner H. Brain magnetic resonance imaging and neuropsychologic evaluation of patients with idiopathic dilated cardiomyopathy. Stroke 1991; 22:195–199.

92. Aronson MK, Ooi WL, Morgenstern H, et al. Women, myocardial infarction and dementia in the very old. Neurology 1990; 40:1102–1106.

93. Fisher CM. Dementia in cerebral vascular disease. In: Siekert RG, Whisnant JP eds. Cerebral vasculature diseases. Transactions of the six Princeton Conference. New York, London: Grune & Stratton, 1968, pp 232–236.

94. Wade PH, Wong W, Barnett HJM, Vandervoort P. Bilateral occlusion of the internal carotid arteries. Presenting symptoms in 74 patients and a prospective study of 34 medically treated patients. Brain 1987; 110:667–682.

95. Guo Z, Viitanen M, Fratiglioni L, Winblad B. Low blood pressure and dementia in elderly people: the Kungsholmen project. Br Med J 1996; 312:805–808.

96. Passant U, Warkentin S, Gustafson L. Orthostatic hypotension and low blood pressure in organic dementia: a study of prevalence and related clinical characteristics. Int J Geriatr Psychiatry 1997; 12:395–403.

97. Passant U, Warkentin S, Kalson S, Nilsson K, Edvinson L, Gustafson L. Orthostatic hypotension in organic dementia: relationship between blood pressure, cortical blood flow and symptoms. Clin Autonomi Res 1996; 6:29–36.

98. Kuriyama M, Takahashi K, Yamano T, Hokezu Y, Togo S, Osame M, Igakura T. Low levels of serum apolipoprotein AI and AII in senile dementia. Jpn J Psychiatry Neurol 1994; 48:589–593.

99. Betard C, Robitaille Y, Gee M, Tiberghien D, Larivee D, Roy P, Mortimer JA, Gauvreau D. ApoE allele frequencies in Alzheimer's disease, Lewy body dementia, Alzheimer's disease with cerebrovascular disease and vascular dementia. Neuroreport 1994; 5:1893–1896.

100. Kawamata J, Tanaka S, Shimohama S, Ueda K, Kimura J. Apolpoproteine E polymorphism in Japanese patients with Alzheimer's disease or vascular dementia. J Neurol Neurosurg Psychiatry 1994; 57:1414–1416.

101. Kuriyama M, Hozeku Y, Togo S, Nagata K, Takahashi K, Igakura T, Osame M. Serum lipids, lipoproteins and apolipoproteins in patients with senile dementia. Nippon Ronen Igakkai Zasshi 1992; 29:559–564.

102. Mahieux F, Couderc R, Moulignier A, Bailleul S, Prodabinek N, Laudet J. Isoform

4 of apolipoprotein E and Alzheimer disease. Specificity and clinical study. Rev Neurol 1995; 151:231–239.

103. Stengard JH, Pekkanen J, Sulkava R, Ehnholm C, Erkinjuntti T, Nissinen A. Apolipoprotein E polymorphism, Alzheimer's disease and vascular dementia among elderly Finnish. Acta Neurol Scand 1995; 92:297–298.

104. Scacchi R, de Bernardini L, Mantuano E, Vilardo T, Donini LM, Ruggeri M, Gemma AT, Pascone R, Corbo RM. DNA polymorphisms of apolipoprotein B and angiotensin I-converting enzyme genes and relationships with lipid levels in Italian patients with vascular dementia of the Alzheimer's disease. Dementia Cogn Disord 1998; 9:186–190.

105. Isoe K, Urakami K, Sato K, Takahashi K. Apolipoprotein E in patients with dementia of the Alzheimer type and vascular dementia. Acta Neurol Scand 1996; 93:133–137.

106. Pirttila T, Lehtimaki T, Rinne J, Marrtila K, Frey H, Nikkari T. The frequency of apolipoprotein E4 allele is not increased in patients with probable vascular dementia. Acta Neurol Scand 1996; 93:352–354.

107. Sulkava R, Kainulainen K, Verkkoniemi A, Niinisto L, Sobel E, Davanipour Z, Polvikoski T, Haltia M, Kontula K. APOE alleles in Alzheimer's disease and vascular dementia in a population aged 85+. Neurobiol Aging, 1996; 17:373–376.

108. Helisalmi S, Linnarata K, Lehtovirta M, Mannermaa A, Heinonen O, Ryynanen M, Riekkinen P Sr, Soininen H. Apolipoprotein E polymorphism in patients with different neurodegenerative disorders. Neurosci Lett 1996; 205:61–64.

109. Treves TA, Bornstein NM, Chapman J, Klimovski S, Verchovsky R, Asherov A, Veschev IO, Korcyn AD. APOE-epsilon 4 in patients with Alzheimer disease and vascular dementia. Alzheimer Dis Assoc Disord 1996; 10:189–191.

110. Higuchi S, Arai H, Nakagawa T, Muramatsu T, Sakai H, Trojanowski JQ. The apolipoprotein E gene in Binswanger's disease and vascular dementia. Clin Genet 1996; 50:459–461.

111. Slooter AJ, Tang MX, van Duijn CM, Stern Y, Ott A, Bell K, Breteler MM, van Broeckhoven C, Tatemichi TK, Tycko B, Hofman A, Mayeux R. Apolipoprotein E epsilon 4 and the risk of dementia with stroke. A Population-based investigation. JAMA 1997; 277:818–821.

112. Bergem AL, Lannfelt L. Apoliporotein E type epsilon4 allele, heritability and age at onset in twins with Alzheimer disease and vascular dementia. Clin Genet 1997; 52:408–413.

113. Hofman A, Ott A, Breteler MM, Bots ML, Slooter AJ, van Harskamp F, van Duijn CN, van Broeckhoven C, Grobbee DE. Atherosclerosis, apolipoprotein E, and prevalence of dementia and Alzheimer's disease in the Rotterdam Study. Lancet 1997; 349:151–154.

114. Katzman R, Zhang MY, Chen PJ, Gu N, Jiang S, Saitoh T, Chen X, Klauber M, Thomas RG, Liu WT, Yu ES. Effects of apolipoprotein E on dementia and aging in the Shanghai Survey of Dementia. Neurology 1997; 49:779–785.

115. Palumbo B, Parnetti L, Nocentini G, Cardinali L, Brancorsini S, Riccardi C, Senin U. Apolipoprotein E genotype in normal aging, age-associated memory impairment, Alzheimer's disease and vascular dementia. Neursoci Lett 1997; 231:59–61.

116. Burlinson S, Burns A, Mann D, Pickering-Brown S, Owen F. Effect of apolipopro-

tein E status on clinical features of dementia. Int J Geriatr Psychiatry 1998; 13: 177–185.

117. Ji Y, Urakami K, Adachi Y, Maeda M, Isoke K, Nakashima K. Apolipoprotein E polymorphism in patients with Alzheimer's disease, vascular dementia and ischemic cerebrovascular disease. Dementia Geriatr Cognit Disord 1998; 9:243–245.

118. Kalman J, Juhasz A, Csaszar A, Kanka A, Rimanoczy A, Janka Z, Rasko I. Increased apolipoprotein E4 allele frequency is associated with vascular dementia in the Hungarian population. Acta Neurol Scand 1998; 98:166–1668.

119. Tilvis RS, Strandberg TE, Juva K. Apolipoprotein E phenotypes, dementia and mortality in a propsective population sample. J Am Geriatr Soc 1998; 46:712–715.

120. Scacchi R, De Bernardini L, Mantuano EW, Donini LM, Vilardo T, Corbo RM. Apolipoprotein E (APOE) allele frequencies in late-onset sporadic Alzheimer's disease, mixed dementia and vascular dementia: a lack of association of epsilon 4 allele with AD in Italian octogenarian patients. Neursci Lett 1995; 201:231–234.

121. Marin DB, Breuer B, Marin ML, Silverman J, Schmeidler J, Greenberg D, Flynn S, Mare M, Lantz M, Libow L, Neufeld R, Alstiel L, Davis KL, Mohs RC. The relationship between apolipoprotein E, dementia and vascular illness. Atherosclerosis 1998; 140:173–180.

122. Inagaki T, Shikimi T, Ishino H, Okunishi H, Takaori S. Changes in the ratio of urinary alpha-1 microglobulin to ulinastatin levels in patients with Alzheimer-type dementia and vascular dementia. Psychiatry Clin Neurosci 1995; 49:287–290.

123. Cooper JK, Mungas D. Risk factor and behavioral differences between vascular and Alzheimer's dementias: the patwhay to end-stage disease. J Geriatr Psychiatry Neurol 1993; 6:29–33.

124. Pasquier F, Leys D. Why are stroke patients prone to develop dementia? J Neurol 1997; 244:135–142.

125. Brun A. Pathology and pathophysiology of cerebrovascular dementia: pure subgroups of obstructive and hypoperfusive etiology. Dementia 1994; 5:145–147.

126. Alafuzoff I, Adolfson R, Grundke-Iqbal I, Winblad B. Perivascular deposition of serum proteins in cerebral cortex in casuclar dementia. Acta Neuropathol 1985; 66:292–298.

127. Elovara I, Seppala I, Palo J, Sulkava R, Erkinjubtti T. Oligoclonal bands in cerebrospinal fluid of patients with Alzheimer's disease and vascular dementia. Acta Neurol Scand 1988; 77:397–401.

128. Mecocci P, Parnetti L, Reboldi GP, Santucci C, Gaiti A, Ferri C, Gernini I, Romagnoli M, Cadini D, Senin U. Blood-brain barrier in a geriatric population: barrier function in degenerative and vascular dementias. Acta Neurol Scand 1991; 84:210–213.

129. Lopez OL, Rabins BS, Huff FJ, Rezek D, Reinmuth OM. Serum autoantibodies in patients with Alzheimer's disease nd vascular dementia and in nondemented control subjects. Stroke 1992; 23:1078–1083.

130. Olsson Y, Brun A, Englund E. Fundamental pathological lesions in vascular dementia. Acta Neurol Scand 1996; 168(suppl):31–38.

131. Meyer JS, Muramatsu K, Mortel KF, Obara K, Shirai T. Prospective CT confirms differences between vascular and Alzheimer's dementia. Stroke 1995; 26:735–742.

132. Watanabe M, Takahashi A, Hashizume Y, Yoshida Y. Difference of cerebral arte-

riolosclerosis between the deep and subcortical white matter in normal aging and vascular dementia of Binswanger type. Rinsho Shinkeigaku 1994; 34:16–21.

133. Choi JY, Morris JC, Hsu CY. Aging and cerebrovascular disease. Neurol Clin, 1998; 16:687–711.

134. Ross GW, Petrovic H, White LR, Masaki KH Li CY, Curb JD, Yano K, Rodriguez BL, Foley DJ, Blanchette PL, Havlik R. Characterization of risk factors for vascular dementia: the Honolulu-Asia Aging study. Neurology 1999; 53:337–343.

135. Seux ML, Thijs L, Forette F, Staessen JA, Birkenhager WH, Bulpitt CJ, Girerd X, Jaaskivi M, Vanhanen H, Kivinen P, Yodfat Y, vanska O, Antikainen R, Laks T, Webster JR, Hakamaki T, Lehtomaki E, Lilov E, Grigorov M, Janculova K, Halonen K, Kohonen-Jalonen P, Kermova R, Nachev C, Tuomilehto Correlates of cognitive status of old patients with isolated systolic hypertension: the Syst-Eur Vascular dementia project. Hypertens 1998; 16:963–969.

136. Tournier-Lasserve E, Ibazizen Mt, Romero N, Bousser MG. Autosomal dominant syndrome with stroke-like episodes adn leukoencephalopathy. Stroke 1991; 22: 1297–1302.

137. Lin RT, Lai CL, Tai CT, Liu CK, Howng SL. Cranial computer tomography in ischemic stroke patients with and without dementia-a prospective study. Kao-Hsiung i Hsueh Tsa Chih 1998; 14:203–211.

138. Hennerici MG, Oster M, Cohen S, Schwartz A, Motsch L, Daffertshofer M. Are gait disturbances and white matter degeneration early indicators of vascular dementia? Dementia 1994; 5:197–202.

139. Ishii N, Nishihara Y, Imamura T. Why do frontal lobe symptoms predominate in vascular dementia with lacunes. Neurology 1986; 36:340–345.

140. Cummings JL, Miller B, Hill MA, Neshkes R. Neuropsychiatric aspects of multi-infarct dementia and dementia of the Alzheimer type. Arch Neurol 1987; 44:389–393.

141. Almqvist O. Neuropsychological deficits in vascular dementia in relation to Alzheimer's disease: reviewing evidence for functional similarity or divergence. Dementia 1994; 5:203–209.

142. Caplan LR, Schoene WC. Clinical features of subcortical arteriosclerotic encephalopathy (Binswanger disease). Neurology 1978; 28:1206–1215.

143. Erkinjuntti T, laaksonen R, Sulkava R, Syrjalainen R, Palo J. Neuropsychological differentiation between normal aging, Alzheimer's disease and vascular dementia. Acta Neurol Scand 1986; 74:393–403.

144. Kotsoris H, Barclay LL, Kheyfets S, Hulyakar A, Dougherty J. Urinary and gait disturbances as markers foe early multi-infarct dementia. Stroke 1987; 18:138–141.

145. Cummings JL. Vascular subcortical dementias: the clinical aspects. Dementia 1994; 5:177–180.

146. Sjogren M, Wallin A, Edman A. Symptomatological characteristics distinguish between frontotemporal dementia and vascular dementia with a dominant frontal lobe syndrome. Int J Geriatr Psychiatry 1997; 12:656–661.

147. Mendez MF, Cherrier MM, Perryman KM. Differences between Alzheimer's disease and vascular dementia on information processing measures. Brain Cognit 1997; 34:301–310.

148. Binetti G, Bianchetti A, Padovani A et al. Delusions in Alzheimer's disease and multi-infarct dementia. Acta Neurol Scand 1993; 88:5–9.
149. Harris Y, Gorelick PB, Cohen D, Dollear W, Forman H, Freels S. Psychaitric symptoms in dementia associated with stroke: a case-control analysis among predominantly African-American patients. JAMA 1994; 86:697–702.
150. Meguro K, Yamaguchi S, Yamazaki H, Itoh M, Yamaguchi T, Matsui H, Sasaki H. Cortical glucose metabolism in psychiatric wandering patients with vascular dementia. Psychiatry Res 1996; 67:71–80.
151. Cummings JL. Depression in vascular dementia. Hillside J Clin Psychiatry 1988; 10:209–231.
152. Ballard C, Bannister C, Solis M, Oyebode F, Wilcock G. The prevalence, associations and symptoms of depression among dementia sufferers. J Affect Disord 1996; 36:135–144.
153. Laplane D, Levasseur M, Pillon B et al. Obsessive-compulsive and other behavioral disorders changes after bilateral basal ganglia lesions. Brain 1989; 112:699–725.
154. Simpson S, Allen H, Tomenson B, Bursn A. Neurological correlates of depressive symptoms in Alzheimer's disease and vascular dementia. J Affect Disord 1999; 53:129–136.
155. Payne JL, Lyketsos CG, Steele C, Baker L, Galik E, Kopunek S, Steinberg M, Warren A. Relationship of cognitive and functional impairment to depressive features in Alzheimer's disease and other dementias. J Neuropsychiatry Clin Neurosci 1998; 10:440–447.
156. Ballard CG, Cassidy G, Bannister C, Mohan RN. Prevalence, symptom profile, and aetiology of depression in dementia sufferers. J Affect Disord 1993; 29:1–6.
157. Verhey FR, Ponds RW, Rozendal N, Jolles J. Depression, insight, and personality changes in Alzheimer's disease and vascular dementia. J Geriatr Psychiatry Neurol 1995; 8:23–27.
158. Tsai SJ, Hwang JP, Yang CH, Liu KM, Lo Y. Capgras' syndrome in a patient with vascular dementia: a case report. Kao-Hsiung iHusch Ko Huseh Tsa Chih 1997; 13:639–642.
159. Wagner MT, Spangenberg KB, Bachman DL, O'Connell P. Unawareness of cognitive deficit in Alzheimer disease and related dementias. Alzheimer's Disease Asooc Disord 1997; 11:121–122.
160. Bowler JV, Eliasziw M, Steenhuis R, Munoz DG, Fry R, Merskey H, Hachinsky VC. Comparative evalution of Alzheimer disease, vascular dementia and mixed dementia. Arch Neurol 1997; 54:697–703.
161. Lafosse JM, Reed BR, Mungas D, Sterling SB, Wahbeh H, Jagust WJ. Fluency and memeory differences between ischemic vascular dementia and Alzheimer's disease. Neuropsychology 1997; 11:514–522.
162. Bentham PW, Jones S, Hodges JR. A comparison of semantic memory in vascular dementia and dementia of the Alzheimer's type. Int J Geraitri Psychiatry 1997; 12:575–580.
163. Cherrier MM, Mendez MF, Perryman KM, Pachana NA, Miller BL, Cummings JL. Frontotemporal dementia versus vascular dementia: differential features on mental status examination. J Am Geratr Soc 1997; 45:579–583.
164. Hassing L, Beckmn L. Episodic memory functioning in population-based samples

of very old adults with Alzheimer's disease and vascular dementia. Dementia Geriatr Cognit Disord 1997; 8:376–383.

165. Mazzoni M, Moretti P, Lucchini C, Vista M, Muratorio A. Category-specific semantic disorders in Alzheimer's disease. Riv Neurol 1991; 61:77–85.

166. Matsubara E, Amari M, Shoji M, Yamaguchi H, Okamoto K, Hirai S. Serum concentrations of alpha-1-antichymotrypsin is elevated in patients with senile dementia of the Alzheimer type. Prog Clin Biol Res 1989; 317:707–714.

167. Laine M, Vuorinen E, Rinne JO. Picture naming deficits in vascular dementia and Alzheimer's disease. J Clin Exp Neuropsychol 1997; 19:126–140.

168. Gonzalez Montalvo JI, Del Ser Quijano T, Berejo Pareja F. Arq Neurobiol 1990; 53:162–170.

169. Cherrier MM, Mendez MF, Dave M, Perryman KM. Performance on the Rey-Osterreith Complex Figure Test in Alzheimer disease and vascular dementia. Neuropsychiatry Neuropsychol Behav Neurol 1999; 12:95–101.

170. Barr A, Brandt J. Word-list generation deficits in dementia. J Clin Exp Neuropsychol 1996; 18:810–822.

171. Lukatela K, Malloy P, Jenkins M, Cohen R. The naming deficit in early Alzheimer's disease and vascular dementia. Neuropsychology 1998; 12:565–572.

172. Lamar M, Podell K, Carew TG, Cloud BS, Resh R, Kennedy C, Goldberg E, Kaplan E, Libon DJ. Perseverative behavior in Alzheimer's disease and subcortical ischemic vascular dementia. Neuropsychology 1997; 11:523–534.

173. Perez Trullen JM, Modegro Pardo PJ, Iniguez C, Vazqeuz Andre ML. Emotional components of language in multi-infarct dementia. Med Clin 1994; 102:537–539.

174. Powell AL, Cummings JL, Hill MA, Benson DF. Speech and language alterations in multi-infarct dementia. Neurology 1988; 38:717–719.

175. Matsuda O, Saito M Sugishita M. Cognitive deficits of mild dementia: a comparison between dementia of the Alzheimer's type and vascular dementia. Psychiatry Clin Neurosci 1998; 52:87–91.

176. Ricker JH, Keenan PA, Jacobson MW. Visuoperceptual-spatial ability and visual memory in vascular dementia and dementia of the Alzheimer type. Neuropsychologia 1994; 32:1287–1296.

177. Hogan DB, Ebly EM. Primitive reflexes and dementia: results from the Canadian Study of health and aging. Age Aging 1995; 24:375–381.

178. Tanaka A, Okuzumi H, Kobayashi I, Murai N, Meguro K, Nakamura T. Gait disturbance of patients with vascular and Alzhemier-type dementia. Percept Motor Skills 1995; 80:735–738.

179. Vreeling FW, Houx PJ, Jolles J, Verhey FR. Primitive reflexes in Alzheimer's disease and vascular dementia. J Geriatr Psychiatry Neurol 1995; 8:11–117.

180. Bennet DA, Gilley DW, Lee, Cochran EJ. White matter changes: neurobehavioral manifestations of Binswanger's disease and clinical correlates in Alzheimer's disease. Dementia 1994; 5:148–152.

181. Leys D, Pasquier F, Lucas C, Pruvo JP. Résonance magnétique dans la démence vasculaire. J Mal Vasc 1995; 20:194–202.

182. Meyer JS, Shirai T, Akiyama H. Neuroimaging in differentiating vascular from Alzheimer's dementias. Cerebrovasc Brain Metab Revi 1996; 8:1–10.

183. Kuwabara Y, Ichiya Y, Otsuka M, Masuda K, Ichiyama A, Fujishima M. Cerebrovascular responsiveness to hypercapnia in Alzheimer's dementia and vascular dementia of the Binswanger type. Stroke 1992; 23:1534–1535.

184. Pirttila T, Kim KS, Mehta PD, Frey H, Wisniewski HM. Soluble amyloid beta protein in the cerebrospinal fluid from patients with Alzheimer's disease, vascular dementia and controls. J Neurol Sci 1994; 127:90–95.

185. Ihara Y, Hayabara T, Sasaki K, Fujisawa Y, Kawada R, Yamamoto T, Nakashima Y, Yoshimuro S, Kawai M, Kitaba M, Kuroda S. Free radicals and superoxide dismutase in blood of patients with Alzhiemer's disease and vascular dementia. J Neurol Sci 1997; 153:76–81.

186. Foy CJ, Passmore AP, Vahidassr MD, Young IS, Lawson JT. Plasma chain-breaking antioxydants in Alzheimer's disease, vascular dementia and Parkinson's disease. Q J Med 1999; 92:39–45.

187. Rosengren LE, Karlsson JE, Sjogren M, Blennow K, Wallin A. Neurfilament protein levels in CSF are increased in dementia. Neurology 1999; 52:1090–1093.

188. Tekin S, Aykut C, Ozgun S, Aktan S. The role of autoimmunity in vascular dementia. Dementia 1996; 7:91–94.

189. Matsubara E, Hirai S, Amari M, Shoji M, Yamaguchi H, Okamoto K, Ishiguro K, Harigaya Y, Wakabayashi K. Aplha 1 antichymotrypsin as a possible biochemical marker for Alzheimer-type dementia. Ann Neurol 1990; 28:561–567.

190. Licastro F, Parnetti L, Morini MC, Davis LJ, Cucinotta D, Gaiti A, Senin U. Acute phase reactant alpha-1 antichymotrypsin is increased in cerebrospinal fluid and scrum of patients with probable Alzhemier's disease. Alzheimer's Dis Assoc Disord 1995; 9:112–118.

191. Nagao T, Hamamoto M, Hagiwara M, Kanda A, Ichiseki H, Miyazaki T, Isse K, Tanaka K, Ogura M, Tsushima T Serum alpha 1 antichymotrypsin in senile dementia. Nippon Ronen Igakkai Zasshi 1992; 29:778–782.

192. Kurita K, Manaka H, Kato T, Katagiri T, Sasaki H. A case of Creutzfeldt-Jakob disease with markedly elevated ubiquitin concentration in the cerbrospinal fluid. Rinsho Shinkeigaku 1991; 31:666–668.

193. Isoe K, Urakami K, Ji Y, Adachi Y, Nakashima K. Presenilin-1 polymorphism inpatients with Alzheimer's disease, vascular dementia and alcohol-associated dementia in Japanese population. Acta Neurol Scand 1996; 94:326–328.

194. Blennow K, Davisdson P, Wallin A, Gottfries CG, Svennerholm L. Ubiquitin in cerebrospinal fluid in Alzheimer's disease and vascular dementia. Int Psychogeriatr, 1994; 6:13–22.

195. Blennow K, Davidsson P, Wallin A, Ekman R. Chromagranin A in cerebrospinal fluid: a biochemical marker for synaptic degeneration in Alzheimer's disease? Dementia 1995; 6:306–311.

196. Mari D, Parnetti L, Coppola R, Bottasso B, Reboldi GP, Senin U, Mannucci PM. Hemostasis abnormalities in patients with vascuar dementia and Alzhmeier's disease. Thrombo Hemostas 1996; 75:216–218.

197. Van Kooten F, Ciabattoni G, Koudstaal PJ, Grobbee DE, Kluft C, Patrono C. Increased thromboxane biosynthesis is associated with poststroke dementia. Stroke 1999; 30:1542–1547.

198. Moroney JT, Tang MX, Berglund L, Small S, Merchant C, Bell K, Stern Y, Mayeux

R. Low-density lipoprotein cholesterol and the risk of dementia with stroke. JAMA 1999; 282:254–260.

199. Kario K, Matsuo T, Hoshide S, Umeda Y, Shimada K. Effect of thrombin inhibition in vascular dementia and silent cerebrovascular disease. An MR spectroscopy study. Stroke 1999; 30:1033–1037.

200. Tilvis RS, Erkinjuntti T, Sulkava R, Miettinen TA. Fatty acid of plasma lipids, red cells and platelets in Alzheimer's disease and vascular dementia. Atherosclerosis 1987; 65:237–245.

201. Mecocci P, Ekamn R, Parnetti L, Senin U. Antihistone and anti-dsDNA autoantibodies in Alzhemeier's disease and vascular dementia. Biol Psychiatry 1993; 34: 380–385.

202. Mecocci P, Parnetti L, Romano G, Scarelli A, Chionne F, Cecchetti R, Polidori MC, Palumbo B, Cherubini A, Senin U. Serum anti-GFAP and anti-S100 autoantibodies in brain aging, Alzhemeier's disease and vascular dementia. J Neuroimmunol 1995; 57:165–170.

203. Mecocci P, Parnettti L, Donato R, Santucci A, Cadini D, Foa E, Cecchetti R, Senin U. Serum autoantibodies against glial fibrillary acid protein in brain aging and senile dementia. Brain Behav Immun 1992; 6:286–292.

204. Kira J, Hamada T, Kawano Y, Okayama M, Yamasaki K. An association of human T-cell lymphotropic virus type I infection with vascular dementia. Acta Neurol Scand 1997; 96:305–309.

205. Yarnada K, Kono K, Umenagi H, Yamada K, Iguchi A, Fukatsu T, Nakashima N, Nishiwaki H, Shimada Y, Sugita Y. Decreased interleukin-6 levels in the cerebrospinal fluid of patients with Alzheimer-type dementia. Neurosci Lett 1995; 186: 219–221.

206. Cacaabelos R, Alvarez XA, Fernandez-Novoa L, Franco A, Mangues R, Pellicer A, Nishimura T. Brain interleukin-1 beta in Alzheimer's disease and vascular dementia. Methods Findings Exp Clin Parmacol 1994; 16:141–151.

207. Wakutani Y, Urakami K, Shimomura T, Takahashi K. Heat shock protein 70 mRNA levels in mononuclear blood cells from patients with dementia of the Alzheimer type. Dementia 1995; 6: 301–305.

208. Wallin A, Blennow K, Rosengren LE. Glial fibrillary acidic protein in the cerebrospinal fluid of patients with dementia. Dementia 1996; 7:267–272.

209. Martinez M, Frank A, Diez-Tejedor E, Hernanz A. Amino-acid concentrations in cerebrospinal fluid and serum in Alzhemier's disease and vascular dementia. J Neural Transm 1993; 6:1–9.

210. Gottfries CG, Blennow K, Karlsson I, Wallin A. The neurochemistry of vascular dementia. Dementia 1994; 5:163–167.

211. Mashige F, Takai N, Matsushima Y, Takano M, Tsuchiya E, Kanazawa H, Nagata Y, Shinozuka N, Wada H. Simultaneous determination of cathecolamines, serotonin, and their precursors and metabolites in body fluid by an HPLC system with multi-electrode electrochemical dtetector. Rinsho Byori 1994; 42:591–599.

212. Fukuda H, Nakamura S, Hara K, Udaka F, Kameyama M. Study on the concentration of 5-hydroxyidoleacetic acid (5HIAA) in the lumbar cereberospinal fluid (CSF) in neurological diseases. Rinsho Shinkeigaku 1989; 29:1192–1194.

213. Wallin A, Blennow K, Edman A, Mansson JE. Decreased lumbar cerebrospinal

fluid levels of monoamine metabolites on vascular dementia. Int Psychogeriatr 1996; 8:425–436.

214. Tohgi H, Ueno M, Abe T, Takahashi S, Nozaki Y. Concentrations of monoamines and their metabolites in the cerebrospinal fluid from patients with senile dementia of the Alzheimer type and vascular dementia of the Binswanger type. J Neural Transm 1992; 4:69–77.

215. Tohgi H, Abe T, Kimura M, Saheki M, Takahashi S. Cerebrospinal fluid acetylcholine and choline in vascular dementia of Binswanger and multiple small infarct types as compared with Alzheimer-type dementia. J Neural Transm 1996; 103: 1211–1220.

216. Ohara K, Kondo N, Xie D, Tanabe K, Yamamoto T, Kosaka K, Miyasato K, Ohara K. Normal sequences of muscarinic acetylcholine receptors (m1 and m2) in patients with Alzheimer's disease and vascular dementia. Neurosci Lett 1994; 178:23–26.

217. Szilagyi AK, Nemeth A, Martini E, Lendvai B, Venter V. Serum and CSF cholinesterase activity in vasrious kinds of dementia. Eur Arch Psychiatry Neurol Sci 1987; 236:309–311.

218. Yoshinaga J, Sasaki T, Ideshita H, Hikiji A, Kuwaki T. Acetylcholinesterase activity in CSF in senile dementia of Alzheimer type, vascular dementia and Parkinson's disease. Rinsho Shinkeigaku 1989; 29:376–378.

219. Yamamoto Y, Nakano S, Kawashima S, Nakamura S, Urakami K, Kato T, Kameyama M. Plasma and serum G4 isoenzyme of acetylcholinesterase in patients with Alzheimer-type dementia and vascular dementia. Ann Clin Biochem 1990; 27:321–326.

220. Heilig M, Sjogren M, Blennow K, Ekman R, Wallin A. Cerebrospinal fluid neuropetides in Alzheimer's disease and vascular dementia. Biol Psychiatry 1995; 38: 210–216.

221. Gomez JM, Aguilar M, Navarro MA, Ortola J, Soler J. Secretion of growth hormonc and thyroidstimulating hormone in patients with dementia. Clin Invest 1994; 72:489–493.

222. Parnetti L, Palumbo B, Cardinali L, Loretti F, Chionne F, Cecchetti R, Senin U. Cerebrospinal fluid neuron-specific enolase in Alzhemiemr's disease and vascular dementia. Neurosci Lett 1995; 183:43–45.

223. Blennow K, Wallin A, Ekman R. Neuron specific enolase in cerebrospinal fluid: a biochemical marker for neuronal degeneration in dementia disorders? J Neural Transm 1994; 8:183–191.

224. Sulkava R, Viinikka L, Erkinjuntti T, Roine R. Cerebrospinal fluid neuron-specific enolase is decreased in multi-infarct dementia but unchanged in Alzheimer's disease. J Neurol Neurosurg Psychiatry 1988; 51:549–551.

225. Tohgi H, Abe T, Takahashi S, Kikuchi T. The urate and xanthine concentrations in thc cerebrospinal fluid in patients with vascular dementia of the Binswanger type, Alzheimer type dementia and Parkinson's disease. J Neural Transm 1993; 6: 119–126.

226. Wada H. Blood-brain barrier permeability of the demented elderly as studied by cerebrospinal fluid-serum albumin ratio. Int Med 1998; 37:509–513.

227. Tohgi H, Abe T, Nakanishi M, Hamato F, Sasaki K, Takahashi S. Concentrations

of alpha-tocopherol and its quinone derivative in cerebrospianl fluid from patients with vascular dementia of the Bisnwanger type and Alzheimer's disease. Neurosci-Lett 1994; 174:73–76.

228. Szilagyi AK, Martini E, Venter V. Function of blood-cerebrospinal fluid barrier and selected biochemical cerebrospinal fluid components in senile dementias of various types. Psychiatrie Neurol Med Psychol, 1986; 38:1–8.

229. Wallin A, Blennow K, Fredman P, Gottfries CG, Karlsson I, Svennerholm L. Blood brain barrier function in vascular dementia. Acta Neurol Scand 1990; 81:318–322)

230. Pantoni L, Inzitari D, Pracucci G, Lolli F, Giordano G, Bracco L, Amaducci L. Cerebrospinal fluid proteins in patients with leukoaraiosis: possible abnormalities in blood-brain barrier. J Neurol Sci 1993; 115:125–131.

231. Yoshida F, Sadoshima S, Fuji K, Iino K, Fujishima M. Regional cerebral blood flow in chronic stroke patients with dementia Jpn J Med, 1988; 27:172–176.

232. Mielke R, Heiss WD. Positron emission tomography for the diagnosis of Alzheimer's disease and vascular dementia. J Neural Transm 1998; 53:237–250.

233. Pavics L, Grunwald F, Reichmann K, Horn R, Kitschenberg A, Hartmann A, Menzel C, Schomburg AG, Overbeck B, Csernay L, Biersack HJ. Regional cerebral blood flow single-photon emission tomography with 99mTc-HMPAO and the acetazolamide test in the evaluation of vascular and Alzheimer's dementia. Eur J Nucl Med 1999; 26:239–245.

234. Reference deleted.

235. Velakoulis D, Lloyd JH. The rôle of SPECT scanning in a neuropsychiatric unit. Aust NZ J Psychiatry 1998; 32:511–522.

236. Talbot PR, Lloyd JJ, Snowden JS, Neary D, Testa HJ. A clinical role for 99mTc-HMPAO SPECT in the investigation of dementia. J Neurol Neurosurg Psychiatry 1998; 64:306–313.

237. Pullicino P, Benedict RH, Capruso DX, Vella N, Withiam-Letich S, Kwen Pl. Neuroimaging criteria for vascular dementia. Arch Neurol 1996; 53:723–728.

238. Sabri O, Ringelstein EB, Hellwig D, Schneider R, Schreckenberger M, Kaiser HJ, Mull M, Buell U. Neuropsychological impairment correlates with hypoperfusion and hypometabolism but not with severity of white matter lesions on MRI in patients with cerebral microangiography. Stroke 1999; 30:556–566.

239. De Reuck J, Decoo D, Hasenbroeckx MC, Lamont B, Santens P, Goethals P, Strijckmans K, Lemahieu I. Acetazolamide vasoreactivity in vascular dementia: a positron emission tomographic study. Eur Neurol 1999; 41:31–36.

240. Tohgi H, Abe T, Yamazaki K, Murata T, Isobe C, Ishizaki E. The cerebrospinal fluid oxidized NO metabolites, nitrite and nitrate, in Alzhemier's disease and vascular dementia of Binswanger's type and multiple small infarct type. J Neural Transm 1998; 105:1283–1291.

241. Tohgi H, Abe T, Takahashi S, Kimura M. A selective reduction of excitatory amino-acids in cerebrospinal fluid of patients with Alzheimer type dementia compared with vascular dementia of the Binswanger type. Neurosci Lett 1992; 141:5–8.

242. Garcia JH, Brown GG. Vascular dementia: neuropathologic alterations and meatbolic brain changes. J Neurol Sci 1992; 109:121–131.

243. Szelies B, Mielke R, Herholz K, Heiss WD. Quantitative topographical EEG compared to FDG PET for classification of vascular and degenerative dementia. Electroencephalogr Clin Neurophysiol 1994; 91:131–139.

244. Signorino M, Pucci E, Belardinelli N, Nolfe G, Angeleri F. EEG spectral analysis in vascular and Alzheimer dementia. Electroencephalogr Clin Neurophysiol 1995; 94:313–325.

245. Tomlinson BE, Blessed G, Roth M. Observations of the brain of demented old people. J Neurol Sci 1970; 11:205–242.

246. Del Ser T, Bermejo F, Portera A et al. Vascular dementia: a clinico-pathological study. J Neurol Neurosurg Psychiatry 1990; 96:1–17.

247. Forette F, Amery A, Staessen J, Strasser T, Thijs L, Beevers DG, Bert P, Clement D, Cox J, de Leeuw PW et al. Is prevention of vascular dementia possible? The Syst-Eur Vascular Dementia Project. Aging 1991; 3:373–382.

248. Fischhof PK, Moslinger-Gehmayr R, Herrmann WM, Friedmann A, Russmann DL. Therapeutic efficacy of vincamine in dementia. Neuropsychobiology 1996; 34:29–35.

249. Molto JM, Falip R, Martin R, Insa R, Pastor I, Matias Guiu J. Comparative study of nicardipine vesrus placebo in the prevention of cognitive deterioration in patients with transient ischemic attacks. Rev Neurol 1995; 23:54–58.

250. Anonymous An experimental, randomized, double-blind, placebo-controlled clinical trial to investigate the effect of nicardipine on cognitive functions in patients with vascular dementia. Rev D Neurol, 1999; 28:835–845.

251. Saletu B, Paulus E, Linzmayer L, Anderer P, Semlistch IIV, Grunberger J, Wicke L, Neuhold A, Podreka I. Nicergoline in senile dementia of Alzheimer type and multi-infarct dementia: a double-blind, placebo-controlled, clinical and EEG/ERP mapping study. Psychopharmacology 1995; 117:385–395.

252. Blume J, Ruhlmann KU, de la Haye R, Rettig K. Treatment of chronic cerebrovascular disease in elderly patients with pentoxyfylline. J Med 1992; 23:417–432.

253. Kittner B, Rossner M, Rother M. Clinical trials in dementia with propentofylline. Ann NY Acad Sci 1997; 82:307–316.

254. Mielke R, Kittner B, Ghaemi M, Kessler J, Szelies B, Herholz K, Heiss WD. Propentofylline improves regional cerebral glucose metabolism and neuropsychologic performance in vascular dementia. J Neurol Sci 1996; 141:59–64.

255. Mielke R, Moller HJ, Erkinjuntti T, Rosenkrantz B, Rother M, Kittner B. Propentofylline in the treatment of vascular dementia and Alzheimer-type dementia: overview of phase I and phase II clinical trials. Alzheimer Dis Assoc Disord 1998; 12(suppl 2):S29–S35.

256. Rother M, Erkinjuntti T, Roessner M, Kittner B, Marcusson J, Karlsson I. Propentofylline in the treatment of Alzheimer's disease and vascular dementia: a review of phase III trials. Dementia Geriatr Cognit Disord 1998; 9(suppl 1):36–43.

257. Black RS, Barclay LL, Nolan KA, Thaler HT, Hardimann ST, Blass JP. Pentoxyfylline in cerebrovascular dementia. J Am Geriatri Soc 1992, 40:237–244.

258. Rainer M, Brunnbauer M, Dunky A, Ender F, Goldsteiner H, Holl O, Kotlan P, Paulitsch G, Reiner C, Stossl J, Zachhuber C, Mossler H. Therapeutic results with cerebrolysin in the treatment of dementia. Wien Med Wochenschr, 1997; 147:426–431.

259. Schneider LS, Olin JT. Overview of clinical trials of hydergine in dementia. Arch Neurol 1994; 51:787–798.
260. Cucinotta D, Aveni Casucci MA, Pedrazzi F, Ponari O, Capodaglio M, Valdina P, Toxiri I, Bartorelli L, Granata Q, Franzini C. Multicentre clinical placebo-controlled study with buflomedil in the treatment of mild dementia of vascular origin. J Int Med Res 1992; 20:136–149.
261. Lechner H. Status of treatment of vascular dementia. Neuropeidemiology 1998; 17:10–13.
262. Ditzler K. Efficacy and tolerability of memantine in patients with dementia syndrome. A double-blind placebo-controlled trial. Arzneim-Forschung 1991; 41:773–780.
263. Di Perri R, Coppola G, Ambrosio LA, Grasso A, Puca FM, Rizzo M. A multicentre trial to evaluate the efficacy and tolerability of alpha-glycerophosphocholine versus cytosine diphosphocholine in patients with vascular dementia. J Int Med Res 1991; 19:330–341.
264. Grossmann WM, Standt A, May U, van Laak HH, Hirche H. Naftidrofuryl in the treatment of midl senile dementia. A double-blind study. Pharmacopsychiatry 1990; 23:265–273.
265. Tohgi H, sasaki K, Chiba K, Nozaki Y. Effect of vinpocetine on oxygen release of hemoglobin and erythrocyte organic polyphosphate concentrations in patients with vascular dementia of the Binswangers' type. Arzneim-Forschung 1990; 40:640–643.
266. Nadeau SE, Malloy PF, Andrew ME. A crossover trial of bromocriptine in the treatment of vascular dementia. Ann Neurol 1988; 24:270–272.
267. Gillis JC, Benefield P, Mc Tavish D. Idebenone: a review of its pharamacodynamic and pharmacokinetic properties, and therapeutic use in age-related cognitive disorders. Drug Aging 1994; 5:133–152.

10
Pharmacological and Cell-Based Therapies for Stroke Recovery

Dileep R. Yavagal
Massachusetts General Hospital and
Harvard Medical School, Boston, Massachusetts

Seth P. Finklestein
Massachusetts General Hospital and Harvard Medical School, and
ViaCell Neuroscience, Boston, Massachusetts

I. INTRODUCTION

Stroke is a major cause of disability in the United States and around the world. In the last decade, exciting new therapies have become available for treatment of the acute phase of ischemic stroke, giving hope to patients for better treatment. Even then, a large majority of patients come to medical attention too late or are not candidates for acute therapies. There exists a huge potential to modify the recovery phase after acute stroke to improve outcome and lessen disability. Such recovery therapies have been in intense development in laboratories and clinics around the globe. This chapter summarizes various pharmacological and cell-based modalities for enhancement of the process of recovery from stroke.

II. DRUGS ENHANCING STROKE RECOVERY

The natural process of stroke recovery may be amenable to pharmacological enhancement. Several pharmacological strategies and drugs, based on the physiological mechanisms of repair in the brain after stroke, are being intensely studied at present. Three promising groups of pharmacological agents for enhancement of recovery after stroke are discussed below.

263

III. GROWTH FACTORS

Neuronal sprouting and new synapse formation may represent important reparative mechanisms after stroke (1). Growth factors most likely are crucial in this
reparative process. They are naturally occurring polypeptides that act through
high-affinity receptors on neuronal cells to promote neuronal survival and outgrowth of neuronal processes (2,3). They also appear to protect against hypoxia,
decreased glucose, and exogenous toxins in vitro. Growth factor "superfamilies"
important to the nervous system include neurotrophins, fibroblast growth factors
(FGF), transforming growth factors (TGFs), and platelet-derived growth factors
(PGDFs) among others. A few hours after cerebral infarction several growth factors are upregulated in peri-infarct territory. The neuroprotective role is suggested
by the timing of this expression and has been validated with respect to some of
these growth factors in animal studies (4,5). Indeed basic fibroblast growth factor
(bFGF) given within a few hours of acute focal ischemia decreases infarct volume
as compared to controls. Also, some growth factors are highly expressed in the
peri-infarct region throughout the course of sensorimotor recovery (6), most
likely playing a crucial role in the physiological processes underlying repair.
Exogenous administration of three such growth factors, bFGF, osteogenic pro-
tein-1 (OP-1), and nerve growth factor (NGF), has been shown to enhance recovery.

A. Basic Fibroblast Growth Factor

Basic fibroblast growth factor is a 154-amino-acid, 18-kDa polypeptide (7). It is
named for its ability to promote fibroblast proliferation in vitro. It acts through
high-affinity tyrosine kinase receptors on cells initiating a cascade of phosphory-
lation reactions. It is distributed widely in the mammalian body with relatively
high concentrations in the brain. In the mature brain it is largely cell associated
within a few select neuronal populations as well as scattered astroglial cells.
It supports neuronal survival and axonal outgrowth along with angiogenic and
gliotrophic actions. Following mechanical brain injury or ischemia, levels of
bFGF mRNA, and protein are markedly upregulated in the tissue surrounding
wounds or infarcts (6). This observation and bFGF's neuroprotective role against
hypoxia in vitro have formed the rationale for its use as a neuroprotective agent
after acute stroke. Given within the first few hours after acute permanent or reversible focal ischemia, bFGF markedly reduced the infarct size as compared to
controls (4,5). Intravenously administered bFGF appears to cross the damaged
blood-brain barrier (BBB) after stroke (5). Moreover, there appears to be an active
transport system for bFGF across the intact BBB as well (8). bFGF appears to
reduce infarct size via upregulation of anti-apoptotic molecules in the ischemic
penumbra after stroke (9).

Basic FGF's role in stroke recovery was examined by Kawamata et al. (10). Exogenous administration of this growth factor enhanced behavioral recovery in an animal model of stroke. Basic FGF, 0.5–1 μg, was administered intracisternally 24 hr after permanent proximal middle cerebral artery occlusion and then biweekly for 4 weeks. Control animals were treated with vehicle. The intracisternal route ensured access to both the injured and the intact brain. The animals were tested for recovery of the impaired limb contralateral to the infarcts, using limb placement, beam balance, and postural reflex tests. The bFGF-treated animals did significantly better as compared to the vehicle-treated animals. There was no difference in infarct volume between the two groups. This suggests a mechanism of action for the bFGF other than neuroprotection for the enhancement of recovery. Indeed, there is increased neuronal sprouting in the intact contralateral brain, which correlates with improvement in recovery. This is evidenced by increased immunoreactivity to GAP-43, a growth cone protein on the neuronal membrane in the contralateral cortex in the bFGF-treated animals (11). Further data to support this mechanism come from an experiment where antisense oligonucleotide to GAP-43 blocked the recovery-enhancing properties of bFGF along with blocking of increased immunoreactivity of GAP-43 in the contralateral cortex (12). The enhancement of recovery correlating with increased neuronal sprouting in the contralateral cortex fits with the observed activation of contralateral cortical areas during stroke recovery in human PET and fMRI studies (13).

At the dose of 1μg of bFGF, significant weight loss was the main adverse effect, which was eliminated in subsequent studies using a 0.5-μg dose (11). Moreover, in subsequent studies, as few as two doses of intracisternal bFGF (0.5 μg at 1 and 3 days after stroke) were sufficient to enhance behavioral recovery (12). No tumors or histopathological abnormalities were observed in the bFGF-treated animals in these studies.

B. Osteogenic Protein-1

Osteogenic protein-1 (OP-1), also known as bone morphogenic protein-7 (BMP-7), is a member of the BMP subfamily of the transforming growth factor-β (TGF-β) superfamily. It is 35-kDa homodimeric glycoprotein, which was initially identified by its ability to promote new bone formation in bone. It is also expressed in the developing and mature brain (14,15). OP-1 exerts its actions by binding to type I and II high-affinity serine and threonine kinase receptors. In culture, OP-1 selectively promotes the outgrowth of dendritic processes from both peripheral and central neurons (16,17). This is a unique property of OP-1 as most identified neurotrophic factors largely support axonal growth. Given the potential importance of dendritic sprouting in functional recovery after stroke, OP-1 may be useful as a pharmacological agent in recovery. Indeed, exogenous administration of OP-1 beginning at 1 day after acute ischemic stroke significantly enhances recovery in animal studies. Kawamata, Finklestein, et al. used human recombinant OP-1 in doses of 1–10 μg injected into the cisterna magna of mature male rats at 1 and 4 days after focal cerebral infarction induced by MCA occlusion (18). OP-1-treated animals showed marked enhancement of recovery of impaired forelimb and hindlimb function as assessed by limb placement tests at 1 month after the ischemic stroke. This effect was dose-dependent, with a trend toward greater enhancement of recovery at a dose of 10 μg than 1 μg/injection. No adverse effects were noted. To define the time window for starting the injections, a further study was done, which showed that there is enhancement of recovery if OP-1 treatment is initiated at 1 or 3 days, but not at 7 days, after stroke (19). Also, even a single injection of OP-1 enhances recovery (20). There was no difference in infarct volume among the OP-1-treated and control animals, suggesting a mechanism affecting the repair process rather than neuroprotection leading to recovery enhancement. This may be due to stimulation of new dendritic sprouting and synapse formation in uninjured regions of brain.

C. Nerve Growth Factor

Nerve growth Factor (NGF) belongs to the neurotrophin superfamily, which includes BDNF, NT-3, and NT4/5. It is a 26-kDa homodimer that binds to tyrosine kinase A (trkA) receptor and has trophic action on cholinergic neurons in the intact mature brain. In vitro, it protects PC-12 cells against death from anoxia, hypoglycemia, and free radical–induced death (21). In models of forebrain global ischemia in gerbils and rats, intracerebroventricular administration of NGF (2–10 μg) beginning just before or after onset of ischemia has been shown to reduce death of CA-1 hippocampal neurons (22,23). NGF has been shown to have a crucial role in neuronal plasticity process in unlesioned animals housed in an enriched environment (24,25).

Exogenous administration of NGF seems to improve functional recovery after stroke (26). Kolb et al. administered NGF or vehicle intraventricularly after unilateral cortical devascularization causing an infarct. The NGF-treated rats showed attenuation of behavioral symptoms assessed by forelimb reaching tasks, beam traversing tasks, and spatial navigation tasks. Analysis of dendritic arborization showed reversal of lesion-induced atrophy of dendritic fields in pyramidal motor neurons as well as reversal of lesion-induced reduction in spine density in NGF-treated rat brains. The mechanism of this enhanced recovery seems to be due to NGF-mediated plastic changes in the ipsilateral cortical neurons correlating with recovery from sensorimotor deficits.

D. Other Growth Factors in Stroke Recovery

Other growth factors that have been shown to be upregulated during recovery from focal ischemia include platelet-derived growth factor (PGDF), ciliary neurotrophic factor (CNTF), and transforming growth factor-β-1 (TGF-β1) (27). This suggests a role for these factors in facilitating functional recovery and possibilities for pharmacological use. Exogenous administration experiments in models of stroke recovery have not yet been done for these factors.

IV. AMPHETAMINES

Drugs increasing monoamine release at synaptic terminals have been shown in animal and human studies to promote functional recovery after stroke. This benefit is seen when drugs are administered in combination with physical therapy. Amphetamine is the best studied among these drugs. Mailing and Achaieson, in 1946, reported temporary alleviation of symptoms of cortical injury after administration of amphetamine (28). This effect was further studied in rats recovering from cortical injury by Feeney et al. in 1982 (29). Amphetamine, 2 mg, was given intraperiotoneally 24 hr after sensorimotor cortex ablation. At 5 days, the hemiplegic animals receiving amphetamine showed superior improvement on beam-walking test scores when compared to animals given placebo. Furthermore this effect was shown to be dose dependent (30). Rats receiving amphetamine, 4 mg intraperitoneally, recovered fully at 14 days as compared to 26 days for rats receiving 2 mg.

These encouraging preclinical data for amphetamine in stroke recovery have been borne out in preliminary human studies. Amphetamine combined with physical therapy has been shown to significantly improve recovery as compared to physical therapy alone. In one double-blinded study of amphetamine in stroke, patients were given amphetamine, 10 mg orally, coupled with physical therapy within 10 days of ischemic hemiplegia (31). The day after treatment, the four patients receiving amphetamine with physical therapy showed significantly higher gains on the Fugl-Myer scale of sensorimotor function as compared to four controls. In another study, amphetamine was given to hemiparetic subjects in a single-blinded manner at a dose of 10 mg orally every fourth day, 16–30 days after onset of stroke (32). The five patients receiving active drug showed improved motor function on the Fugl-Myer scale compared to patients receiving placebo. This benefit was preserved at 1 week and also at 12 months after drug discontinuation. Use of amphetamine for recovery after aphasia has also been studied in humans with encouraging results (33), indicating a role in improving recovery of cognitive function after stroke.

The mechanism by which amphetamine enhances stroke recovery is not clear. There is supporting experimental evidence for several possible processes. The noradrenergic action of amphetamine may cause disinhibition of inhibiting circuits, facilitating remote alternate pathways to mediate the sensorimotor function impaired by injury (34,35). Another mechanism thought to play a role is the general increase in cortical metabolism after administration of amphetamine (36).

Stroemer et al. (37) showed evidence of increased neurite growth and synaptogenesis in rat brains correlating with enhanced recovery after treatment with amphetamine. This suggests selective upregulation of neurite growth by the drug leading to its benefits in recovery. Yet another mechanism felt to be important is the effects of amphetamine on long-term potentiation and learning (38).

The overall preclinical and clinical data, although limited in number, hold truly promising prospects for larger-scale studies and potentially wider clinical use of monoaminergic agonists in stroke recovery.

V. CELL-BASED THERAPY

Another burgeoning area of stroke recovery therapeutics envisages neural cell transplantation to augment the process of repair after stroke. The modern era of neural transplantation began with the pioneering experiments of Stenevi et al. (39–41) and Lund and Hauschka in 1976 (42). The field has progressed rapidly since then and the functional success of fetal neural grafting has been demonstrated. The limited supply of fetal tissue and ethical concerns are major obstacles to large-scale application of this technology. Cell-based therapies have rapidly emerged as exciting alternatives for CNS repair. Table 1 shows the different types of cell-based therapies being developed both in the laboratory and in human phase I clinical trials.

A. Neural Stem Cells

Neural stem cells (NSCs) are pleuripotent progenitors that can generate into mature neuronal and glial phenotypes after manipulation in cell cultures (43). Transplantation of immortalized NSCs is emerging as a powerful tool for enhancement of CNS recovery after stroke and other injuries. These cells can survive, integrate,

Table 1 Types of Cell-Based Therapies

A. Neural stem cells
    Immortalized neural stem cells
    Endogenous activation
    Autologous neural stem cells
    Neural stem cells as delivery systems
B. Clonal neuronal cell lines
C. Xenogenic cell transplants

---

and differentiate into both neurons and glia after transplantation to the intact or damaged brain. One technique involves "immortalization" prior to transplantation, to ensure a genetically homogenous and large supply of cells (44). This is achieved by incorporation of different isoforms of oncogenes into the NSCs. More recently, temperature-sensitive alleles of SV40 large tumor antigens are being used to permit "conditional" immortalization; the cells proliferate in vitro when cultured at a temperature permissive for SV40 tumor antigen expression (33°C). They exit the cell cycle and differentiate when subsequently switched to a temperature not permissive for SV40 tumor antigen expression (39°C), which corresponds to the mammalian core body temperature. The CRE-Lox-P system allows removal of the immortalizing gene prior to transplantation (45). After transplantation, immortalized NSCs can migrate over extended distances, differentiate in a site-specific manner into neuronal and glial species, and fully integrate into regional microenvironment in vivo (46). Immortalized NSC transplantation into ischemia-lesioned hippocampus in rats improved water maze tasks. Postmortem study of the implanted rat brains indicated that the transplanted cells migrate to the region of damage, adopt both neuronal (pyramidal) and glial phenotypes in vivo, and reconstitute the normal laminated appearance of the CA1 cell field (47).

Endogenous activation of NSCs and autologous transplantation are exciting alternative strategies for enhancement of CNS recovery. Although NSCs were initially identified in the fetal neural tube (48), they have been subsequently shown to be present in the periventricular ependymal zone, dentate gyrus, and other areas in the adult vertebrate brain (49,50). These cells have been also been demonstrated in the subependymal zone of the lateral ventricles and hippocampus in adult human brains (51,52). The NSCs from adult brains proliferate and differentiate into neurons and glia in vitro with the same efficiency as fetal stem cells (53,54). In vivo, the proliferation of fetal stem cells can be stimulated by intraventricular administration of epidermal growth factor but only 3% of proliferating cells labeled with bromodeoxyuridine differentiate into neurons (55). One possible explanation is the lack of signaling environment in the adult brain (40). An enriched environment has been shown to promote survival of proliferating neuronal precursor cells in the dentate gyrus in mice (56). Furthermore, neurogenesis is increased in vivo in response to excitotoxic and mechanical lesions in the dentate gyrus in adult rats (57) and after transient global ischemia in gerbils (58). These combined observations suggest the clinical potential for endogenous activation of NSCs with neurotrophic factor stimulation for CNS repair, without actual transplantation and invasive surgery. There is also the exciting potential for autologous transplantation. The latter would involve a limited brain biopsy from the patient, amplification and genetic modification in vitro, and reintroduction into the brain. This would potentially eliminate the need for immunosuppression posttransplantation.

B. Clonal Neuronal Cell Lines

An alternative strategy to neural stem cell transplants involves the use of human clonal postmitotic neuronal cell lines with a committed neuronal phenotype. These cells are not fully mature in vitro but differentiate further into adult-neuron-like cells in vivo after transplantation. Clonal neuronal cell lines have several advantages over other cell-based therapies. They provide a large population of transplantable cells that have a stable phenotype and are well characterized. Therefore, appropriate types of neuronal cell lines may be transplanted according to the location of the central nervous system (CNS) injury. Also, posttransplant visualization of these cells is possible by transfecting cells to express desired characteristics, for example, enzyme transmitters, growth factors, and marker genes.

Retinoic acid induction of human teratocarcinoma cell (Ntera-2) is used to produce postmitotic-neuron-like cells. This technique yields >95% of pure cultures of neuronal cells (59). Cryopreserved human Ntera transplanted intrastriatally into rats with focal cerebral infarcts from MCAO normalized asymmetrical motor behavior as compared with ischemic animals receiving only medium. Immunosuppressive drugs were given to prevent rejection. Histological analysis of grafted brains revealed a positive correlation between number of surviving hNT neurons and degree of functional recovery (60). No neoplastic transformation was noted at 1 year in the transplanted brains. In the first case reported from the human phase I trials, about two million neurons derived from the hNT cell lines were injected close to the site of infarct under CT guidance in a 62-year-old woman with a right hemiparesis and impaired speech. Cyclosporine was used for immunosuppression. Patients are assessed for safety and functional recovery. Sequential MRI is done to assess brain-tissue response, and PET studies to measure regional brain metabolism are planned (61).

C. Cells as Delivery Systems

Since the early 1990s genetically modified cells have been used to deliver trophic molecules to promote regeneration in the damaged CNS (62,63). Fibroblasts serve as relatively inert and easy-to-transfect vehicles. Transplantation of fibroblasts genetically engineered to produce BDNF into partial cervical hemisection cavity promoted the regeneration of the interrupted rubrospinal tract (64). NGF-gene-transfected fibroblasts transplanted 1 week before ischemia resulted in significant attenuation of CA1-CA2 hippocampal loss induced by 10 min of global ischemia (65). Newer strategies use neural stem cells for gene delivery to the CNS given their ability to migrate widely throughout the brain after injection, and to integrate in a functional and nondisruptive manner. In the latter aspects they are superior to nonneural cells. In the MCAO model in rats, neural stem cells secreting NGF transplanted into the striatum, 7 days before ischemia, conferred significant neuroprotection against 30 min of ischemia (66).

D. Xenogenic Cell Transplantation

The relative immunological privilege of the brain may mean good xenograft survival. Porcine fetal neural cell transplantation is being developed for multiple CNS diseases including stroke. Pig neural tissue is considered optimal for xenotransplantation for several reasons, including the physiological similarity to human neurons and similar size and development patterns (67). Also, the ease of breeding and production of large number of embryos per litter lends a production advantage. Recently, the first human xenotransplant for stroke was carried out, as part of a human phase I clinical trial, in which a 39-year-old patient with left arm weakness from a stroke 4 years earlier had porcine cells transplanted into her brain (68). The cells were pretreated with a novel immunomodulator to avoid the use of immunosuppresants. Relults of efficacy and safety are awaited.

VI. CONCLUSION

Increasing attention is being focused on therapies to improve pace and degree of recovery from neurological deficits in stroke patients. A wide spectrum of modalities, from cell transplantation to use of growth factors and already existing pharmacological agents such as amphetamine, are being tested for this purpose. There is promising laboratory evidence and in some cases preliminary clinical evidence for efficacy for these therapies. Given the staggering burden of patients disabled from stroke each year, these modalities will have an immense clinical utility if proven to be beneficial in human trials.

REFERENCES

1. Stroemer RP, Kent TA, Hulsebosch CE. Neocortical neural sprouting, synaptogenesis, and behavioral recovery after neocortical infarction in rats. Stroke 1995; 26(11): 2135–2144.
2. Kawamata T, Speliotes EK, Finklestein SP. The role of polypeptide growth factors in recovery from stroke. Adv Neurol 1997; 73:377–382.
3. Finklestein SP, et al. Growth factor expression after stroke. Stroke 1990; 21(suppl 11):III122–III124.
4. Koketsu N, et al. Pretreatment with intraventricular basic fibroblast growth factor decreases infarct size following focal cerebral ischemia in rats. Ann Neurol 1994; 35(4):451–457.

5. Fisher M, et al. Delayed treatment with intravenous basic fibroblast growth factor reduces infarct size following permanent focal cerebral ischemia in rats. J Cereb Blood Flow Metab 1995; 15(6):953–959.

6. Speliotes EK, et al. Increased expression of basic fibroblast growth factor (bFGF) following focal cerebral infarction in the rat. Brain Res Mol Brain Res 1996; 39(1–2):31–42.

7. Baird AKM. The fibroblast frowth factor family. Ann NY Acad Sci 1991; 3:239–243.

8. Wagner JP, Black IB, DiCicco-Bloom E. Stimulation of neonatal and adult brain neurogenesis by subcutaneous injection of basic fibroblast growth factor. J Neurosci 1999; 19:6006–6016.

9. Ay I, Sugimori H, Finklestein SP. Basic fibroblast growth factor (bFGF) decreases DNA fragmentation and increases bcl-2 expression following stroke in rats (abstr.). Stroke 2000; 31:282.

10. Kawamata T, et al. Intracisternal basic fibroblast growth factor (bFGF) enhances behavioral recovery following focal cerebral infarction in the rat. J Cereb Blood Flow Metab 1996; 16(4):542–547.

11. Kawamata T, Dalton-Dietrich W, Schallert T, Gotts JE, Cocke RR, Beneowiz LI, Finklestein SP. Intracisternal basic fibroblastic growth factor enhances functional recovery and upregulates the expression of a molecular marker of neuronal sprouting following focal cerebral infarction. Proc Natl Acad Sci USA 1997; 94(15):8179–8184.

12. Kawamata T, et al. Intracisternal antisense oligonucleotide to growth associated protein-43 blocks the recovery-promoting effects of basic fibroblast growth factor after focal stroke. Exp Neurol 1999; 158(1):89–9612.

13. Cramer SC, Nelles G, Benson RR, Kaplan JD, Parker RA, Kwong KK, Kennedy DN, Finklestein SP, Rosen BR. A functional MRI study of subjects recovered from hemiparetic stroke. Stroke 1997; 28(12):2518–2527.

14. Ozkaynak E, et al. OP-1 cDNA encodes an osteogenic protein in the TGF-beta family. Embo J 1990; 9(7):2085–2093.

15. Sampath TK, et al. Bovine osteogenic protein is composed of dimers of OP-1 and BMP-2A, two members of the transforming growth factor-beta superfamily. J Biol Chem 1990; 265(22):13198–13205.

16. Lein P, et al. Osteogenic protein-1 induces dendritic growth in rat sympathetic neurons. Neuron 1995; 15(3):597–605.

17. Withers GS, et al. Bone morphogenetic protein-7 enhances dendritic growth and receptivity to innervation in cultured hippocampal neurons. Eur J Neurosci 2000; 12(1):106–116.

18. Kawamata T, et al. Intracisternal osteogenic protein-1 enhances functional recovery following focal stroke. Neuroreport 1998; 9(7):1441–1445.

19. Ren J, et al. Time window of intracisternal osteogenic protein-1 in enhancing functional recovery after stroke. Neuropharmacology 2000; 39(5):860–865.

20. Kawamata T, Finklestein SP. Single administration of OP-1 improves recovery following stroke. Soc Neurosci Abstr 1998.

21. Ke Chen SPF. Neurotrophic factors. In: Cy H, ed. Ischemic Stroke: From basic concepts to new drug development. Basel: Kraeger, 1998, pp 116–126.

22. Shigeno T, et al. Amelioration of delayed neuronal death in the hippocampus by nerve growth factor. J Neurosci 1991; 11(9):2914–2919.

23. Tanaka K, et al. Effect of NGF on delayed neuronal death after cerebral ischemia. Acta Neurochir 1994; 129:64–71.

24. Olsson T, Donaldson LF, Henriksson BG, Seckl JR. Glucocorticoid receptor and NGF I-A gene expression are induced in the hippocampus after environmental enrichment in adult rats. Mol Brain Res 1998; 23:349–353.

25. Dahlqvist P, et al. Environmental enrichment alters nerve growth factor-induced gene A and glucocorticoid receptor messenger RNA expression after middle cerebral artery occlusion in rats. Neuroscience 1999; 93(2):527–535.

26. Kolb B, et al. Nerve growth factor treatment prevents dendritic atrophy and promotes recovery of function after cortical injury. Neuroscience 1997; 76(4):1139–1151.

27. Johansson BB. Neurotrophic factors and transplants. In: Goldstein LB, ed. Restorative Neurology: Advances in Pharmacotherapy for Recovery after Stroke. Armkonk, NY: Futura Publishing Co., 1998.

28. Mailing HM, Achaieson G. Righting and other postural activity in low-decerebrate and spinal cats after D-amphetamine. J Neurophys 1946; 9:379–386.

29. Feeney DM, Gonzalez A, Law WA. Amphetamine, haloperidol, and experience interact to affect rate of recovery after motor cortex injury. Science 1982; 217(4562): 855–857.

30. Hurwitz BE, et al. Amphetamine promotes recovery from sensory-motor integration deficit after thrombotic infarction of the primary somatosensory rat cortex. Stroke 1991; 22(5):648–654.

31. Crisostomo EA, et al. Evidence that amphetamine with physical therapy promotes recovery of motor function in stroke patients. Ann Neurol 1988; 23(1):94–97.

32. Walker-Batson D, et al. Amphetamine paired with physical therapy accelerates motor recovery after stroke. Further evidence. Stroke 1995; 26(12):2254–2259.

33. Walker-Batson. Pharmacotherapy in treatment of aphasia. In: Restorative Neurology: Advances in Pharmacotherapy for Recovery after Stroke. Armonk, NY: Futura Publishing Co, 1998.

34. Sutton RL. Intracerebral chromaffin cell autografts accelerate functional recovery in adult cats with unilateral frontal cortex ablation. Brain Dys 1989; 2:201–209.

35. Boyeson MG, Feeney DM. Intraventricular norepinephrine facilitates motor recovery following sensorimotor cortex injury. Pharmacol Biochem Behav 1990; 35(3): 497–501.

36. Dietrich WD, et al. Influence of amphetamine treatment on somatosensory function of the normal and infarcted rat brain. Stroke 1990; 21(suppl 11):III147–III150.

37. Stroemer RP, Kent TA, Hulsebosch CE. Enhanced neocortical neural sprouting, synaptogenesis, and behavioral recovery with D-amphetamine therapy after neocortical infarction in rats [see comments]. Stroke 1998; 29(11):2381–2393; discussion 2393–2395.

38. Gold PE, Delanoy RL, Merrin J. Modulation of long-term potentiation by peripherally administered amphetamine and epinephrine. Brain Res 1984; 305(1):103–107.

39. Stenevi U, Bjorklund A, Svendgaard NA. Transplantation of central and peripheral monoamine neurons to the adult rat brain: techniques and conditions for survival. Brain Res 1976; 114(1):1–20.

40. Bjorklund A, Stenevi U, Svendgaard N. Growth of transplanted monoaminergic neurones into the adult hippocampus along the perforant path. Nature 1976; 262(5571): 787–790.

41. Svendgaard NA, Bjorklund A, Stenevi U. Regeneration of central cholinergic neurones in the adult rat brain. Brain Res 1976; 102(1):1–22.

42. Lund RD, Hauschka SD. Transplanted neural tissue develops connections with host rat brain. Science 1976; 193(4253):582–584.

43. McKay R. Stem cells in the central nervous system. Science 1997; 276(5309):66–71.

44. Martinez-Serrano A, Bjorklund A. Immortalized neural progenitor cells for CNS gene transfer and repair. Trends Neurosci 1997; 20(11):530–538.

45. Westerman KA, Leboulch P. Reversible immortalization of mammalian cells mediated by retroviral transfer and site-specific recombination. Proc Natl Acad Sci USA 1996; 93(17):8971–8976.

46. Lundberg C, et al. Conditionally immortalized neural progenitor cell lines integrate and differentiate after grafting to the adult rat striatum. A combined autoradiographic and electron microscopic study. Brain Res 1996; 737(1–2):295–300.

47. Sinden JD, et al. Recovery of spatial learning by grafts of a conditionally immortalized hippocampal neuroepithelial cell line into the ischaemia-lesioned hippocampus. Neuroscience 1997; 81(3):599–608.

48. Goslin K, et al. Development of neuronal polarity: GAP-43 distinguishes axonal from dendritic growth cones. Nature 1988; 336(6200):672–674.

49. Palmer TD, et al. Fibroblast growth factor-2 activates a latent neurogenic program in neural stem cells from diverse regions of the adult CNS. J Neurosci 1999; 19(19): 8487–8497.

50. Palmer TD, Takahashi J, Gage FH. The adult rat hippocampus contains primordial neural stem cells. Mol Cell Neurosci 1997; 8(6):389–404.

51. Kirschenbaum B, et al. In vitro neuronal production and differentiation by precursor cells derived from the adult human forebrain. Cereb Cortex 1994; 4(6):576–589.

52. Johansson CB, et al. Neural stem cells in the adult human brain. Exp Cell Res 1999; 253(2):733–736.

53. Johe KK, et al. Single factors direct the differentiation of stem cells from the fetal and adult central nervous system. Genes Dev 1996; 10(24):3129–3140.

54. Roy NS, et al. In vitro neurogenesis by progenitor cells isolated from the adult human hippocampus [see comments]. Nat Med 2000; 6(3):271–277.

55. Craig CG, et al. In vivo growth factor expansion of endogenous subependymal neural precursor cell populations in the adult mouse brain. J Neurosci 1996; 16(8):2649–2658.

56. Kempermann G, Kuhn HG, Gage FH. More hippocampal neurons in adult mice living in an enriched environment. Nature 1997; 386(6624):493–495.

57. Gould E, Tanapat P. Lesion-induced proliferation of neuronal progenitors in the dentate gyrus of the adult rat. Neuroscience 1997; 80(2):427–436.

58. Liu J, et al. Increased neurogenesis in the dentate gyrus after transient global ischemia in gerbils. J Neurosci 1998; 18(19):7768–7778.

59. Kleppner SR, et al. Transplanted human neurons derived from a teratocarcinoma

cell line (NTera-2) mature, integrate, and survive for over 1 year in the nude mouse brain. J Comp Neurol 1995; 357(4):618–632.

60. Borlongan CV, et al. Viability and survival of hNT neurons determine degree of functional recovery in grafted ischemic rats. Neuroreport 1998; 9(12):2837–2842.

61. Bonn D. First cell transplant aimed to reverse stroke damage [news]. Lancet 1998; 352(9122):119.

62. Rosenberg MB, et al. Grafting genetically modified cells to the damaged brain: restorative effects of NGF expression. Science 1988; 242(4885):1575–1578.

63. Fisher LJ, et al. Survival and function of intrastriatally grafted primary fibroblasts genetically modified to produce L-dopa. Neuron 1991; 6(3):371–380.

64. Liu Y, et al. Transplants of fibroblasts genetically modified to express BDNF promote regeneration of adult rat rubrospinal axons and recovery of forelimb function. J Neurosci 1999; 19(11):4370–4387.

65. Pechan PA, et al. Genetically modified fibroblasts producing NGF protect hippocampal neurons after ischemia in the rat. Neuroreport 1995; 6(4):669–672.

66. Andsberg G, et al. Amelioration of ischaemia-induced neuronal death in the rat striatum by NGF-secreting neural stem cells. Eur J Neurosci 1998; 10(6):2026–2036.

67. Nairne SP. Animal-to-Human Transplants: The Ethics of Xenotransplantation. London: Nuffield Council on Bioethics, 1996.

68. Diacrin. Fetal pig cells implanted in stroke patient. Press release. September 22, 1999.

11
Cost-Benefit Issues

Graeme J. Hankey
Royal Perth Hospital and University of Western Australia,
Perth, Western Australia, Australia

I. THE INCREASING NEED FOR ECONOMIC EVALUATION OF STROKE CARE

Increasingly, modern health care provision and utilization requires consideration and evaluation of the economic aspects. This is no more evident than in the care of stroke patients, where costs are not only high but also rising, owing to a combination of factors. These include the current high annual incidence of stroke and prevalence of disabled stroke survivors, the rising absolute number of incident cases of stroke and prevalent disabled survivors as the population ages, and the rapid development and application of new and expensive diagnostic technologies (e.g., magnetic resonance imaging) and treatments (e.g., tissue plasminogen activator, clopidogrel, carotid endarterectomy, and stenting) for stroke patients. These high and rising costs have prompted a search for greater efficiency in the delivery of stroke care. Not only do research grant funding bodies now encourage an economic evaluation of new health technologies and treatments (1), but in some countries there is now a need to actually demonstrate relative cost-effectiveness of new health technologies and treatments. In Australia, economic evaluation is a requirement for public sector funding of new drugs (2), and in the American state of Oregon, economic evaluation has been used to define what services should be included in Medicare (3).

II. TYPES OF ECONOMIC EVALUATION

Programs funded by the public sector have primarily been evaluated by a cost-benefit analysis, which has measured costs and benefits (outcomes) in monetary terms. Other forms, such as cost-effectiveness and cost-utility analysis, have been developed to analyze outcomes that are measured in health-related terms, such as disability after stroke or quality adjusted life years (QALY) (4). The results of such studies are usually expressed as ratios of cost to outcome. Because of the increasing demand for economic evaluation of health care, coupled with several difficulties associated with the definition, measurement and valuation of costs, benefits, effectiveness, and utility, there have been recent efforts to standardize the methods of economic evaluation (5,6).

   In the field of stroke care, there remains a need for standardized methods of evaluating the economic burden of stroke (7,8). Among 18 studies from eight countries published between 1990 and 1998 on the economic burden of stroke worldwide, the majority of studies (83%) based the calculation of total costs of stroke on the number of prevalent stroke cases in one year, and half of the studies reported the cost of stroke care in terms of national direct costs (9). Discounting was applied in a minority of cases (22%) while sensitivity analyses were performed in only three studies (17%). Few studies provided sufficient detail to allow critical appraisal of the cost calculations, and generally accepted aspects of health economic methodology were neglected in many studies. Consequently, it is difficult, if not impossible, to compare the national stroke costs because of the use of different study methodologies, as well as variations in stroke epidemiology and treatment patterns. For example, estimates of the cost of stroke are influenced by the functional status and prognosis for long-term survival of patients and carers before the stroke, the type and severity of the stroke, and the long-term outcome and requirements of patients and carers (which, in turn, can be influenced by specific interventions/treatments) (10). Nevertheless, the well-conducted burden-of-illness studies can provide reasonably robust estimates of national stroke expenditure that may assist local decision makers in allocating resources. The data from published studies are presented below.

III. THE COST OF STROKE

A. Types of Costs

There are several types of costs of stroke, such as the total costs, direct costs, indirect costs, and lifetime costs of first stroke, that are important to distinguish.

   The direct costs are related to the diagnosis and treatment (including rehabilitation) of stroke, and include not only hospital costs but also direct costs related to long-term care of disabled survivors.

The indirect costs are related to the economic and social impact upon patients, their caregivers, and the nation, such as loss of family income and national productivity, which dominate the lifetime costs of stroke.

B. Total Costs of Stroke

Current data suggest that stroke accounts for 3.4–4.6% of the total cost of health care throughout the world (9,11–19).

In the United States, the total cost of stroke in 1997 was estimated to be US$40.9 billion; and in 1998 it was estimated to be US$43.3 billion (20,21). In Australia, the total cost of stroke in 1993–1994 was estimated to be Aus$1.7 billion. The cost (direct and indirect) of each stroke was estimated to average about Aus$40,000, which is about Aus$50,000 currently (Table 1) (22).

Table 1 Estimated Direct and Indirect Costs of Stroke in Australia (22)

Direct costs	No. patients	Cost ($ million)
Acute care	29,556	175
Nursing homes (new admissions)	10,735	418
Rehabilitation	5,911	72
Other	3.1 million	77
Outpatient attendances		
GP visits		
Allied health interventions		
Hospital transport		
Home modifications		
District nursing		
Home help		
Meals on wheels		
Community health care		
Respite care		
Total direct costs		742
Indirect costs		Cost ($ million)
Lost earnings of patient due to premature morbidity		582
Lost earnings of spouses/partner due to morbidity of patient		345
Total indirect costs		927
TOTAL	41,477	$1669 million
Cost per stroke		$40,243

C. Direct Costs of Stroke

Most studies that have attempted to define the costs of stroke care have focused on direct hospital costs because it is difficult to quantify the indirect costs related to loss of productivity and reorganization of family life (12,23–28). In general, the direct costs have been reported to account for between 42% and 90% of total stroke costs (9). In the United States, the direct cost of stroke is about $26.2 billion per year, which is about two-thirds of the total costs, and represents an average cost per case of about US$50,000 (20,21). In Australia, the direct cost of stroke is about Aus$742 million, which is about 45% of the total costs of stroke, and represents an average cost per case of about Aus$18,500 (22).

1. Hospital Costs

As a considerable proportion of the direct costs are related to inpatient hospital costs, the estimates of direct costs vary from country to country depending on the proportion of patients admitted to hospital, the nature and intensity of hospital care, and the length of stay in hospital (including rehabilitation hospital) and nursing homes (9). For example, in the United Kingdom, only 55% of acute stroke patients are admitted to hospital, whereas in Australia (Perth) and Italy (Perugia) about 80% are admitted, and in Sweden about 95% (29). The average length of stay in hospital is relatively short in the United States (particularly since the introduction of managed care), and less so in the Netherlands (27 days), when compared with countries such as Sweden (59 days) and Scotland (65 days) (16).

The cost of hospitalization in the acute phase of stroke has been estimated to amount to about 20% of the total direct cost of stroke management in the United States (13), whereas in Europe and other parts of the world, with longer lengths of hospital stay, it absorbs 25–85% of the sums spent during the first year postictus (10,12,23,24,30).

In one analysis of individual hospital expenses (in the United Kingdom), nursing costs accounted for about 81% of the inpatient hospital costs of stroke, while 19% covered the remaining costs (of which 40% was for instrumental examinations, 31% for general treatment, 19% for physicians, and 10% for specific drugs) (31).

Very little information is available on rehabilitation unit costs, and all is based on isolated experiences. Similarly, the cost of nursing home care, which can be substantial for disabled stroke patients, is not reflected in most studies. In 1990 in the United States, there were 101,900 nursing home admissions attributable to stroke, and the mean length of stay was 432 days resulting in a net current cost of about US$30,000 per patient admission (32). The mean length of stay is similar in the Netherlands (470 days).

Very few cost-of-illness studies have evaluated which patient and physician factors influence the cost of stroke, although these may dictate whether and which

expensive diagnostic tools and treatments are used (25–28). In the United States, the inpatient costs of subarachnoid hemorrhage are estimated to be twice as great as those of parenchymal haemorrhage and four times as great as those of ischemic stroke (25). Among ischemic strokes, severe cases that survive cost significantly more than milder cases (25,30). Indeed, the lifetime costs of caring for disabled stroke survivors coupled with loss of productivity far exceed the costs of care in the first year. Furthermore, because survivors of recurrent stroke tend to be more disabled than survivors of first-ever stroke, the costs of recurrent-stroke survivors are greater than those of first-stroke survivors (33). With regard to the specialty of the attending physician, one study found that neurologists treating stroke patients were significantly more expensive (in terms of direct costs) than other physicians but their patients achieved significantly better outcomes (34).

D. Indirect Costs

Indirect costs account for a consistent part of the lifetime cost for all types of stroke and are related not only to the patient's condition but also to the lives of the family and caregiver.

In the United States, the indirect cost of stroke in 1997 was estimated to be US$14.7 billion, mainly due to loss of output (20). Although loss of productivity is a major indirect cost, it is difficult to evaluate, and has therefore been reported in only about half of all studies (9). In these studies, only a minority (about 20%) of patients of working age return to work, and not always to the same job, often needing to readapt to their disabilities and the new conditions (35,36).

Another indirect cost is reduced quality of life due to loss of social activity, lack of social support, functional disability, and depression among patients. Other determinants of quality of life include age, social class, and cardiovascular diseases. However, in one study the most important factor related to quality of life in long-term stroke survivors, ahead of health and functional status, was the satisfaction of the next-of-kin (37). Frequently, the next-of-kin is the caregiver. In the Perth community stroke study, 43% of stroke patients had survived more than 1 year and were living at home dependent on a caregiver. More than half (55%) of the caregivers of these patients were emotionally distressed, particularly if the patients were affected by dementia or abnormal behavior. The feeling expressed by caregivers included anxiety (58%), depression (50%), fear (35%), frustration (32%), resentment (29%), impatience (25%), and guilt (36%) (38).

E. Lifetime Costs

In 1996, the lifetime cost of stroke per person was estimated to be US$103,576 (32). However, the lifetime cost per person was higher for patients with subarach-

noid hemorrhage because of not only the higher direct cost but also the greater indirect costs as a result of the earlier mean age of onset (32).

A more recent estimate has been based on a stroke economic model derived from short-term clinical trial data and several Markov submodels predicting patient transitions among various locations over time (10). The cost of managing a stroke over the first 12 weeks was estimated to be about US$13,650 per patient on average, of which hospitalization accounted for about 73%, rehabilitation center another 16%, outpatient services 7%, and nursing home the remaining 4% (10). For patients who survived to the end of the trials, the remaining lifetime costs of stroke were estimated to be about US$125,000 if there remains a major impairment at 12 weeks compared with about US$46,000 when there is only a minor impairment (10). The average lifetime costs of stroke for all patients treated initially, accounting for patients who died within the first 2 weeks, is estimated to be about US$66,000 (10). When short-term costs are included, the total lifetime cost of managing a stroke patient increases to nearly US$82,000. Thus long-term costs account for more than 80% of the total stroke costs. Institutional care is estimated to account for 26% of the total stroke costs (hospital 18.4%, nursing home 3.2%, and rehabilitation center 4.3%) (10). Most of the lifetime costs (88%) were accounted for by patients who went home or to a retirement home (10). Although this may seem counterintuitive, most of the patients who suffer a stroke return home, and although nursing homes are expensive, their patients tend to die earlier and therefore stop contributing to the costs.

IV. THE INCREASING NEED TO PREVENT STROKE AND OPTIMIZE ACUTE AND LONG-TERM CARE

The burden of stroke, measured in terms of social and economic impact, highlights the need to minimize it, and thus contain the costs of stroke. It is not only crucial to reduce the incidence of stroke, particularly as the population ages (by effective primary and secondary prevention strategies), but also to reduce the major direct costs of stroke (hospital care, particularly for disabled stroke survivors). This involves not only a rational allocation of available resources but also the active adoption of evidence-based, efficient, and cost-effective interventions, and implementation as part of an organized and uniform approach to stroke care (e.g., critical pathways) (39,40).

V. DELAYED AND INCOMPLETE APPLICATION OF EFFECTIVE INTERVENTIONS INTO PRACTICE

An emerging issue is stroke prevention is that interventions shown to be effective in clinical trials are not being used, or are being used suboptimally (41). There

are many possible explanations for this underuse, such as the failure of new research results to reach practicing clinicians.

VI. THE IMPACT OF RESOURCES AND COSTS ON CLINICAL DECISIONS AND VICE VERSA

Another important reason why treatment patterns are slow to change relates to resources and cost, ranging from concerns about inappropriate use of societal resources to more immediate concerns of organizations and individuals about their financial well-being. The decisions by a formulary committee to make a new treatment available, by a clinician to recommend it to a patient, and by a patient to use it have different cost implications for different decision makers. At one end of the spectrum, the patient is concerned about out-of-pocket expenses. At the other end, the insurance company is concerned about incurring definite short-term drug costs to possibly, but not definitely, realize a long-term savings from diminishing morbidity and mortality of disease. Assessing the cost impact of a new treatment, and thus the financial incentives faced by decision makers, is difficult but nevertheless pivotal to understanding and influencing real-world treatment decisions (41).

VII. WHEN IS AN INTERVENTION GOOD VALUE?

Assessing whether an intervention is good value for money depends on the perspective taken (e.g., whose values and whose money?) and how value is measured. Three key areas are relevant: evidence of effectiveness, equity, and patient choice (42).

> Effectiveness means the extent to which the intervention (e.g., an acute stroke treatment) achieves the desired effect (e.g., the proportion of patients who survived free of a disability). Clearly, ineffective interventions should not be purchased or provided. However, clinicians are usually faced with making decisions where evidence is insufficient, and thus they vary in their practice, often basing decisions on the likely effectiveness, taking into account the quality of the evidence.
>
> Equity: the basic principle of equity is that equals should be treated equally, with no discrimination on any grounds.
>
> Patient choice: evidence for the effectiveness of interventions must be in the form of improvements in outcome measures that are important to patients. If such evidence is available, then patients should not be able to choose an ineffective intervention (as this would deny another patient

access to an effective treatment) but they can choose between interventions of similar efficiency.

"Value" is a judgment on how valuable the desired effect is in the relevant individual(s) relative to the value of other interventions. Three factors are particularly relevant to the value of an intervention: the additional length of life (and particularly quality of life) that the intervention brings, the contribution that the intervention makes to the patient's well-being, and the level of need of those who benefit from the intervention.

VIII. WHAT ACUTE STROKE INTERVENTIONS ARE GOOD VALUE?

The acute stroke interventions for which there is reasonable evidence of effectiveness (and ineffectiveness) include stroke units, aspirin, thrombolysis, and heparin; the evidence for all other acute medical therapies, specific rehabilitation therapies, and surgery for primary intracerebral hemorrhage (PICH) is inadequate.

A. Stroke Units

Compared with conventional care in a general medical ward, organized care in a stroke unit reduces death and dependency at 1 year after stroke from 62.0% to 56.4% (Table 2) (44). This is a relative risk reduction (RRR) of 9% [95% confidence interval (CI): 4–14%] and an absolute risk reduction (ARR) of 5.6%. The ARR of 5.6% means that treating 1000 acute stroke patients in a stroke unit would prevent about 56 patients from dying or becoming dependent compared to treating 1000 patients in a general ward. The number needed to treat (NNT) in a stroke unit to prevent one from dying or becoming dependent is 18.

The potential impact in the population depends not just on the effectiveness of stroke units, but also on their availability and accessibility. About 80% of acute stroke patients are admitted to hospital in Australia (Perth) and Europe (Perugia, Italy) but, as stated above, rates vary from as low as 55% (United Kingdom) to as high as 95% (Sweden) (29). If stroke units are available to accommodate all—say 80%—of acute stroke patients who present to hospital in the population then they would avoid about 8.3% of all people who die or become dependent each year after stroke in the population (45).

There are insufficient data on the cost of stroke unit care but at least it does not seem to increase length of stay (44). Because the main costs of inpatient stroke care are due to "hotel" and staffing costs, length of stay is a reasonable surrogate measure of costs, assuming staffing levels are relatively constant (31).

Table 2 Summary of the Effectiveness and Cost of Acute Treatment for Stroke Patients

Intervention	Target population (% of all strokes)	Death or dependency,		Relative risk reduction (RRR) (95% CI)	Absolute risk reduction (ARR)	No. deaths/dependents avoided per 1000 patients treated	No. patients needed to treat to avoid one death or dependency (NNT)	Approximate cost per death or dependency avoided (Aust$)
		Control	Intervention					
Stroke unit	<80%	62.0%	56.4%	9% (4–14%)	5.6%	56	18	? Nil additional
Aspirin	80%	47.0%	45.8%	3% (1–5%)	1.2%	12	83	$83
Thrombolysis	<10%	62.7%	56.4%	10% (5–15%)	6.3%	63	16	$36,000 (tissue plasminogen activator) $3,200 (streptokinase)

If so, the cost of stroke unit care should not be any more than care in a general ward, and may even be less.

B. Aspirin

Aspirin, 160–300 mg daily, reduces death and dependency from 47.0% to 45.8% (46–48), a RRR of 3% (95% CI: 1–5%) and an ARR of 1.2% (Table 2). Therefore, treating 1000 ischemic stroke patients prevents about 12 dying or becoming dependent. The NNT is 83.

In the general population, about 85% of all stroke patients have an *ischemic* stroke each year. As aspirin may be contraindicated or not tolerated in about 5% of patients, it could be given to about 95% of ischemic stroke patients each year, and save about 1.2% from death or dependency, which is about 1.8% of all people who die or become dependent each year after stroke (45).

The cost of treating acute stroke patients with 300 mg aspirin daily for 2 weeks is about Aus$1 per patient (7), which totals Aus$83 to prevent one from dying or becoming dependent.

C. Thrombolysis

Intravenous thrombolysis within 6 hr of onset of ischemic stroke reduces death and dependency from 62.7% to 56.4% (49), a RRR of 10% (95% CI: 5–15%) and an ARR of 6.3% (Table 2). If so, treating 1000 ischemic stroke patients prevents about 63 from dying or becoming dependent. The NNT is 16. For patients presenting within 3 hr, intravenous (IV) tPA reduces death and dependency from 71.6% to 57.7%, a RRR of 19.4% and ARR of 13.9% (49). Treating 1000 patients prevents 139 from death or dependency. The NNT is 7.

However, thrombolysis is also hazardous. The risk of early death (within 14 days of stroke) is increased from 11.8% (control) to 20.9% (thrombolysis), a 9.1% absolute excess [odds ratio (OR): 2.0, 95% CI: 1.6–2.5] among all patients treated within 6 hr. This is because of an excess of early symptomatic intracranial hemorrhage [2.5% (control) vs. 9.4% (thrombolysis); OR: 3.5, 95% CI: 2.8–4.4], and fatal intracranial hemorrhage [1.1% (control) vs. 5.8% (thrombolysis); OR: 4.1, 95% CI: 2.9–5.9] (49).

In North America tPA has been approved in a dose of 0.9 mg/kg within 3 hr of acute ischemic stroke. International trials are planned to identify the clinical and imaging characteristics of the minority of patients who are harmed (about 9%) and helped (about 15%), and the majority whose outcome is not influenced by thrombolysis.

At present, thrombolysis is likely to be accessible to, and appropriate for, only about 2–3% of all acute stroke patients (i.e., those who present to an appropriate facility within a few hours of onset, are competently assessed, and have no contraindication to thrombolysis, including a CT scan that rules out intracranial hemorrhage). Indeed, a recent audit in Cleveland, 1 year after the FDA approved IV tissue plasminogen activator (tPA), found that only 1.1% of stroke patients actually received it (50). Assuming very optimistically that 10% of stroke patients really can be treated with thrombolysis, this will save about only 1.2% of patients who die or become dependent each year after stroke (45).

Treating 16 patients with r-tPA, at Aus$2250 per 50 mg vial, totals about Aus$36,000 to prevent one from dying or becoming dependent. If streptokinase is as effective as tPA, then the cost, at Aus$200 per 1.5 million i.u. injection (45), totals Aus$3,200 to prevent one from dying or becoming dependent.

D. Heparin

The most recent systematic review of heparin or heparinoid in acute ischemic stroke indicates that routine treatment does not reduce the risk of death or dependency (RRR: 1%, 95% Cl: −5–6%), despite significantly reducing the odds of deep vein thrombosis (OR: 0.21, 95% Cl: 0.15–0.39) and pulmonary embolism (OR: 0.61, 95% Cl: 0.45–0.83) (51,52).

E. Neuroprotection

Trials of neuroprotective agents (e.g., selfotel, aptiganel, chlormethiazole, tirila-d, lubeluzole) have failed to identify a favorable treatment effect, and some e revealed dose-limiting intolerance and systemic adverse effects, such as essive sedation and hypertension (53). Trials of other agents (e.g., magne-) are in progress.

ther Medical Treatments

lution, corticosteroids, and glycerol have not been proven effective.

gery for Primary Intracerebral Hemorrhage

r PICH is associated with a nonsignificant increase in odds of death ency at 6 months (OR: 1.23, 95% Cl: 0.77–1.98) (54). Further evi-ongoing trials is awaited.

SECONDARY STROKE PREVENTION ENTIONS ARE GOOD VALUE?

roke prevention interventions for which there is reasonable evi-eness have been discussed elsewhere (55,56).

X. CONCLUSION

Although limited, the available evidence suggests that the cost of organized, multidisciplinary care in a stroke unit is not any greater than conventional general medical ward care. Stroke unit care is therefore likely to be a highly cost-effective initiative, given that it has a similar absolute treatment effect as thrombolysis, and is appropriate for so many more acute stroke patients. The development of an organized approach to stroke care must therefore be the major priority in any endeavor to deliver a stroke service and this itself will facilitate the best use of thrombolysis and randomized controlled trials of other promising interventions. Although aspirin has only a very modest effect, it is extremely cost-effective (about $83 to prevent one death or dependent stroke survivor) because it is widely applicable and accessible, inexpensive, and relatively safe. Thrombolysis is less cost-effective, but an accurate analysis requires considerably more data than from a total of only about 5000 patients in 17 trials (49).

The highest priority for providers of a stroke service must be to establish a stroke unit and multidisciplinary team that delivers organized stroke care. Acute ischemic stroke patients should be immediately started on aspirin, 300 mg daily, and—if possible—many entered into further trials of thrombolysis and other promising treatments. After the acute phase, aspirin should be continued in a lower dose, 75 mg daily; smoking discouraged; high blood pressure treated initially with a diuretic; and fibrillating ischemic stroke/TIA survivors anticoagulated long term with warfarin, or given aspirin if anticoagulation is not sensible (55). Statins are probably indicated in patients who already have symptomatic coronary heart disease. Adding dipyridamole to aspirin, substituting clopidogrel for aspirin, and carotid endarterectomy are all expensive interventions to prevent stroke, but if ways could be found to focus them on those patients at particularly high risk of stroke, they would become more affordable.

REFERENCES

1. Drummond MF. Economic Analysis Alongside Controlled Trials. Leeds: NHS utive, 1994.
2. Commonwealth of Australia. Guidelines to the Pharmaceutical Industry on the aration of Submissions to the Pharmaceutical Benefits Advisory Committee ing Submissions Involving Economic Analysis. Canberra: Department of Housing, and Community services, 1992.
3. Tengs TO. An evaluation of Oregon's Medicaid rationing algorithms. He 1996; 5:171–181.
4. Palmer S, Byford S, Raftery J. Types of economic evaluation. Br Med J 1349.
5. Drummond MF, Jefferson TO, on behalf of the BMJ economic Evaluation

Party. Guidelines for authors and peer reviewers of economic submissions to the BMJ. Br Med J 1996; 313:275–283.

6. Raftery J. Economic evaluation: an introduction. Br Med J 1998; 316:1013–1014.

7. Holloway RG, Benesch CG, Rahilly CR, Courtright CE. A systematic review of cost-effectiveness research of stroke evaluation and treatment. Stroke 1999; 30:1340–1349.

8. Ebrahim S. Systematic review of cost-effectiveness research of stroke evaluation and treatment. Stroke 1999; 30:2759–2760.

9. Perri LR. A review of the economic burden of stroke. Stroke 2000; 31:313 (abstract P85).

10. Caro JJ, Huybrechts KF, for the Stroke Economic Analysis Group. Stroke treatment economic model (STEM). Predicting long-terms costs from functional status. Stroke 1999; 30:2574–2579.

11. Drummond MF, Ward GH. The financial burden of stroke and the economic evaluation of treatment alternatives. In: Rose FC, ed. Stroke: Epidemiological, Therapeutic and Socioeconomic Aspects. London: Royal Society of Medicine Services Ltd, 1986.

12. Bergman L, van der Meulen JHP, Limburg M, Habbema JDF. Costs of medical care after first-ever stroke in the Netherlands. Stroke 1995; 26:1830–1836.

13. Dobkin B. The economic impact of stroke. Neurology 1995; 45:S6–S9.

14. Evers SMAA, Engel GL, Ament AJHA. Cost of stroke in the Netherlands from a societal perspective. Stroke 1997; 28:1375–1381.

15. Forbes JF. Cost of stroke. Scott Med J 1993; 38:S4–S5

16. Isard PA, Forbes JF. The cost of stroke to the National Health Service in Scotland. Cerebrovasc Dis 1992; 2:47–50.

17. Scott WG, Scott H. Ischaemic stroke in New Zealand: an economic study. NZ Med J 1994; 107:443–446.

18. Weill C, Schneider T. The cost of cerebrovascular accidents in France in 1982. In. In: Rose FC, ed. Stroke: Epidemiological, Therapeutic and Socioeconomic Aspects. London: Royal Society of Medicine Services Ltd, 1986, pp 147–162.

19. Porsdal V, Boysen G. Cost-of-illness studies of stroke. Cerebrovascular Diseases 1997; 7:258–63.

20. American Heart Association. Heart and Stroke Facts Statistics: 1997 Statistical Supplement. Dallas: American Heart Association, 1997.

21. American Heart Association. Economic cost of cardiovascular diseases. URL: http://www.americanheart.org/scientific/ HSstats98/10econom.html.

22. National Health and Medical Research Council (NHMRC) Quality of Care and Health Outcomes Committee. Clinical Practice Guidelines: Prevention of Stroke— The Role of Anticoagulants, Antiplatelet Agents and Carotid Endarterectomy. NHMRC, Canberra 1996, p. 4.

23. Thorngren M, Westling B. Utilisation of health care resources after stroke: a population-based study of 258 hospitalised cases followed during the first year. Acta Neurol Scand 1991; 84:303–310.

24. Smurawska LT, Alexandrov AV, Bladin CF, Norris JW. Cost of acute stroke care in Toronto, Canada. Stroke 1994; 25:1628–1631.

25. Holloway RG, Witter DM, Lawton KB, Lipscomb J, Samsa G. Inpatient costs of

specific cerebrovascular events at five academic medical centres. Neurology 1996;
46:854–860.

26. Leibson CL, Hu T, Brown RD, Hass SL, O'Fallon WM, Whisnant JP. Utilisation
    of acute care services in the year before and after first stroke: a population-based
    study. Neurology 1996; 46:861–869.

27. Jorgensen HS, Nakayama H, Raaschou HO, Olsen TS. Acute stroke care and rehabil-
    itation: an analysis of the direct cost and its clinical and social determinants. The
    Copenhagen Stroke Study. Stroke 1997; 28:1138–1141.

28. Mamoli A, Censori B, Casto L, Sileo C, Cesana B, Camerlingo M. An analysis of
    the costs of ischaemic stroke in an Italian stroke unit. Neurology 1999; 53:112–116.

29. Sudlow CLM, Warlow CP. Comparable studies of the incidence of stroke and its
    pathological subtypes. Results from an International Collaboration. Stroke 1997; 28:
    491–499.

30. Terent A, Marke LA, Asplund K, Norrving B, Jonsson E, Wester PO. Costs of stroke
    in Sweden: a national perspective. Stroke 1994; 25:2363–2369.

31. Dennis M, Wellwood I, McGregor K, Dent J, Forbes J. What are the major compo-
    nents of the cost of caring for stroke patients in hospital in the UK? Cerebrovasc
    Dis 1995; 5:243.

32. Taylor TN, Davis PH, Torner JC, Holmes J, Meyer JW, Jacobsen MF. Lifetime cost
    of stroke in the United States. Stroke 1996; 27:1459–1466.

33. O'Brien JA, Pierce D, Caro JJ. The importance of additional events in estimating
    the costs of stroke. Stroke 2000; 31:324 (abstract P136).

34. Mitchell JB, Ballard DJ, Whisnant JP, Ammering CJ, Samsa GP, Matchar DB. What
    role do neurologists play in determining the costs and outcomes of stroke patients?
    Stroke 1996; 27:1937–1943.

35. Cornes P, Roy CW. Vocational Rehabilitation Index assessment of rehabilitation
    medicine service patients. Int Disabil Stud 1991; 13:5–8.

36. Angeleri F, Angeleri VA, Foschi N, Giaquinto S, Nolfe G. The influence of depres-
    sion, social activity, and family stress on functional outcome after stroke. Stroke
    1993; 24:1478–1483.

37. King RB. Quality of life after stroke. Stroke 1996; 27:1467–1472.

38. Anderson CS, Linto JRN, Stewart-Wynne EG. A population-based assessment of
    the impact and burden of caregiving for long-term stroke survivors. Stroke 1995;
    26:843–849.

39. Bowen J, Yaste C. Effect of a stroke protocol on hospital costs of stroke patients.
    Neurology 1994; 44:1961–1964.

40. Wentworth DA, Atkinson RP. Implementation of an acute stroke program decreases
    hospitalisation costs and length of stay. Stroke 1996; 27:1040–1043.

41. Sudlow M, Thomson R, Thwaites B, Rodgers H, Kenny RA. Prevalence of atrial
    fibrillation and eligibility for anticoagulants in the community. Lancet 1998; 352:
    1167–1171.

42. Matchar DB. The value of stroke prevention and treatment. Neurology 1988;
    51(suppl 3):S31–S35.

43. Hope T, Hicks N, Reynolds DJM, Crisp R, Griffiths S. Pationing and the health
    authority. Br Med J 1998; 317:1067–1069.

44. Stroke Unit Trialists' Collaboration. Organised in-patient (stroke unit) care after stroke (Cochrane Review). In: The Cochrane Library. Oxford: Update Software, Issue 1, 2002.

45. Hankey GJ, Warlow CP. Hankey GJ, Warlow CP. Treatment and secondary prevention of stroke: evidence, costs, and effects on individuals and populations. Lancet 1999; 354:1457–1463.

46. International Stroke Trial Collaborative Group. The International Stroke Trial (IST): a randomised trial of aspirin, subcutaneous heparin, both or neither among 19435 patients with acute ischaemic stroke. Lancet 1997; 349:1569–1581.

47. CAST (Chinese Acute Stroke Trial) Collaborative Group. CAST: a randomised placebo-controlled trial of early aspirin use in 20,000 patients with acute ischaemic stroke. Lancet 1997; 349:1641–1649.

48. Chen ZM, Sandercock PAG on behalf of the CAST and IST Collaborative Groups. Indications for early aspirin use in acute ischaemic stroke: A combined analysis of over 40,000 randomised patients (abstract). Stroke 1999; 30:243.

49. Wardlaw JM, del Zoppo G, Yamaguchi T. Thrombolysis for acute ischaemic stroke (Cochrane Review). In: The Cochrane Library. Oxford: Update Software, Issue 1, 2002.

50. Katzan IL, Furlan AJ, Way LE, Frank JI, Harper DL, Hinchey JA, Sila CA. A systematic audit of IV tPA in Cleveland Area Hospitals (abstract). Stroke 1999; 30: 266.

51. Gubitz G, Counsell C, Sandercock P, Signorini D. Anticoagulants for acute ischaemic stroke (Cochrane Review). In: The Cochrane Library. Oxford: Update Software, Issue 4, 1999.

52. Sandercock PAG, Gubitz G, Counsell C, Signorini D. Immediate anticoagulant therapy for acute ischaemic stroke. Part 1. A systematic review of 21 randomised trials of anticoagulant vs control, including 23,374 patients. (abstract). Stroke 1999; 30: 248.

53. Lees KR. Does neuroprotection improve stroke outcome? Lancet 1998; 351:1447–1448.

54. Hankey GJ, Hon C. Surgery for primary intracerebral haemorrhage: is it safe and effective? A systematic review of case series and randomised trials. Stroke 1997; 28:2126–2132.

55. Hankey GJ, Warlow CP. Treatment and secondary prevention of stroke: evidence, costs, and effects on individuals and populations. Lancet 1999; 354:1457–1463.

56. Hankey GJ. Health care issues, benefits, and costs. In: Bogousslavsky J, ed. Drug Therapy for Stroke Prevention. London: Taylor and Francis, 2001, 275–292.

12

Sphincter Disturbances in Stroke Patients

K. Diserens
University of Lausanne and Centre Hospitalier Universitaire Vaudois, Lausanne, Switzerland

A. T. Al-Khodairy
Clinique Romande de Réadaptation, Sion, Switzerland

I. INTRODUCTION

Cerebrovascular disease is the third most common cause of death and one of the most common causes of disability in the United States and Europe. Based on health interviews, it is estimated that 3.3 million Americans, representing 1.3% of the population, have symptomatic cerebrovascular disease, 39.4% of whom are limited in their daily activities (36). The prevalence of stroke in persons older than 65 years of age is estimated at approximately 60 per 1000, and, in persons older than 75, 95 per 1000 (35). The prevalence is also much higher in blacks than in whites (66). The annual incidence has been estimated at 6–12 per 1000 in individuals of 65–74 years and at 40 per 1000 in those over 85 years. Thrombosis, occlusion, and hemorrhage are the most common causes leading to variable-sized areas of ischemia and infarction in the brain, usually around the internal capsule (63). The highest risk factor for stroke is age, with 70% of all strokes occurring in individuals over the age of 65. Other risk factors include hypertension, cardiac disease, atrial fibrillation, diabetes mellitus, cigarette smoking, alcohol abuse, and hyperlipidemia (11,24,34).

Urinary incontinence affects 5–15% of elderly patients living in the community and over 50% of patients in institutions (46). After a stroke it was estimated that 38–60% of the patients present with urinary incontinence in the early recovery period (7,10,24) and that 28–29% of the survivors from cerebral and brainstem stroke will remain incontinent at 12 weeks (4,14,48). Stroke, a major cause of handicap in the adult population, may occur at an age when the patient may suffer from other causes of genitourinary problems such as benign hypertrophy of the prostate in the male patient or weakness of the pelvic floor in the female patient. It was estimated that 17% of stroke victims had preexisting urinary incontinence (7,14). The prevalence of fecal incontinence is 0.5–1.5% in the general population and approximately 10% in the elderly institutionalized patients (33,55). Forty percent of stroke victims present anorectal disturbances (23)

Management of incontinence is costly. It is estimated that $400 million is spent on adult diapers in the United States each year, whereas a total of $1–10 billion is spent annually in caring for patients with urinary incontinence (33,42,50). Neurogenic bladder and bowel can lead to medical complications including urinary tract infection, skin excoriation, development of renal and bladder calculi, and renal failure. Incontinence often results in embarrassment and a feeling of lost autonomy with serious social and psychological repercussion. The presence of bowel and bladder dysfunction is often a major factor in determining whether or not the patient may be discharged.

II. ANATOMY AND PHYSIOLOGY

A. Central Pathways (Fig. 1)

Stimulation studies in animals and the analysis of the effects of ablation and tumors in humans have revealed a number of areas in the brain with an influence on micturition (19). Developments in neurological investigation using electrical (53) or magnetic stimulation (5,28) of the motor cortex have helped in the further understanding of the relationship between the vesicourethral apparatus and the somatically innervated pelvic floor.

Since micturition is subject to social constraint, the cortical control of lower autonomic centers is highly developed in social animals. The areas involved in humans are the superior frontal gyrus and the adjacent anterior cingulate gyrus, which lie in the territory of the anterior cerebral and pericallosal arteries. Ischemic or hemorrhagic lesions in these territories diminish the awareness of vesical events, allowing the lower centers to act autonomously and thus promote incontinence. Local tumors may have the same effect, and similar manifestations occur in more generalized cerebral disorders such as cerebral atrophy and hydrocephalus. Lesions more posteriorly in the frontal region (paracentral lobule) may result in spasticity of the striated sphincters and levator ani, producing urinary retention (43).

The principal subcortical areas involved in the control of micturition are the septal region, the anterior hypothalamus, the pontine reticular formation, and

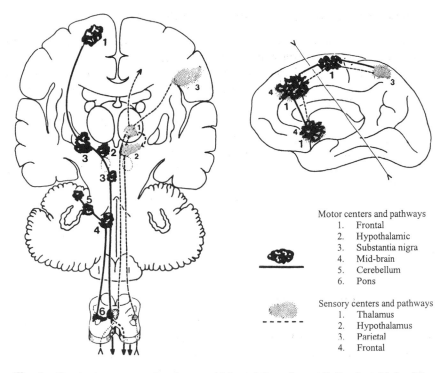

Fig. 1   Cerebral centers and pathways. (Adapted from Lacert P, Perrigot M. In: Maury M, ed. La paraplégie chez l'adulte et chez l'enfant. Paris: Flammarion Médecine-Sciences, 1981, p 198.)

the cerebellum. These areas are controlled not only by the frontal cortex but also by the limbic system, explaining why bladder function is so influenced by emotion. Balanced facilitation and inhibition between the various cortical and subcortical areas of the brain are necessary for coordinated bladder function. The interaction between these areas is summarized diagrammatically in Fig. 1.

Efferent fibers from the reticular formation of the brainstem, concerned with bladder control, pass caudally in relation to the lateral corticospinal tract (43). Kuru (38) suggests that in animals fibers conveying vesicoconstriction and vesicorelaxation outflow run separately in the lateral and ventral reticulospinal tracts, respectively. In humans the position may be laterally close to the insertion of the dentate ligaments (29) or medially between the lateral corticospinal tract and the intermediolateral gray matter of the cord. The fact that tract localization in the cord is difficult may suggest individual variability, or perhaps that the tracts are not localized (43).

B. Anatomy of the Lower Urinary Tract (Fig. 2)

The bladder wall consists primarily of the detrusor muscle, which is composed of intertwined smooth-muscle bundles arranged in three layers: an outer and inner longitudinal layer and a circular intermediate layer (8,16,21). Distally it tapers into the bladder neck and urethra. The latter is composed of inner and outer smooth-muscle layers separated in the male by the prostate gland. Two distinct sphincter mechanisms facilitate continence. The internal urinary sphincter is formed by the outer smooth-muscle layer of the urethra. It allows closure of the bladder neck and the proximal urethra. The external sphincter is composed of two layers of skeletal striated voluntary muscle fibers. The first periurethral layer surrounds the distal urethra. The second layer is a reflection downward from the pelvis floor musculature. Passive continence during bladder filling is secured by the internal sphincter. Active voluntary continence and urinary stream interruption is secured by the external sphincter and thus helps prevent leakage of urine at inappropriate times.

C. Neural Control of Micturition

The lower urinary tract is controlled by three nerves (21) (Fig. 2). The hypogastric nerves transmit the sympathetic outflow originating from the intermediolateral cell column of the dorsolumbar spinal cord at levels T11–L2. Activation of the beta-adrenergic receptors in the bladder wall results in detrusor relaxation and thus facilitates bladder filling. Activation of the alpha-1-adrenergic receptors in the internal urinary sphincter results in its constriction and thus ensures continence during the filling phase. When leakage of urine is to be prevented, somatic voluntary activity is mediated through the pudendal nerves originating from the ventral horn of the sacral spinal segments at levels S2–S4. It results in the contraction of the external urinary sphincter and the pelvic floor. During filling parasympathetic afferent nerve fibers convey information to the pelvic nuclei located in the intermediolateral cell column of the sacral spinal cord at levels S2–S4. Detrusor sensory axons in the spinal cord synapse with the neurons of the pontine-mesencephalic portion of the brainstem reticular formation (9). The output of these nuclei is modulated by neural signals generated in the anterior vermis and fastigial nucleus of the cerebellum. Information is transmitted from these nuclei to and from the frontal part of cerebral cortex through pathways receiving contributions from the basal ganglia and thalamus. When the bladder is full and the situation for voiding is acceptable, inhibition from the cerebral cortex is released and parasympathetic activity originating in the sacral nuclei is conveyed through the erector nerves and insures contraction of the detrusor and bladder emptying.

During micturition, the parasympathetic system is activated while the sympathetic and somatic systems are inhibited. Bladder and sphincter activity is coor-

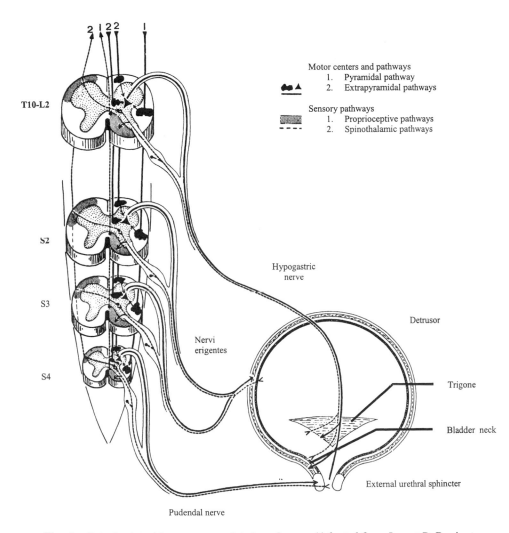

Fig. 2 Spinal micturition centers and their pathways. (Adapted from Lacert P, Perrigot M. In: Maury M, ed. La paraplégie chez l'adulte et chez l'enfant. Paris: Flammarion Méde-cine-Sciences, 1981, p 197.)

dinated so that when the bladder contracts, the internal and external sphincters relax in a coordinated fashion.

III. MICTURITION DISTURBANCES AFTER STROKE

Previous studies have shown an association between the development of urinary incontinence and the presence of certain neurological deficits, including moderate or severe motor deficits (7), aphasia (7), hemiparesis (47), and the combination of hemiplegia, proprioceptive deficits, and visual neglect. However, the studies have not specifically determined whether these deficits might be directly responsible for incontinence, independent of bladder dysfunction. Pelissier et al. (44) compared 32 stroke patients with micturition disturbances to 65 stroke patients without micturition disturbances. He concluded that the correlation between stroke and urinary incontinence depends essentially on the importance of motor deficit rather than the localization of the lesion or the neuropsychological dysfunction. Others found no correlation with the side of stroke, sex, age, hemianopsis (47), and history of stroke (10,14,40,56).

Gelber et al. (24) and Brocklehurst et al. (10) hypothesized that in some stroke patients urinary incontinence may be directly due to stroke-related cognitive or language deficits rather than to the selective dysfunction of the neuromicturition pathways. Gelber et al. (24) conclude that there are three major mechanisms responsible for urinary incontinence after stroke:

1. Disruption of the neuromicturition pathways, resulting in bladder hyperreflexia and urgency incontinence.
2. Stroke-related cognitive and language deficits resulting in incontinence with normal bladder function.
3. Concurrent neuropathy or medication use, resulting in bladder hyporeflexia and overflow incontinence.

A. Clinical Presentation

Urinary frequency and urgency are frequently associated with frontoparietal and basal ganglia—internal capsular infarctions involving motor pathways; incontinence is frequently associated with urinary frequency and urgency (57). Sakakibara et al. (47) studied histories and performed urodynamic, CT, and MRI studies in 72 acute hemispheric stroke patients. Within 3 months from the onset, 53% of the patients had urinary symptoms including irritation as well as obstruction, and the most common symptom was nocturnal urinary frequency in 36%, which was followed by urge urinary incontinence in 29% and difficulty of voiding in 25% of the patients. Micturition disturbance was more common in lesions of the frontal lobe than in those of the occipital lobe. Brain CT or MRI in symptomatic patients showed lesions of anterior and medial surface of the frontal lobe, anterior edge of the paraventricular white matter, genu of the internal capsule, and large lesions of the putamen or thalamus. Perrigot et al. (45) analyzed 3014 hemiplegic cases and found that almost 50% of patients presented some form of urinary disturbance, which was considered clinically important in 20% of the cases. When the lesion was in the territory of the Sylvian or the vertebrobasilar trunk, 70% of the patients presented incontinence and urgency and 30% presented retention. When the lesion was in the territory of the anterior cerebral artery, 90% of the patients presented incontinence and urgency versus 10% with retention.

The lesion may cause frequency and urgency when the patient is awake and incontinence when asleep (2). These patients may be aware that they need to urinate but cannot suppress bladder contraction. The result is uncontrolled bladder emptying. During the first 7–10 days after a large infarct or hemorrhage, there may be associated mental confusion, depression of the level of consciousness, and awareness of the need to urinate or defecate leading to incontinence (41). Incontinence is situational when the patients feel the need to pass urine but are unable to do so independently. They might be unable to call for assistance or to reach the toilet or handle and manipulate clothes, a bedpan, or urinal because of impaired upper-limb function. They cannot suppress urination even though they are aware of the need to urinate and know what to do. So, during the early phases of stroke recovery, incontinence may be a combination of neural dysfunction, decreased awareness, immobility, and dependency. Factors associated with urinary incontinence at 4 weeks after stroke were impaired mobility, severity of motor deficit, mental impairment, and dysphasia (14). Among factors that may contribute to urinary incontinence are communication problems, urinary infection often without other symptoms, fecal impaction, excess urinary flow due to high fluid intake, diuretics, and poorly controlled diabetes, too few carers/nurses, and underestimation of the importance of maintaining continence by the carers/nurses (61).

Some continent stroke victims sense the urge to void and are often considered as being normal. Garrett et al. showed that incomplete bladder emptying occurred in more than half of the 85 patients they studied (22). Gelber et al. (24) noted bladder hyporeflexia in 17–25% of poststroke patients. This raises the possibility of overflow incontinence as another cause of urinary incontinence in stroke patients.

Sakakibara et al. (48) showed that 3 months after brainstem stroke 21% of the patients presented urinary retention. These patients demonstrate a significantly higher rate of urinary infection.

B. Urodynamic Findings

Urodynamic evaluation and measurement of the postvoidal residual urine are essential in the diagnosis of neurogenic bladder, and findings often determine the therapeutic approach.

1. The Bladder

Detrusor hyperreflexia with decreased bladder capacity is the most common cystometric finding in the incontinent stroke victims who present with urinary frequency and urgency (35,44,47,57). It was noted mostly in lesions of the frontal lobe (55). Patients with basal ganglia damage, brain atrophy, and lesion of the putamen may have poor bladder contractions leading to retention (35,44,57). Thirty-eight out of seventy-seven hemiplegic patients were studied by uroflowmetry. Thiry et al. (54) concluded that retention was exclusively caused by a mechanical outlet obstacle. Kahn et al. (34,35) found uninhibited relaxation of the external urethral sphincter during involuntary bladder contractions in patients with cerebral cortex and/or internal capsule lesions, and normal sphincter function in patients with lesions only in the basal ganglia or the thalamus. Two of their patients had normal CT scans, suggesting that their urinary trouble was not related to the stroke. Sakakibara et al. (47) found uninhibited sphincter relaxation in the frontal lobe only. Some patients may present an early need to void with urgency without other cystometric anomaly (44).

Hypertonic bladder seems related to lesions more than 40 mm in diameter (17). The most favorable prognostic factors for urinary continence are a nonhypertonic bladder and absence of extensive brain lesions (17).

Urodynamic studies in patients suffering from brainstem stroke showed that detrusor hyperreflexia was present in 73% of patients, low compliance bladder in 9%, atonic bladder in 27%, detrusor-sphincter dyssynergia in 45%, and uninhibited sphincter relaxation in 27% (56). Brain MRI images of the lesions in the symptomatic patients were concentrated in the dorsolateral pons including pontine reticular nucleus and the reticular formation adjacent to the medial parabrachial nucleus and the locus ceruleus.

In the acute phase, measurement of the postvoidal residual urine volume in the apparently continent patient can be achieved either by catheterization or by ultrasound investigation. Retention is considered when this volume exceeds 50 mL. It can be caused by an hypoactive bladder or by mechanical obstruction.

2. The External Urethral Sphincter

The urethral pressure profile gives information on the external urethral sphincter length and pressures. Thiry and al. (54) found that urethral pressure was equally normal, decreased, or increased in the 77 patients he studied regardless of whether or not they were continent. Others (57), found that in patients presenting bladder hyperactivity with urgency, the sphincter activity either may be normal and well coordinated with bladder activity or may be uncoordinated (detrusor-sphincter dyssynergia), in which case patients presented retention. Detrusor-sphincter dyssynergia, rather common in spinal cord injury, seems related to bilateral infarcts and in basal ganglia lesions (34,47). When left untreated, patients are at high risk to develop serious urological complications such as vesicoureteral reflux, hydronephrosis, urolithiasis, and sepsis (6). Sometimes, uninhibited relaxation of the external urethral sphincter may be present in frontal lobe lesions (47).

As mentioned earlier, measurement of the postvoidal residual urine volume and uroflowmetry, which require patient collaboration, are valuable tools, when practicable, to evaluate mechanical bladder outlet obstruction, which may be produced by an uncoordinated sphincter activity or an enlarged prostate in the male patient. Electromyography and pressure measurement of the external urinary sphincter help to further differentiate these two entities. In the former, instead of electric silence and decrease of sphincter pressure during contraction of the bladder and voiding, the electric activity and sphincter pressure increase.

C. Management

Continence and the severity of hemiparesis exert independent effects on the likelihood of returning home or survival, the degree of bladder control being the more powerful predictor (3,4,58). Subjects whose urinary incontinence persisted throughout their rehabilitation program made less improvement in rehabilitation and exhibited lower functional recovery and recovery of independent mobility functional status at discharge (26). Therapeutic decisions and treatment strategies should be based on the knowledge of abnormal voiding physiology, as demonstrated by urodynamic study (23,24).

Treatment should aim to reestablish continence and personal dignity. In the acute phase, whatever the urinary problem, an indwelling catheter may be considered to facilitate management. If the initial presentation is retention, a long-term indwelling catheter should be reserved for the last option (27) and intermittent catheterization (32) should be considered rapidly within the first week. This has the advantage of reducing the risk of urinary infection. When incontinence is the initial presentation and assuming the patient did not have any urinary problem before stroke, clamping of the indwelling catheter should be attempted by the end of the second week to check whether or not the desire to void returns and at what bladder capacity. Some patients will be able to void voluntarily and others will not. For these, the indwelling catheter should be shut off periodically to distend the bladder to a normal capacity to make certain that it is not allowed to contract. Management should be discussed, whenever possible, with the patient. Pharmacotherapy can influence the different structures of the lower urinary tract:

bladder, bladder neck, external urethral sphincter and the prostate gland (12,65). In high-pressure bladder hyperreflexia one might consider administrating a smooth-muscle-relaxing drug such as probantheline, flavoxate, trospium, or emepronium to reduce uninhibited detrusor contractions and to obtain a low-pressure reservoir. Should these drugs fail, one may consider prescribing more powerful anticholinergic drugs such as oxybutinin and tolderodine in combination with intermittent catheterization. Anticholinergic medication should not be used for long periods unless absolutely necessary, especially in elderly men with an enlarged prostate, since these drugs may cause acute and chronic urinary retention. For those patients with low-pressure bladder outlet and urinary sphincter, one may consider sympathomimetic drugs such as phenyl propanolamine and ephedrine. In the male patient with benign hypertrophy of the prostate, a selective alpha-1 sympathetic drug to reduce the obstruction may be considered. One should be aware that urinary infection, spasticity, and constipation may influence bladder function and these should be investigated and treated appropriately.

Persisting sphincter dyssynergia may be treated by injection of botulinum toxin type A (15,49). This drug offers a time-limited effect (2–3 months) and can predict the outcome of sphincterotomy. Often, treatment of infravesical obstruction due to external sphincter spasticity, the prostate gland, or urethral anatomical anomaly decreases detrusor pressure.

Whenever possible, a pragmatic approach using continence charts and bladder training or biofeedback often results in improvement of continence and should be attempted (24). A typical program involves offering the patient a urinal or bedpan, or placing him or her on the commode on a regularly scheduled basis. Such a program should include the recording of fluid intake and losses. In incontinent male patients, a condom catheter can be an option (23) provided there is no concomitant hypertonic bladder and bladder outlet obstruction.

D. Outcome Associations and Predictive Factors

Following an acute stroke, urinary retention is common. With time, this usually resolves and then incontinence becomes the most problematic urological manifestation. Urinary incontinence is an important cause of distress to patients and carers, increases the risk of pressure sores, often interferes with rehabilitation by interrupting physiotherapy sessions, and influences the patient's requirements for ongoing nursing care, discharge, and the long-term outcome (60). Incontinence has been identified as being indicative of a poor prognosis after a stroke (23). Outcome after stroke is much better in those who remain or become dry and it seems possible that recovery of continence may promote morale and self-esteem, which could actually hasten overall recovery (11,35).

Of 639 registered stroke patients studied by Taub et al. (52), 392 without previous disability survived and were assessed for disability at 3 months. The results showed that 34 (9%) were severely disabled and another 60 (15%) were moderately disabled. In both instances, initial incontinence was the best single predictor of disability with a sensitivity of 60% and a specificity of 78%. At 12 months, 11% still had moderate or severe disability with initial incontinence again being the single best predictor of disability. Wade and Hewer (58) studied 532 patients shortly after the onset of an acute stroke. The presence of urinary incontinence in the first 7 days after the stroke was a poor prognostic factor for survival because more than half of the incontinent patients died within 6 months of suffering a stroke. Urinary incontinence at 3 weeks was also shown to predict a higher chance of dying and less chance at regaining mobility (11). Therefore, urinary incontinence early after stroke can indentify a subset of patients who are at risk for a poor recovery. Such patients must be given the special care needed to optimize the potential for a successful recovery (11).

Aggressive treatment of urinary incontinence reduces long-term costs of hospitalization (64). Understanding which factors may be associated with the recovery of urinary incontinence and how urinary incontinence is associated with overall functional outcome is of value since early recognition of these factors may assist in the rehabilitative management of stroke patients, particularly in triage to the appropriate treatment setting and in improving their longer-term outcome. The prospective study of Wccn ct al. (63) tried to identify these factors and concluded that urinary incontinence on admission was associated with severe functional impairment with large infarctions and was probably caused by general severity rather than specific impairment of neurological micturition control. Patients with less impairment (admission Functional Independence Measure > 60) and small-vessel strokes were likely to recover continence. Furthermore, urinary incontinence on admission had a negative impact on outcome, regardless of the severity of the stroke.

IV. BOWEL DISTURBANCES AFTER STROKE

The ability to respond to the conscious sensation of rectal filling by retaining fecal matter and defecation is initiated as a voluntary act. Its cortical representation has been mapped, but the higher-level processes concerned with suppression and initiation of reflex and voluntary defecation in humans are unknown (51). The descending pathways through the brainstem anterior pons (62) and spinal cord are thought to be closely related to those subserving micturition described previously. Control of defecation, continence, is lost in the presence of diffuse lesions of the brain, especially those associated with frontal or bifrontal dysfunction (7).

Cerebrovascular events are followed less frequently by disturbances in the control of defecation. It was estimated that 40% of hemiplegic patients present some form of anorectal disturbance (35). In unilateral or bilateral ACA occlusion fecal incontinence occurs less frequently and less severely than urinary incontinence (2,66). Anterior or posterior pontine lesions have been shown to be associated with delayed colonic transit (19,62).

A. Fecal Incontinence

The incidence of fecal incontinence was estimated at 23% within 1 year, with three-quarters occurring within the first 2 weeks and most of it clearing during the first year (10). Perhaps the fact that feces are not fluid accounts for there being less incontinence of feces, and the fact that the rectum fills less frequently than the bladder accounts for there being less frequency of defecation (2). Fecal incontinence, which is not associated with severe cognitive problems, is almost always remediable by dealing with constipation or diarrhea (60).

B. Constipation

The most common bowel problem after stroke is constipation (10,41). Its incidence was estimated at 15–17% (39). Central dysfunction, depressed conscious level, difficulty of communication, and immobility after stroke may precipitate constipation. Constipation may be aggravated by poor fluid and food intakes, change in alimentary habits, constipating analgesics, and lack of privacy.

C. Management

The frequency of bowel movements should be monitored. Simple monitoring will detect constipation and diarrhea and may help to establish the pattern of any fecal incontinence. Patients should not be allowed to go beyond 3 days without moving their bowels in which case they must be checked for fecal impaction (41). When diarrhea occurs without obvious reason it may be occasionally useful to culture the stool to exclude infection. More often, when the patient has fecal incontinence associated with diarrhea one should check carefully for fecal impaction by manual per rectum examination or suitable proctoscopic examination. Plain X-ray of the abdomen is often of much help. More detailed investigation is usually not required unless there are persistent unexplained problems.

Bowel regularity can be achieved by adequate fluid and fiber intake, taking the patient to the toilet, or putting him on a bedpan on a regular basis and preferably after meals, and offering privacy. Bulk laxatives, stool softeners, stimulants acting on the mucosa of the colon, peristaltic activators, and enemas might be necessary to obtain bowel emptying and should be used carefully.

Achieving continence of feces is often a crucial step in discharging the patient.

V. CONCLUSION

Urinary and bowel disturbances are common manifestations after stroke and in relationship with the localization of the lesion. Urinary and/or fecal incontinence is often a burden on the patient and the nursing staff. Achieving continence is often a crucial step to recovery and in discharging the patient. Whenever urodynamic facility is available, patients should be evaluated and prompt management should be undertaken.

REFERENCES

1. Abrams P, Blaivas JG, Stanton SL, Andersen JT. The standardisation of terminology of the lower urinary tract function. Scand J Urol Nephrol 1988; Supplementum 114(suppl): 5–19.
2. Andrew J, Nathan PW. Lesions of the anterior frontal lobes and disturbances of micturition and defaecation. Brain 1964; 87:233–282.
3. Barer DH, Mitchell JRA. Predicting the outcome of acute stroke: do multivariate models help? Q J Med 1989; 70(261):27–39.
4. Barer DH. Continence after stroke: useful predictor or goal of therapy? Age Ageing 1989; 18:183–191.
5. Barker AT, Jalinow R, Freeston JL. Non-invasive magnetic stimulation of human motor cortex. Lancet 1985; 1:1106–1107.
6. Blaivas JG. Neurological dysfunction. In: Yalla SV, McGuire EJ, Elbadawi A, Blaivas JG, eds. Neurourology and Urodynamics: Principles and Practice. New York: Macmillan, 1988, pp 343–357.
7. Borrie MJ, Campbell AJ, Caradoc-Davies TH, Spears GFS. Urinary incontinence after stroke: a prospective study. Age Ageing 1986; 15:177–181.
8. Brading A. Physiology of bladder smooth muscle. In: Torrens M, Morrison JFB, eds. The Physiology of the Lower Urinary Tract. New York: Springer Verlag, 1987, pp 161–191.
9. Bradley WE, Timm GW, Scott FB. Cystometry: central nervous system organization of detrusor reflex. Urology 1975; 5(4):578–580.
10. Brocklehurst JC, Andrews K, Richards B, Laycock PJ. Incidence and correlates of incontinence in stroke patients. J Am Geriatr Soc 1985; 33(8):540–542.
11. Burney Tracy L, Senapati M., Desai S, Choudhary ST, Badlani GH. Effects of cerebrovascular accident on micturition. Urol Clin North Am 1996: 23(3):483–490.
12. Caine M, ed. The Pharmacology of the Urinary Tract. Heidelberg: Springer Verlag, 1984.
13. Caplan LR, Zervas NT. Speech arrest in a dextral with a right mesial frontal astrocytoma. Arch Neurol 1978; 35:252.
14. Codine PH, Pelissier J, Manderscheit JC, Costa P, Enjalbert M, Perrigot M. Les troubles urinaires au cours des hémiplégies vasculaires. In: Pelissier J, ed. Hémiplégie vasculaire et médecine de rééducation. Paris: Masson, 1988, pp 261–269.
15. Dykstra DD, Sidi AA. Treatment of drtusor-sphincter dyssynergia with botulinum A toxin: a double-blind study. Arch Phys Med Rehabil 1990; 71:24–26.

16. Elbadawi A. Neuromuscular mechanisms of micturition. In: Yalla SV, McGuire EJ, Elbadawi A, Blaivas JG, eds. Neurourology and Urodynamics: Principles and Practice. New York: Macmillan, 1988, pp 3–35.

17. Feder M, Heller L, Tadmor R, Snir D, Solzi P, Ring H. Urinary continence after stroke: association with cystometric profile and computerized tomography findings. Eur Neurol 1987; 27:101–105.

18. Fletcher TF, Bradley WB. Neuroanatomy fo the bladder-urethra. J Urol 1978; 119: 153–160.

19. Fukuda H, Fukai K, Yamane M, Okada H. Pontine reticular responses to pelvic nerve and colonic mechanical stimulation in dog. Brain Res 1981; 207:59–71.

20. Furlan AJ. Central nervous system causes of urinary incontinence in the elderly. In: Zawada ET, Sica DA, eds. Geriatric Nephrology and Urology. Littleton: PSG Publishing Company, 1985, pp 329–333.

21. Galeano C, Corcos J, Schick E. Anatomie simplifiée de l'unité fonctionnelle vésico-urétrale. In: Corcos J, Schick E, eds. Les vessies neurogènes de l'adulte. Paris: Masson, 1996, pp 1–10.

22. Garrett VE, Scott JA, Costich J, Aubrey DL, Gross J. Bladder emptying assessment in stroke patients. Arch Phys Med Rehabil 1989; 70:41–43.

23. Gelber D.: Neurogenic bladder and bowel. In: Lazar R. Principles of Neurologic Rehabilitation. New York: McGraw-Hill, Vol 18, pp 289–294.

24. Gelber DA, Good DC, Laven LJ, Verhilst SJ. Causes of urinary incontinence after acute hemispheric stroke. Stroke 1993; 24:378–382.

25. Giaquinto S, Buzzelli S, Di Francesco L, Lottarini A, Montenero P, Tonin P, Nolfe G. On the prognosis of outcome after stroke. Acta Neurol Scand 1999; 100:202–208.

26. Gross JC. Urinary incontinence and stroke outcomes. Arch Phys Med Rehabil 2000; 81:22–27.

27. Hanson S, Degraba TJ, Villar-Cordova, Yatsu FM. Medical complications of stroke. In: Barnett HJM, Mohr JP, Stein BM, Yatsu FM, eds. Stroke: Pathophysiology, Diagnosis and Management. Philadelphia: Churchill Livingstone, 1998, pp 1125–1126.

28. Hess CW, Mills KR, Murray NM Measurement of central motor conduction in multiple scleroris by magnetic brain stimulation. Lancet 1986; 2:355–358.

29. Hitchcock E, Newsam D, Salama M. The somatotrophic representation of the micturition pathways in the cervical cord of man. Br J Surg 1974; 61:395–401.

30. Ho H, Goh HS. Anorectal physiological parameters in chronic constipation of unknown actiology and of cerebravascular accidents. Ann Acad Med Singapore 1995; 24:376–378.

31. Hu T. Impact of urinary incontinence on health-care costs. J Am Geriatr Soc 1990; 38:292–295.

32. Hunt GM, Oakeshott P, Whitaker RH. Intermittent catheterisation: simple, safe, and effective but underused. Br Med J 1996; 312:103–107.

33. Jorge JM, Wexner SD. Etiology and management of fecal incontinence. Dis Colon Rectum 1993; 36:77–97.

34. Khan Z, Hertanu J, Yang WC, Meman A, Leiter E. Predictive correlation of urodynamic dysfunction and brain injury after cerebrovascular accident. J Urol 1981; 126: 86–88.

35. Khan Z, Starer P, Yang WC, Bhola A. Analysis of voiding disorders in patients with cerebrovascular accidents. Urology 1990; 35(3):265–270.
36. Krayenbühl H, Yasargil MG. Das normale Hirngefässsystem im angiographischen Bild. In: Gänshirt H, ed. Der Hirnkreislauf. Stuttgart: Georg Thieme, 1972, pp 161–200.
37. Kuntzer T, Waeber B.: Peripheral nerve, muscle, and autonomic changes. In: Bogousslavsky J, Caplan L, eds. Stroke Syndromes. Cambridge: Press Syndicate of the University of Cambridge, 1995, vol 21, pp 205–206.
38. Kuru M. Nervous control of micturition. Physiol Rev 1965; 45:425–494.
39. Labat J-J, Costa P. Les maladies cérébro-vasculaires et tumorales cérébrales. In: Corcos J, Schick E, eds. Les vessies neurogènes de l'adulte. Paris: Masson, 1996, pp 59–64.
40. Lorenze EJ, Simon HB, Lienden JL, Plain W. Urologic problems in rehabilitation of hemiplegic patients. JAMA 1959; 169:1042–1046.
41. Millikan CH, McDowell F, Easton JD. Rehabilitation from stroke. In: Millikan CH, McDowell F, Easton JD, eds. Stroke. Philadelphia: Lea & Febiger, 1987, pp 208–210.
42. Ouslander JG, Kane RL, Abrass IB. Urinary incontinence in elderly nursing home patients. JAMA 1982; 248:1194–1198.
43. Parson KF, Feneley DDI, Forren SMJ. Rehabilitation and management of the neuropathic bladder. In: lllis LS, ed. Neurological Rehabilitation. Oxford: Blackwell Scientific Publications, 1994, pp 352–355.
44. Pelissier J, Costa P, Miermont JC, Leroux JL, Brun V, Navratil H. Les troubles mictionnels lors d'hémiplégies vasculaires: éssai de classification. Ann Réadapt Méd Physi 1985; 28:279–289.
45. Perrigot M, Veaux-Renault V, Fackcas C, Pichon J. Les troubles mictionnels chez l'hémiplégique. J Réadapt Méd 1981; 1(5):145–148.
46. Resnick NM, Yalla SV. Management of urinary incontinence in the elderly. N Engl J Med 1985; 13:800–805.
47. Sakakibara R, Hattori T, Yasuda K, Yamanishi T. Micturitional disturbances after acute hemispheric stroke: analysis of the lesion site by CT and MRI. J Neurol Sci 1996; 137:47–56.
48. Sakakibara R, Hattori T, Yasuda K, Yamanishi T. Micturitional disturbances and the pontine tegmental lesion: urodynamic and MRI analyses of vascular cases. J Neurol Sci 1996; 141:105–110.
49. Schurch B, Hodler J, Rodic B. Botulinum A toxin as a treatment of detrusor-sphincter dyssynergia in patients with spinal cord injury: MRI controlled transperineal injections. J Neurol Neurosurg Psychiatry 1997; 63:474–476.
50. Sier H, Ouslander J, Orzeck S. Urinary incontinence among geriatric patients in an acute-care hospital. JAMA 1987; 257:1767–1771.
51. Swash M, Henry M. The colon and anal sphincters. In: Swash M, Oxburg J, eds. Clinical Neurology. London: Churchill Livingstone, 1991, pp 614–623.
52. Taub NA, Wolfe CD, Richardson E., Burney PG: Predicting the disability of first-time stroke suffers at one year. 12-month follow-up of a population-based cohort in southeast England. Stroke 1994; 25:352–357.
53. Thiry AJ, Deltenre PF. Neurophysiological assessment of the central motor pathway to the external urethral sphincter in man. Br J Urol 1989; 63:515–519.

54. Thiry AJ, Demol O, Demeurisse G, Robaye E. Etiologie des troubles sphinctériens urinaires secondaires aux accidents vasculaires cérébraux. Sem Hôp Paris 1983; 59(31):2173–2177.

55. Tobin GW, Brockelhurst JC. Faecal incontinence in residential homes for the elderly: prevalence, aetiology and management. Age Ageing 1986; 15:41–46.

56. Trebinjac S, Buljina A, Radoje R. Fréquence des troubles vésico-sphinctériens dans la phase avancée de la rééducation à la suite d'un accident vasculaire cérébral. J Réadapt Méd 1990; 10:5–8.

57. Tsuchida S, Noto H, Yamaguchi O, Itoh M. Urodynamic studies on hemiplegic patients after cerebrovascular accident. Urology 1983; 21:315–318.

58. Wade DT, Hewer RL. Functional abilities after stroke: measurement, natural history and prognosis. J Neurol Neurosurg Psychiatry 1987; 50:177–182.

59. Wade DT, Hewer RL. Outlook after an acute stroke: urinary incontinence and loss of consciousness compared in 532 patients. Q J Med 1985; 56:601–608.

60. Warlow CP, Dennis MS, van Gijn J, Hankey GJ, Sandercock PAG, Bamford JM, Wardlaw J. Faecal incontinence and constipation. In: Warlow CP, Dennis MS, van Gijn J, Hankey GJ, Sandercock PAG, Bamford JM, Wardlaw J, eds. Stroke: A Practical Guide to Management. Oxford: Blackwell Science, 1996, pp 493.

61. Warlow CP, Dennis MS, van Gijn J, Hankey GJ, Sandercock PAG, Bamford JM, Wardlaw J. Urinary problems. In: Warlow CP, Dennis MS, van Gijn J, Hankey GJ, Sandercock PAG, Bamford JM, Wardlaw J, eds. Stroke: A Practical Guide to Management. Oxford: Blackwell Science, 1996, pp 491–493.

62. Weber J, Denis P, Mohout B, Muller JM, Blanquart F, Galmiche JP, Simon P, Pasquis P. Effect of brain-stem lesion on colonic and anorectal motility: study of three patients. Dig Dis Sci 1985; 30:419–425.

63. Ween JE, Alexander MP, D'Esposito M, Roberts M. Incontinence after stroke in a rehabilitation setting: outcome associations and predictive factors. Neurology 1996; 47(3):659–663.

64. Wein AJ. Clinical neuropharmacology of the lower urinary tract. In: Yalla SV, McGuire EJ, Elbadawi A, Blaivas JG eds. Neurourology and Urodynamics: Principles and Practice. New York: Macmillan, 1988, pp 377–398.

65. Wein AJ. Neuromuscular dysfunction of the lower urinary tract and its treatment. In: Walsh PC, Retik AB, Vaughan ED, Wein AJ, eds. Campbells's Urology, 7th ed. Philadelphia: WB Saunders Company, 1998, vol 29, pp 954–1006.

66. Wolf PA, Kannel WB, D'Agostino RB. Epidemiology of stroke. In: Ginsberg MD, Bogousslavsky J, eds. Cerebrovascular disease—Pathophysiology, Diagnosis and Management. Oxford: Blackwell Science, Vol 59, pp 834–849.

Index

About the Editor

JULIEN BOGOUSSLAVSKY is Professor and Chairman of the Department of Neurology, University of Lausanne and Centre Hospitalier Universitaire Vaudois, Switzerland. The author of more than 600 journal articles and book chapters, he is president-elect of the International Stroke Society, former chairman of the European Stroke Council, and an elected Trustee of the World Federation of Neurology. He received the M.D. degree (1983) from the University of Geneva, Switzerland.

ISBN 0-8247-0624-2